AF352232

1996
YEAR BOOK OF
UROLOGY®

Statement of Purpose

The YEAR BOOK Service

The YEAR BOOK series was devised in 1901 by practicing health professionals who observed that the literature of medicine and related disciplines had become so voluminous that no one individual could read and place in perspective every potential advance in a major specialty. In the final decade of the 20th century, this recognition is more acutely true than it was in 1901.

More than merely a series of books, YEAR BOOK volumes are the tangible results of a unique service designed to accomplish the following:

- to *survey* a wide range of journals of proven value
- to *select* from those journals papers representing significant advances and statements of important clinical principles
- to provide *abstracts* of those articles that are readable, convenient summaries of their key points
- to provide *commentary* about those articles to place them in perspective

These publications grow out of a unique process that calls on the talents of outstanding authorities in clinical and fundamental disciplines, trained literature specialists, and professional writers, all supported by the resources of Mosby, the world's preeminent publisher for the health professions.

The Literature Base

Mosby and its editors survey nearly 1,000 journals published worldwide, covering the full range of the health professions. On an annual basis, the publisher examines usage patterns and polls its expert authorities to add new journals to the literature base and to delete journals that are no longer useful as potential YEAR BOOK sources.

The Literature Survey

The publisher's team of literature specialists, all of whom are trained and experienced health professionals, examines every original, peer-reviewed article in each journal issue. More than 250,000 articles per year are scanned systematically, including title, text, illustrations, tables, and references. Each scan is compared, article by article, to the search strategies that the publisher has developed in consultation with the 270 outside experts who form the pool of YEAR BOOK editors. A given article may be reviewed by any number of editors, from one to a dozen or more, regardless of the discipline for which the paper was originally published. In turn, each editor who receives the article reviews it to determine whether or not the article should be included in the YEAR BOOK. This decision is based on the article's inherent quality, its probable usefulness to readers of that YEAR BOOK, and the editor's goal to represent a balanced picture of a given field in each volume of the YEAR BOOK. In addition, the editor indicates when to include figures and tables from the article to help the YEAR BOOK reader better understand the information.

Of the quarter million articles scanned each year, only 5% are selected for detailed analysis within the YEAR BOOK series, thereby assuring readers of the high value of every selection.

The Abstract

The publisher's abstracting staff is headed by a seasoned medical professional and includes individuals with training in the life sciences, medicine, and other areas, plus extensive experience in writing for the health professions and related industries. Each selected article is assigned to a specific writer on this abstracting staff. The abstracter, guided in many cases by notations supplied by the expert editor, writes a structured, condensed summary designed so that the reader can rapidly acquire the essential information contained in the article.

The Commentary

The YEAR BOOK editorial boards, sometimes assisted by guest commentators, write comments that place each article in perspective for the reader. This provides the reader with the equivalent of a personal consultation with a leading international authority—an opportunity to better understand the value of the article and to benefit from the authority's thought processes in assessing the article.

Additional Editorial Features

The editorial boards of each YEAR BOOK organize the abstracts and comments to provide a logical and satisfying sequence of information. To enhance the organization, editors also provide introductions to sections or individual chapters, comments linking a number of abstracts, citations to additional literature, and other features.

The published YEAR BOOK contains enhanced bibliographic citations for each selected article, including extended listings of multiple authors and identification of author affiliations. Each YEAR BOOK contains a Table of Contents specific to that year's volume. From year to year, the Table of Contents for a given YEAR BOOK will vary depending on developments within the field.

Every YEAR BOOK contains a list of the journals from which papers have been selected. This list represents a subset of the more than 1,000 journals surveyed by the publisher and occasionally reflects a particularly pertinent article from a journal that is not surveyed on a routine basis.

Finally, each volume contains a comprehensive subject index and an index to authors of each selected paper.

The 1996 Year Book Series

Year Book of Allergy, Asthma, and Clinical Immunology: Drs. Rosenwasser, Borish, Gelfand, Leung, Nelson, and Szefler

Year Book of Anesthesiology and Pain Management: Drs. Tinker, Abram, Chestnut, Roizen, Rothenberg, and Wood

Year Book of Cardiology®: Drs. Schlant, Collins, Engle, Gersh, Kaplan, and Waldo

Year Book of Chiropractic®: Dr. Lawrence

Year Book of Critical Care Medicine®: Drs. Parrillo, Balk, Calvin, Franklin, and Shapiro

Year Book of Dentistry®: Drs. Meskin, Berry, Kennedy, Leinfelder, Roser, Summitt, and Zakariasen

Year Book of Dermatologic Surgery®: Drs. Swanson, Glogau, and Salasche

Year Book of Dermatology®: Drs. Sober and Fitzpatrick

Year Book of Diagnostic Radiology®: Drs. Federle, Clark, Gross, Latchaw, Madewell, Maynard, and Young

Year Book of Digestive Diseases®: Drs. Greenberger and Moody

Year Book of Drug Therapy®: Drs. Lasagna and Weintraub

Year Book of Emergency Medicine®: Drs. Wagner, Dronen, Davidson, King, Niemann, and Roberts

Year Book of Endocrinology®: Drs. Bagdade, Braverman, Horton, Kannan, Landsberg, Molitch, Morley, Nathan, Odell, Poehlman, Rogol, and Ryan

Year Book of Family Practice®: Drs. Berg, Bowman, Davidson, Dexter, and Scherger

Year Book of Geriatrics and Gerontology®: Drs. Beck, Burton, Rabins, Reuben, Roth, Shapiro, and Whitehouse

Year Book of Hand Surgery®: Drs. Amadio and Hentz

Year Book of Hematology®: Drs. Spivak, Bell, Ness, Quesenberry, Wiernik, and Blume

Year Book of Infectious Diseases®: Drs. Keusch, Barza, Bennish, Klempner, Skolnik, and Snydman

Year Book of Infertility and Reproductive Endocrinology: Drs. Mishell, Lobo, and Sokol

Year Book of Medicine®: Drs. Bone, Cline, Epstein, Greenberger, Malawista, Mandell, O'Rourke, and Utiger

Year Book of Neonatal and Perinatal Medicine®: Drs. Fanaroff and Klaus

Year Book of Nephrology, Hypertension, and Mineral Metabolism: Drs. Coe, Curtis, Favus, Henderson, Kashgarian, Luke, and Myers

Year Book of Neurology and Neurosurgery®: Drs. Bradley and Wilkins

Year Book of Neuroradiology: Drs. Osborn, Eskridge, Grossman, Hudgins, and Ross

Year Book of Nuclear Medicine®: Drs. Gottschalk, Blaufox, McAfee, Wackers, and Zubal

Year Book of Obstetrics and Gynecology®: Drs. Mishell, Herbst, and Kirschbaum

Year Book of Occupational and Environmental Medicine®: Drs. Emmett, Frank, Gochfeld, and Hessl

Year Book of Oncology®: Drs. Simone, Bosl, Cohen, Glatstein, Ozols, and Tallman

Year Book of Ophthalmology®: Drs. Cohen, Augsburger, Eagle, Flanagan, Grossman, Laibson, Maguire, Nelson, Rapuano, Sergott, Tasman, Tipperman, and Wilson

Year Book of Orthopedics®: Drs. Sledge, Cofield, Dobyns, Griffin, Poss, Springfield, Swiontkowski, Wiesel, and Wilson

Year Book of Otolaryngology–Head and Neck Surgery®: Drs. Paparella, and Holt

Year Book of Pain: Drs. Gebhart, Haddox, Jacox, Janjan, Marcus, Rudy, and Shapiro

Year Book of Pathology and Laboratory Medicine: Drs. Mills, Bruns, Gaffey, and Stoler

Year Book of Pediatrics®: Dr. Stockman

Year Book of Plastic, Reconstructive, and Aesthetic Surgery®: Drs. Miller, Cohen, McKinney, Robson, Ruberg, and Whitaker

Year Book of Podiatric Medicine and Surgery®: Dr. Kominsky

Year Book of Psychiatry and Applied Mental Health®: Drs. Talbott, Ballenger, Breier, Frances, Meltzer, Schowalter, and Tasman

Year Book of Pulmonary Disease®: Drs. Bone and Petty

Year Book of Rheumatology®: Drs. Sergent, LeRoy, Meenan, Panush, and Reichlin

Year Book of Sports Medicine®: Drs. Shephard, Drinkwater, Eichner, Torg, Col. Anderson, and Mr. George

Year Book of Surgery®: Drs. Copeland, Bland, Deitch, Eberlein, Howard, Luce, Seeger, Souba, and Sugarbaker

Year Book of Thoracic and Cardiovascular Surgery®: Drs. Ginsberg, Wechsler, and Williams

Year Book of Ultrasound®: Drs. Merritt, Carroll, and Fleischer

Year Book of Urology®: Drs. DeKernion and Howards

Year Book of Vascular Surgery®: Dr. Porter

1996

The Year Book of UROLOGY®

Editors

Jean B. DeKernion, M.D.
Director, Division of Urology, UCLA School of Medicine, Los Angeles, California

Stuart S. Howards, M.D.
Professor of Urology and Physiology, University of Virginia School of Medicine, Charlottesville, Virginia

Mosby

St. Louis Baltimore Boston Carlsbad Chicago Naples New York Philadelphia Portland
London Madrid Mexico City Singapore Sydney Tokyo Toronto Wiesbaden

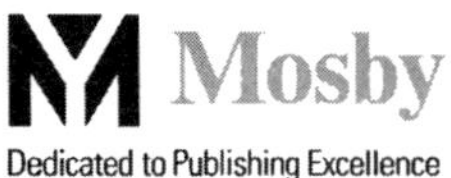

Dedicated to Publishing Excellence

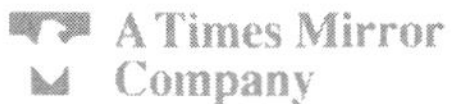

A Times Mirror
Company

Vice President and Publisher, Continuity Publishing: Kenneth H. Killion
Director, Editorial Development: Gretchen C. Murphy
Assistant Developmental Editor, Continuity: Miranda Jackson
Acquisitions Editor: Gina Wright
Manager, Continuity–EDP: Maria Nevinger
Project Specialist, Editing: Denise M. Dungey
Senior Project Manager, Production: Max F. Perez
Freelance Staff Supervisor: Barbara M. Kelly
Illustrations and Permissions Coordinator: Nancy Dunne, R.N.
Director, Editorial Services: Edith M. Podrazik, B.S.N., R.N.
Information Specialist: Kathleen Moss, R.N.
Circulation Manager: Lynn D. Stevenson

1996 EDITION
Copyright © November 1996 by Mosby–Year Book, Inc.

Printed in the United States of America
Composition by Reed Technology and Information Services, Inc.
Printing/binding by Maple–Vail

Mosby–Year Book, Inc.
11830 Westline Industrial Drive
St. Louis, MO 63146

Editorial Office:
Mosby–Year Book, Inc.
161 North Clark Street
Chicago, IL 60601

International Standard Serial Number: 0084–4071
International Standard Book Number: 08151–3484–3

Contributing Editors

Gerald L. Andriole, M.D.
Professor of Urology, Washington University School of Medicine, St. Louis

Zoran Barbaric, M.D.
Professor of Radiology, UCLA School of Medicine; Chief, Abdominal Imaging, UCLA Medical Center, Los Angeles

Arie S. Belldegrun, M.D., F.A.C.S.
Professor of Urology; Chief, Division of Urologic Oncology, Department of Urology, UCLA School of Medicine, Los Angeles

Reginald C. Bruskewitz, M.D.
Professor of Surgery, University of Wisconsin—Madison, Medical School, Madison

E. David Crawford, M.D.
University of Colorado Health Sciences Center, Denver

Michael J. Droller, M.D.
Professor and Chairman, Department of Urology, Mount Sinai Medical Center, New York

Robert C. Flanigan, M.D.
Professor and Chairman of Urology, Department of Urology, Loyola University Medical Center, Maywood, Illinois

Richard S. Foster, M.D.
Associate Professor, Department of Urology, Indiana University Medical Center, Indianapolis

Gerhard J. Fuchs, M.D.
Professor of Urology, UCLA Department of Urology, Los Angeles

Donald P. Griffith, M.D.
St. Luke's Medical Tower, Houston

H. Logan Holtgrewe, M.D.
Associate Professor of Urology, Johns Hopkins University School of Medicine, Baltimore, Maryland

Alan D. Jenkins, M.D.
Associate Professor, Department of Urology, Univerity of Virginia Health Sciences Center, Charlottesville

Steven A. Kaplan, M.D.
Herbert Irving Associate Professor of Urology; Director, Neuro-Urology and The Prostate Center, College of Physicians and Surgeons of Columbia University, New York

Louis R. Kavoussi, M.D.
Associate Professor of Urology; Director, Division of Endourology, The James Buchanan Brady Urological Institute, The Johns Hopkins University School of Medicine, Baltimore, Maryland

Eric A. Klein, M.D.
Head, Section of Urologic Oncology, Department of Urology, Cleveland Clinic Foundation, Cleveland, Ohio

Mark S. Litwin, M.D., M.P.H.
Assistant Professor of Urology and Health Services, UCLA Schools of Medicine and Public Health, Los Angeles

David L. McCullough, M.D.
Professor and Chairman, Department of Urology, Bowman Gray School of Medicine of Wake Forest University, Winston-Salem, North Carolina

Edward J. McGuire, M.D.
Professor and Director, Division of Urology, University of Texas Medical School, Houston

Winston K. Mebust, M.D.
Valk Professor and Chairman, Section of Urologic Surgery, The University of Kansas Medical Center, Kansas City

Brian J. Miles, M.D.
Associate Professor of Urology, Baylor College of Medicine; Chief of Urology, St. Luke's Episcopal Hospital, Houston, Texas

James E. Montie, M.D.
Professor of Surgery, Section of Urology, University of Michigan, Ann Arbor

Judd W. Moul, M.D., LTC, U.S.A.
Director, Center for Prostate Disease Research, Department of Surgery, Uniformed Services University of the Health Sciences; Associate Professor of Surgery, Department of Surgery, Uniformed Services University of the Health Sciences; Urologic Oncologist, Walter Reed Army Medical Center, Bethesda, Maryland

Andrew C. Novick, M.D.
Chairman, Department of Urology, Cleveland Clinic Foundation, Cleveland, Ohio

Anup Patel, M.S., F.R.C.S. (Urol)
Urologic Oncology Fellow, UCLA Department of Urology, Los Angeles

Robert Reiter, M.D.
Assistant Professor Urology, UCLA Department of Urology, Los Angeles

Paul F. Schellhammer, M.D.
Professor and Chairman, Department of Urology; Program Director, Virginia Prostate Center of Eastern Virginia Medical School and Sentara Cancer Institute, Norfolk, Virginia

William A. See, M.D.
Professor, Department of Urology, The University of Iowa, Iowa City

Joel Sheinfield, M.D.
Assistant Attending Surgeon, Urology Service/Department of Surgery, Memorial Sloan-Kettering Cancer Center, New York

Daniel A. Shoskes, M.D., F.R.C.S. (C)
Assistant Professor of Urology, UCLA, Director, Renal Transplantation Program, Harbor-UCLA Medical Center, Torrance, California

William D. Steers, M.D.
J.Y. Gillenwater Professor and Chairman, Department of Urology, University of Virginia Health Sciences Center, Charlottesville

Lynn Stothers, M.D., MHSc, F.R.C.S.C.
Assistant Professor of Urology, University of British Columbia, Vancouver

David A. Swanson, M.D.
Professor and Deputy Chairman, Department of Urology, The University of Texas MD Anderson Cancer Center, Houston

Ian M. Thompson, M.D.

Col, M.C., Chief, Department of Surgery, Brooke Army Medical Center, Fort Sam Houston, Texas

Timothy C. Thompson, Ph.D.

Associate Professor of Urology, Associate Professor of Cell Biology, Associate Professor of Radiology, Director of Research, Scott Department of Urology, Baylor College of Medicine, Houston

E. Darracott Vaughan, Jr., M.D.

James J. Colt Professor of Urology, James Buchanan Brady Foundation, Division of Urology, The New York Hospital-Cornell Medical Center, New York

Thomas M. Wheeler, M.D.

Professor of Pathology and Urology, Baylor College of Medicine; Deputy Chief of Pathology Service, the Methodist Hospital, Houston, Texas

Philippe E. Zimmern, M.D.

Director of the Bladder and Incontinence Center, Associate Professor of Urology, University of Texas Southwestern Medical Center at Dallas, Dallas

Horst Zincke, M.D., Ph.D.

Professor of Urology, Mayo Medical School, Department of Urology, Mayo Clinic, Rochester, Minnesota

Table of Contents

Journals Represented

Mosby and its Editors survey more than 1,000 journals for its abstract and commentary publications. From these journals, the Editors select the articles to be abstracted. Journals represented in this YEAR BOOK are listed below.

Acta Dermato-Venereologica
Acta Neurochirurgica
American Journal of Epidemiology
American Journal of Pathology
American Journal of Physiology
American Journal of Public Health
American Journal of Roentgenology
American Journal of Surgical Pathology
Annals of Oncology
Archives of Environmental Health
British Journal of Radiology
British Journal of Urology
Cancer
Cancer Research
Clin Cancer Res
European Urology
Fertility and Sterility
Human Reproduction
Infection and Immunity
International Journal of Cancer
International Journal of Radiation, Oncology, Biology, and Physics
Journal of Andrology
Journal of Clinical Endocrinology and Metabolism
Journal of Clinical Microbiology
Journal of Clinical Oncology
Journal of Clinical Psychopharmacology
Journal of Computer Assisted Tomography
Journal of Infectious Diseases
Journal of Pediatric Surgery
Journal of Surgical Oncology
Journal of Trauma: Injury, Infection, and Critical Care
Journal of Urology
Journal of the American Geriatrics Society
Journal of the American Medical Association
Journal of the National Cancer Institute
Journal of the Royal College of Surgeons of Edinburgh
Kidney International
Lancet
New England Journal of Medicine
Occupational and Environmental Medicine
Oncology Nursing Forum
Paraplegia
Pediatric Nephrology
Prostate
Radiology
Radiotherapy and Oncology
Scandinavian Journal of Urology and Nephrology

Science
Southern Medical Journal
Transfusion
Transplantation
Transplantation Proceedings
Urological Research
Urology

STANDARD ABBREVIATIONS

The following terms are abbreviated in this edition: acquired immunodeficiency syndrome (AIDS), cardiopulmonary resuscitation (CPR), central nervous system (CNS), cerebrospinal fluid (CSF), computed tomography (CT), deoxyribonucleic acid (DNA), electrocardiography (ECG), health maintenance organization (HMO), human immunodeficiency virus (HIV), intensive care unit (ICU), intramuscular (IM), intravenous (IV), magnetic resonance (MR) imaging (MRI), and ribonucleic acid (RNA).

NOTE

The YEAR BOOK OF UROLOGY is a literature survey service providing abstracts of articles published in the professional literature. Every effort is made to assure the accuracy of the information presented in these pages. Neither the editors nor the publisher of the YEAR BOOK OF UROLOGY can be responsible for errors in the original materials. The editors' comments are their own opinions. Mention of specific products within this publication does not constitute endorsement.

To facilitate the use of the YEAR BOOK OF UROLOGY as a reference tool, all illustrations and tables included in this publication are now identified as they appear in the original article. This change is meant to help the reader recognize that any illustration or table appearing in the YEAR BOOK OF UROLOGY may be only one of many in the original article. For this reason, figure and table numbers will often appear to be out of sequence within the YEAR BOOK OF UROLOGY.

Introduction

Dr. Jean DeKernion and I have reviewed over 3,000 articles to select the most informative and interesting papers which are abstracted in this 1996 YEAR BOOK OF UROLOGY. As in the past, we have decided to augment our areas of expertise with guest editors so that the vast majority of the comments in the YEAR BOOK will be written by experienced analytical experts with appropriate sub-specialties sophistication. We would like to acknowledge the help of our guest editors (see list of Contributing Editors) for their insightful and informative commentary and for their support of this publication.

In this introduction, we would like to highlight some of the most significant manuscripts abstracted in this year's edition of the YEAR BOOK OF UROLOGY.

Imaging

Schuster, Nazos, Lewis, et al. (Abstract 1–1) conducted a study to determine whether or not out-patient excretory urography requires bowel preparation with laxatives and dietary restrictions. They concluded that such preparations are not necessary.

Nephrology

Duclos et al. (Abstract 9–1) reviewed their experience over 15 years with 8 patients who had secreting juxtaglomerular cell tumors. These patients were selected from over 30,000 hypertensive patients. They found that conservative surgery was feasible in all patients.

Renal Failure

Kasiske et al. (Abstract 2–1) studied the long-term effects of reduced renal mass in humans. They found that in normal individuals, unilateral nephrectomy does not cause progressive renal dysfunction, but it may be associated with a small increase in blood pressure.

Transplant

Braun et al. (Abstract 13–1) proposed a new classification of long-term allograft survivals. They found, contrary to some beliefs, that there is no "safe haven" point of time for immunosuppression for allograft recipients. They remain at increased risk for eventual renal allograft dysfunction as well as cardiovascular, neoplastic, infectious, and metabolic diseases.

Stricture

Matanhelia et al. (Abstract 23–1) performed a prospective study to determine whether or not postoperative dilatation is beneficial after internal urethrotomy for urethral stricture. They concluded that short-term postoperative self-dilatation does not prevent recurrent stricture in patients treated with internal urethrotomy.

Adrenals

Nakada et al. (Abstract 8–2) presented the results of enucleation and compared it with the results of adrenalectomy for patients with Conn syndrome due to an adenoma of the adrenal gland. They had excellent results of the enucleation and recommend this as standard treatment.

Infection

Ching et al. (Abstract 4–1) presented their experience with the ligase chain reaction for detection of *Neisseria gonorrhoeae* in urogenital swabs. The test was extremely precise with excellent sensitivity and specificity. It was significantly better than cultures. It appears that this technique will eventually become the diagnostic study of choice.

Renal Cancer

There are several papers relevant to partial nephrectomy for renal cell carcinoma which address the issue of multifocal lesions. Four abstracts analyze the incidence of this problem (Abstracts 10–4 through 10–7) and one abstract reviews an author's experience with intraoperative ultrasonography to detect satellite lesions (Abstract 34–4).

Benign Prostatic Hypertrophy

There are several papers comparing different forms of therapy for BPH, including prospective randomized studies comparing transurethral microwave thermotherapy with TURP (Abstract 20–9), visual laser ablation with TURP (Abstract 20–6), and visual laser ablation with laser evaporation (Abstract 20–13) as well as a retrospective investigation comparing transurethral electrovaporiztion with laser vaporization (Abstract 20–12).

Endourology

Jarret et al. (Abstract 11–2) presented their 9-year experience with the percutaneous management of transitional cell carcinoma of the renal collection system. They concluded that with vigilant follow-up, percutaneous treatment is a reasonable alternative to nephrouroectomy for patients with grade 1 disease and those with grade 2 disease who are at risk for renal insufficiency as well as those individuals with medical contraindications to a major operation. It should be emphasized that this group has extensive experience in that, as they point out, very careful follow-up is necessary.

Incontinence

Trockman et al. (Abstract 15–1) reviewed their experience with a modified Pereyra bladder neck suspension. They performed outcome analysis on 125 patients with a mean follow-up of 10 years. They discovered a very high rate of recurrent stress incontinence after this procedure. Nevertheless, most inpatients were subjectively improved and satisfied with the results of the operation.

Carcinoma of the Penis

Pettaway et al. (Abstract 28–2) reviewed their experience with extended sentinel lymph node dissection for penile carcinoma. They concluded that although extended is a more invasive procedure than standard sentinel node biopsy, it is still associated with a significant false-negative rate of 25%. Therefore, they felt its routine use can no longer be recommended.

Testis Cancer

Baniel, Foster, and Donahue (Abstract 26–1) presented a paper summarizing the surgical anatomy of the lumbar vessels and their implications for retroperitoneal surgery. They noted that the number and course of lumbar vessels are more variable than previously described and emphasized that knowledge of these anatomic variations is important for surgeons operating in this area.

Prostate Cancer

Hugosson et al. (Abstract 21–2) investigated the long-term outcome of patients with deferred treatment of prostatic cancer. They concluded, and of course most urologists would concur, that although early prostate cancer is slow-growing, it is a progressive malignant disease, and if the patient survives long enough, it will kill him.

Bladder Cancer

Lamm et al. (Abstract 19–7) reviewed 22 randomized prospective control studies of almost 4,000 patients treated with intravesical prophylactic chemotherapy for superficial bladder cancer. The long-term results showed no decrease in the incidence of recurrent tumors. Maintenance chemotherapy failed to improve the results. Their conclusion is that prophylactic chemotherapy is probably not indicated in these patients.

Urinary Diversion

Studer et al. (Abstract 16–4) reviewed their experience with over 100 patients who had an ileal low pressure bladder substitute combined with afferent tubular isoperistaltic segment. They had excellent results and highly recommended the use of this technique. Davidsson et al. (Abstract 16–3) reviewed the long-term metabolic effects of urinary diversion on skeletal bone in adults. They did find subtle changes in electrolytes and acid-base hemostasis, but they did not find changes in mineralization of bone over the long-term as had been previously reported in children.

Infertility

Auger et al. (Abstract 22–3) present data from a Paris sperm bank suggesting that sperm counts in Paris have fallen over the last 20 years. This is the most impressive data suggesting a long-term fall in sperm count. However, there have been several papers published since that did not find any fall over long term in sperm counts. Nehra et al. (Abstract 22–5) presented their experience with electroejaculation in vibratory stimulation for patients with spinal cord injury. They found that penile vibratory stimulation is successful in more than half of the patients and recommended it as the first option before going into an electroejaculation protocol. Grasso et al. (Abstract 22–6) Reviewed the results of bilateral varicocelectomy in patients with a clinically significant varicocele on the left side and a grade 1 varicocele on the right. They found no additional benefit from ligating the contralateral spermatic veins.

Peyronie's Disease

Ralph, Al-Akraa, and Pryor (Abstract 27–4) reviewed their experience with the Nesbit procedure in 359 patients with Peyronie's disease. They had excellent results and strongly recommend this procedure.

Impotence

Brant, Ludlow, and Mulcahy (Abstract 25–13) present data to demonstate that one in some instances can immediately replace an infected penile prosthesis. Chen et al. (Abstract 25–7) found that they significantly reduce the pain of prostaglandin E1 injections when they used a new formulation of prostaglandin E1.

Pediatric Oncology

The National Wilms' Tumor Group (Abstract 33–2) looked at the incidence of second malignancies in patients treated for Wilms tumor. They found an 8.4 fold increased incidence over that which would be expected. This obviously is an area of great concern for the long-term survivors and their physicians.

Undescended Testis

Gracia et al. (Abstract 32–5) did a clinical and pathologic study of 2,000 cryptorchid testes. Their opinions were that there is no particular age at which surgery should be performed. This is somewhat at odds with the prevailing wisdom, but is in line with our studies in experimental animals.

Stuart S. Howards, M.D.

1 Imaging

Preparation of Outpatients for Excretory Urography: Is Bowel Preparation With Laxatives and Dietary Restrictions Necessary?
Schuster GA, Nazos D, Lewis GA (Joliet, Ill)
AJR 164:1425–1428, 1995   1–1

Background.—The necessity of bowel cleansing and dietary restriction before excretory urography has never been demonstrated. Nevertheless, both are routinely ordered. The effects of such preparations on radiographic visualization of the urinary tract were studied.

Methods.—One hundred ninety-three outpatients who were undergoing excretory urography were assigned to 1 of 4 groups. Patients in groups 1 and 2 had bowel preparation with cathartics; those in groups 3 and 4 did not. Groups 1 and 3 ate their customary diet before the procedure; groups 2 and 4 consumed a liquid supper the evening before study and then nothing by mouth after midnight. Each set of radiographs was scored for visibility of the urinary tract, with a possible score of 28 if both sides of the system were fully visualized.

Results.—When patients in groups 1 and 3, who ate, were compared with those in groups 2 and 4, who did not, no significant difference was observed in visualization of the urinary tract (mean score, 27.49 for groups 1 and 3; mean score, 27.16 for groups 2 and 4). When patients in groups 1 and 2, who received cathartics, were compared with those in groups 3 and 4, who did not, the difference in visualization, again, was not significant (mean score, 27.45 for groups 1 and 2; mean score, 27.20 for groups 3 and 4). The incidence of pathologic findings was similar among all 4 groups. In addition, no patients vomited during contrast infusion, even those who had eaten.

Conclusion.—Bowel preparation with laxatives and restriction of oral intake before excretory urography do not improve visualization of the urinary tract. Such preparations should be abandoned.

▶ We were very pleased to see this article because it confirms the approach we have long used in our practice. We have never recommended bowel preparation or dietary restrictions before an IV pyelogram. These preparatory measures are even less necessary now since the advent of routine use of higher doses of contrast media and tomography. We occasionally have disagreements with our radiologists regarding this issue; however, the radiologists who routinely do urologic studies agree with our approach. It is reassuring to see our standard technique validated in a prospective study.

S.S. Howards, M.D.

2 Miscellaneous

Long-term Effects of Reduced Renal Mass in Humans
Kasiske BL, Ma JZ, Louis TA, Swan SK (Univ of Minnesota, Minneapolis)
Kidney Int 48:814–819, 1995   2–1

Introduction.—The increasing use of living donors for renal transplantation raises theoretical concerns about the long-term effects of donating a kidney. After many years, hypertension, proteinuria, and renal insufficiency could develop in the donors. The results of studies of the loss of renal mass in human beings have been conflicting. The long-term effects of reduced renal mass in human beings were therefore studied by meta-analysis.

Methods.—Forty-eight studies met the selection criteria, which included an attempt to locate all patients who had a reduction in renal mass from a defined population. The studies included a total of 3,124 patients and 1,703 controls. The median follow-up after reduction in renal mass was nearly 11 years. Multiple linear regression was used to combine the studies and to adjust for differences in follow-up, reason for reduced renal mass, type of controls, age, and sex.

Results.—Unilateral nephrectomy was associated with a mean decline in glomerular filtration rate of 17 mL/min. This parameter tended to improve over time, increasing by 1.4 mL/min/decade of follow-up. For patients who had single kidneys, the level of proteinuria increased by a mean of 76 mg/day/decade; there was no significant change, however, after nephrectomy in trauma patients or kidney donors. Hypertension was no more prevalent in patients who underwent nephrectomy; however, their systolic blood pressure increased by a mean of 2.4 mm Hg and by 1.1 mm Hg/decade. Nephrectomy was followed by a 3.1 mm Hg increase in diastolic blood pressure, but there were no further changes during follow-up.

Conclusions.—Otherwise normal individuals who undergo unilateral nephrectomy do not appear to have progressive renal dysfunction. They may, however, have a slight increase in blood pressure over time. Large follow-up studies are needed to determine whether the increase in blood pressure is clinically relevant and whether patients who have borderline hypertension should be discouraged from donating a kidney.

▶ Ever since Brenner's classic papers, which documented that hyperperfusion after surgical nephrectomy in rats leads to renal failure, there has been controversy regarding whether hyperperfusion injury is a problem in human beings. The literature on this subject is mixed. Many papers have reported no effect of nephrectomy, whereas others have supported the hyperperfusion hypothesis, particularly if more than 50% of the functioning renal mass is removed. This meta-analysis of long-term results is useful and suggests that, in general, there is no significant problem with renal failure after nephrectomy. Of course, the technique of meta-analysis has well-known limitations. The small increase in blood pressure and, particularly, the increase in level of proteinuria with time are somewhat disturbing. Nevertheless, a review of the current literature, along with this additional information, leads to the conclusion that, at least in most instances, unilateral nephrectomy does not shorten life expectancy.

S.S. Howards, M.D.

Ureteroscopy in Pregnancy

Ulvik NM, Bakke A, Høisaeter PÅ (Haukeland Hosp, Bergen, Norway)
J Urol 154:1660–1663, 1995   2–2

Background.—The diagnosis and treatment of pregnant women who have acute symptoms or urinary tract obstruction may be difficult. Conservative, temporizing treatment is often recommended: final diagnosis and treatment are postponed to after delivery, if possible. The use of ureteroscopy in pregnant women was reported.

Methods.—Twenty-four women who had persistent symptoms or ureteral obstruction underwent ureteroscopy for diagnosis and treatment between 1984 and 1994. Ureteroscopy was done with epidural anesthesia in 23 patients, spinal anesthesia in 1, and sedation-analgesia in 1. Standard rigid ureteroscopes of 11.5F were used in most patients.

Findings.—Ureteroscopy was done without great difficulty. In all patients, the ureteroscope was easily introduced into the upper third of the ureter or into the renal pelvis. Ureteral calculi were removed from 13 women. Postoperative complications included fever in 3 patients, perforation of the upper ureter in 1, premature uterine contractions in 1, and spinal headache in 1. Nineteen women had vaginal deliveries, and 2 had cesarean. One infant was born 7 weeks prematurely. All infants were normal but 1, who had a cleft lip and palate. One woman was lost to follow-up before giving birth.

Conclusions.—Ureteroscopy is easy to perform in pregnant women, even during the last weeks of gestation. A total of 29 ureteroscopy procedures, including those in this series, have been reported without serious complications.

▶ This paper documents that ureteroscopy is safe and effective in pregnant women. We have used ureteroscopy, combined with ultrasonography, in this setting. This approach often relieves the problem and is superior to long-term use of a ureteral stent and, of course, more invasive approaches.

S.S. Howards, M.D.

Pathogenesis and Prophylaxis of Postoperative Thromboembolic Disease in Urological Pelvic Surgery
Kibel AS, Loughlin KR (Harvard Med School, Boston)
J Urol 153:1763–1774, 1995

2–3

Introduction.—Thromboembolism is a potentially lethal complication of urologic procedures, particularly pelvic surgery. As many as 51% of patients who undergo pelvic surgery without prophylaxis have deep venous thrombosis, and 2.6% may have pulmonary embolism.

Pathogenesis and Risk Factors.—Patients who are older than 40 years of age, are obese, or have varicose veins are at increased risk of thromboembolism. Additional risk factors include previous thromboembolism, immobility, and the use of estrogen or oral contraceptives. Malignant disease, recent myocardial infarction, and nephrotic syndrome also predispose to this complication, as does a prolonged operating time. Risk factors for venous thromboembolism are additive. Pathophysiologic factors, such as venous stasis, endothelial injury, and hypercoagulability, also contribute to the risk of thromboembolism.

Prevention.—Heparin is an accepted means of preventing venous thromboembolism in patients who undergo urologic surgery, but bleeding, lymphcele formation, and thrombotopenia are potential complications. Low–molecular weight heparin is 1 approach to reducing complication rates; combining heparin with dihydroergotamine is another. Intermittent pneumatic compression stockings have proved effective and entail no risk of bleeding. Properly fitted elastic stockings are also a safe measure but have not proved effective in patients at high risk. Oral anticoagulation with warfarin has long been used to prevent venous thrombosis, but this method may lead to serious bleeding or a hypercoagulable state with cutaneous necrosis. Dextran decreases blood viscosity and inhibits platelet aggregation. Experience with its use in urologic surgery is limited. Aspirin has been used to suppress cyclooxygenase production by platelets, which renders them less able to participate in coagulation.

▶ The risk of postoperative thromboembolic disease is of concern to all urologists who perform major surgery on adults. The authors present a good, focused review of the subject. They point out that, after pelvic surgery, the consensus is that the risks of deep vein thrombosis, pulmonary embolus, and death are 30%, 10%, and 5%, respectively, and that prophylaxis reduces these risks to 10%, 1.5%, and 0.4%. They do not recommend a specific form of prophylaxis. We use intermittent compression stockings and add subcutaneous heparin in special situations. The authors also recommend long-term anticoagulation in patients at high risk.

S.S. Howards, M.D.

Anticoagulant Associated Hematuria: A Prospective Study
van Savage JG, Fried FA (Univ of North Carolina, Chapel Hill)
J Urol 153:1594–1596, 1995   2–4

Introduction.—Urologists are often asked to examine patients who have hematuria and are receiving anticoagulant therapy. As many as 24% of patients who receive warfarin and up to 40% of those who receive heparin may have gross or microscopic hematuria.

Patients.—The records of 32 patients seen consecutively during a 21-month period were reviewed. The patients had no history of trauma or instrumentation. Hematuria was observed while the patients were receiving anticoagulant therapy, which was given for a broad range of indications. None of the patients had bleeding elsewhere, nor did any have prothrombin time greater than 25 seconds or a partial thromboplastin time exceeding 80 seconds.

Results.—Inflammatory and infectious disorders were predominant in the 30 patients evaluated. Lower tract bleeding, usually gross, occurred in 57% of patients, and upper tract bleeding occurred in 40%. In the latter patients, gross hematuria was twice as prevalent as microscopic bleeding. Three patients with microscopic hematuria had nephrolithiasis and underwent lithotripsy. Two of 24 patients who had gross hematuria had neoplastic disease that invaded the bladder. Thirty percent of patients had significant urinary tract disease. Hematuria resolved after treatment in more than 90% of patients. Of the 3 patients in whom it did not resolve, 1 refused treatment, 1 died postoperatively, and 1 had sarcoma invading the bladder.

Conclusions.—All patients who are receiving anticoagulant therapy and have nontraumatic hematuria should undergo a thorough urologic workup. These findings indicate that a large percentage of patients may have significant urologic disease, which raises the possibility of using anticoagulants to unmask such disease.

▶ This paper reconfirms the well-known fact that one cannot accept anticoagulation as an explanation for hematuria and that patients who receive such therapy and have hematuria require a urologic evaluation.

S.S. Howards, M.D.

3 Renovascular Hypertension

Treatment of Renovascular Hypertension: One Year Results of Renal Angioplasty
Jensen G, Zachrisson B-F, Delin K, Volkmann R, Aurell M (Univ of Göteborg, Sweden)
Kidney Int 48:1936–1945, 1995

3–1

Background.—Percutaneous transluminal renal angioplasty is commonly used to treat patients who have hypertension resulting from renal artery stenosis. Renovascular hypertension may account for only 1% to 2% of cases of hypertension. In an older population, however, stenoses of the renal arteries may be a more common cause of hypertension and end-stage renal failure. Percutaneous transluminal renal angioplasty has been performed at 1 medical facility for 10 years. The outcomes of this procedure at 1 year were assessed.

Methods.—Percutaneous transluminal renal angioplasty was performed in 137 patients; 180 procedures were performed during a period of 10 years. The underlying disease was fibromuscular dysplasia in 30 patients and arteriosclerotic vascular disease in 107 patients. The combined clinical, functional, and technical outcome was assessed at 1 year.

Results.—Technical dilatation was successful in 97% of patients who had fibromuscular dysplasia and in 82% of those who had arteriosclerotic vascular disease. Benefits to blood pressure and renal function were observed in both groups. The overall cure and improvement rate for hypertension was 86% in patients who had fibromuscular dysplasia and 64% in those who had arteriosclerotic vascular disease. Total renal function improved significantly in both groups. In 89% of patients who had fibromuscular dysplasia and 74% of those who had arteriosclerotic vascular disease, renal function improved or remained the same; improvement was made by the revascularized kidney. The diagnostic accuracy of outcome as predicted by renal vein renin was excellent. Sensitivity of renal vein renin investigation was 95%, and specificity was 75%. The success rate for patients who had hypertension and renal insufficiency was considerably lower than for the whole group. The recurrence rate was 6.7% for patients who had fibromuscular dysplasia and 15.1% for those who had arteriosclerotic vascular disease. The overall rate of major complications was 5.4%, and the overall rate of minor complications was 5%.

Discussion.—Renal angioplasty is the best first treatment of renovascular hypertension resulting from fibromuscular dysplasia or arteriosclerotic vascular disease. Improvement of renal function is best when renal impairment is moderate and there is a renal parenchymal mass to be preserved. The success of percutaneous transluminal renal angioplasty in these patients was based on a combination of clinical, functional, and technical factors.

▶ It is now accepted that percutaneous transluminal renal angioplasty is the treatment of choice in patients who have fibromuscular hyperplasia. As shown in this paper, however, more patients will have atherosclerotic disease than fibromuscular disease. The authors show an excellent success rate of 64% in patients who have atherosclerotic disease. They do not, however, characterize the nature of the disease in these patients. Many of these patients have osteal stenosis, and the current approach is to use some type of renal artery stent in addition to the angioplasty. With this new technique, the results are better than those previously described.[1]

E.D. Vaughan, Jr., M.D.

Reference

1. MacLeod M, et al: *J Hypertens* 13:791, 1995.

The Contemporary Role of Extra-anatomical Surgical Renal Revascularization in Patients With Atherosclerotic Renal Artery Disease
Fergany A, Kolettis P, Novick AC (Cleveland Clinic Found, Ohio)
J Urol 153:1798–1802, 1995   3–2

Objectives.—All abdominal aortograms done between 1989 and 1993 were reviewed to document the occurrence of significant atherosclerotic disease of the abdominal aorta and visceral arteries in 254 patients who had atherosclerotic renal arterial stenosis. In an additional study, the results of renal revascularization by extra-anatomical bypass, performed from 1980 to 1992 in 171 patients, were examined.

Radiographic Findings.—Loss of renal function secondary to ischemic nephropathy was most likely in patients who had severe bilateral renal artery stenosis or a solitary kidney with a severely stenosed artery. Eighty-one percent of patients in this group had at least moderate atherosclerotic disease of the abdominal aorta. The celiac and common iliac arteries were moderately or severely involved in more than half these patients.

Surgical Results.—The operative mortality rate was 3%. Thrombosis was observed in the repaired renal artery after 7 of 175 revascularization procedures (4%). None of 13 patients with severe hypertension, whose status was followed after revascularization, had graft thrombosis. Hypertension was eliminated in 6 of these patients and improved in the remaining 7. Renal function improved in 50 of 144 patients (35%) who underwent surgery for ischemic nephropathy and remained stable in another 67 (47%). Function deteriorated in 27 of these patients (18%). The best results were achieved when the preoperative serum level of creatinine was less than 2 mg/dL. Hypertension improved or disappeared in 77% of patients who had ischemic nephropathy but remained unchanged in 23%.

Conclusions.—Extra-anatomical bypass is an effective approach in patients who have atherosclerotic renal artery stenosis, especially those in whom ischemic nephropathy develops. When feasible, this procedure is safer than renal revascularization combined with replacement of the aorta.

▶ The Cleveland Clinic group, along with a group at the Lehigh Clinic, have pioneered the notion of avoidance of the aorta in patients who have atherosclerotic renal arterial disease. This paper reviews the extensive experience at the Cleveland Clinic. The other point that should be emphasized is that there are now 2 indications for renal revascularization. The first is classic renovascular hypertension, but the second is the increasingly apparent entity that has been termed "ischemic nephropathy." These patients will have azotemia. They may not have hypertension, and one of the better tests for identifying vascular etiology is Doppler sonography.[1] Patients with a serum level of creatinine between 2 and 4 mg/dL appear to achieve the greatest benefit of either angioplasty or revascularization once the renal arterial disease is delineated.

E.D. Vaughan, Jr., M.D.

Reference

1. Hansen, et al: *Am J Kid Dis* 24:15, 1994.

4 Urinary Tract Infection

Ligase Chain Reaction for Detection of *Neisseria gonorrhoeae* in Urogenital Swabs
Ching S, Lee H, Hook EW III, Jacobs MR, Zenilman J (Abbott Labs, Abbott Park, Ill; Univ of Alabama, Birmingham; Case Western Reserve Univ, Cleveland, Ohio; et al)
J Clin Microbiol 33:3111–3114, 1995   4–1

Introduction.—Currently, gonorrhea is definitively diagnosed by culture on selective medium, which is thought to be 80% to 95% sensitive. The use of DNA amplification methods allows the elimination of problems related to collection and transport of specimens, which may lessen sensitivity. A ligase chain reaction (LCR) DNA amplification assay was used to detect *Neisseria gonorrheae* in swab specimens from the female endocervix and the male urethra.

Methods.—Sterile swabs were used to obtain specimens from patients at 3 geographically disparate sites in the United States. The results of a 4-hour LCR-based assay were compared with those achieved by culture on selective medium. Discordant findings were evaluated by another LCR assay based on *N. gonorrheae*–specific pilin probe sets. A total of 1,539 endocervical and 808 male urethral specimens were assessed.

Results.—Thirty-three specimens were LCR-positive but culture-negative; the reverse findings were noted for 7 specimens. The initial LCR assay was 97% sensitive and 98% specific compared with culture. The specific LCR assay confirmed that 18 of the 23 discordant endocervical specimens initially found to be LCR-positive actually were positive. All initially LCR-negative discordant specimens from both sites were confirmed as positive with the use of the *N. gonorrheae*–specific assay. The final sensitivity of the LCR assay for endocervical specimens was 97% (compared with 84% for culture), and its specificity was 99.6%. Its positive and negative predictive values were 96% and 99.8%, respectively.

Conclusions.—The specific LCR assay is more sensitive than culture for detecting *N. gonorrheae* in endocervical specimens. It also accurately detects infection in swab specimens from the male urethra. This method is highly specific and should prove useful in screening populations with a low prevalence of gonorrheal infection.

▶ There are probably more than 500,000 cases of gonorrhea per year in the United States.[1] Some affected men are seen by urologists. As pointed out in this abstract, the precision of diagnosis by culture is good but not as exact as one would like. The LCR evaluated by the authors has excellent precision, with 97% sensitivity and 98% specificity. In the 1995 YEAR BOOK, we included a paper that described the use of a similar approach in the diagnosis of chlamydial infections. We are beginning to see significant changes in the practice of medicine because of advances in molecular biology. One hopes that, in the not too distant future, more therapeutic options will be available.

S.S. Howards, M.D.

Reference

1. Burczak JD, Ching SF, Hu HY, et al: Ligase chain reaction for the detection of infectious agents, in Wiebrauk D, Farkas DH (eds): *Molecular Methods for Virus Detection.* New York, Academic, 1995, pp 315–327.

Bacterial Infection in Prostatodynia

Lowentritt JE, Kawahara K, Human LG, Hellstrom WJG, Domingue GJ (Tulane Univ, New Orleans, La)
J Urol 154:1378–1381, 1995
4–2

Background.—Prostatodynia is commonly diagnosed and poorly treated. It is differentiated from other prostatitis conditions by a lack of prostatic inflammation and no significant bacteria or leukocytes in prostatic secretions. It is resistant to therapy, and its etiology is unknown. A possible infectious etiology of prostatodynia was explored.

Methods.—Twenty-two patients who had prostatodynia and 16 control individuals were included. Segmented urine specimens were obtained. Bacterial proteins were extracted, and indirect and whole cell enzyme-linked immunosorbent assays were performed.

Results.—Cultures from prostatic secretions were positive in 9 patients. There were 22 bacterial isolates; the most common were coagulase-negative staphylococci, especially *Staphylococcus epidermidis* and *Staphylococcus haemolyticus. Staphylococcus saprophyticus* was also isolated. Prostatic bacteriology was significant compared with that of control individuals. There were no humoral immune differences between patients and control individuals. Antibiotic treatment was individualized and clinically effective.

Conclusions.—The etiology of prostatodynia may be bacterial in some patients. This finding is supported by the response of some patients to antibiotic therapy. Further studies should evaluate host-pathogen interactions and the efficacy of antibiotic therapy. It may be helpful to use molecular techniques to determine whether bacterial nucleic acids remain in prostatic secretions from culture-negative specimens.

▶ The etiology of prostatodynia is unknown, but the findings in this study are provocative. The consensus has been that prostatodynia is not related to bacterial infection. Indeed, one could state that, by definition, prostatodynia is present only in the absence of infection. Also, a recent unpublished investigation that looked at molecular biological evidence found no suggestion of infection as a cause of prostatodynia. The fact that the patients reported a response to antibacterial treatment is difficult to evaluate, because of the well-known placebo effect and the intermittent nature of symptoms in some men who have this disease.

S.S. Howards, M.D.

Minimal Invasive Therapy of Prostatic Abscess by Transrectal Ultrasound-guided Perineal Drainage
Bachor R, Gottfried HW, Hautmann R (Univ of Ulm, Germany)
Eur Urol 28:320–324, 1995   4–3

Background.—Although prostatic abscesses rarely occur, their potential for rupture and sepsis results in a high rate of mortality. Diagnosis is difficult because physical findings and clinical symptoms are variable. The value of transrectal ultrasonography (TRUS) in the diagnosis, treatment, and follow-up of prostatic abscess was determined.

Patients and Methods.—Six patients, aged 29–78 years, were referred to the study institution between April 1992 and November 1993. One patient was receiving maintenance hemodialysis, and 4 had undergone transurethral instrumentation 2–10 days before admission. Fever was present in all patients, and 3 had urinary retention. The prostatic gland was examined with the use of a 7.5-MHz biplanar transrectal probe. Treatment was performed as soon as diagnosis was confirmed. After the administration of local anesthesia, the needle was placed within the abscess and the discharge aspirated. Patients were given oral antibiotics for 2 weeks.

Results.—All abscesses were diagnosed with the use of TRUS after the prostatic gland was examined in longitudinal and transverse direction. Pus was aspirated in all patients. There were no early or late complications, and all patients were free of symptoms within 24 hours. Typical TRUS signs of abscess were the disappearance of the zonal anatomy of the prostatic gland, hypoechoic areas within the enlarged prostate, and a hyperechoic rim. When no abscess was found at follow-up TRUS, usually after 5–7 days, the catheter was removed. No patient has had a recurrent abscess.

Conclusion.—Prostatic abscess should be suspected in patients who have lower urinary tract obstructive symptoms along with unexplained fever and urinary tract infection resistant to treatment. Transrectal ultrasound has many advantages in the diagnosis and treatment of prostatic abscess because it is minimally invasive, easily accessible, and less expensive than CT and MRI. In addition, TRUS does not require ionizing radiation or contrast medium. In this series, prostatic abscesses were successfully drained, and none of the patients has had a recurrence.

Minimally Invasive Treatment of Renal Abscess

Siegel JF, Smith A, Moldwin R (Long Island Jewish Med Ctr, New Hyde Park, NY)
J Urol 155:52–55, 1996   4–4

Background.—Open surgery has been the standard management for renal abscesses, but more recent practice suggests that percutaneous drainage, or even antibiotic therapy, may be effective. The value of conservative treatment was determined, and patients for whom minimally invasive therapy would be appropriate were identified.

Methods.—The records of 52 patients were obtained from 2 hospitals and were examined for discharge diagnoses, radiology files, abscess specimens in the surgical pathology files, and outcome. Also noted were abscess size and location, patient age and gender, clinical symptoms, and laboratory data.

Results.—The average patient age was 47 years, and the male–female ratio was 2:3. Common predisposing factors were renal stones (36%), renal obstruction (29%), diabetes mellitus (25%), and multisystem disease (23%). Most patients had fever, abdominal pain, and/or flank pain, and 92% had pyuria on urinalysis. Symptoms persisted for an average of 22 days before treatment was sought. Abscess size was classified as small (< 3 cm) in 11 patients, medium (3–5 cm) in 17, and large (> 5 cm) in 23. Abscess involvement was perinephric in 19 patients, renal in 27, and renal and perinephric in 6. Average length of hospitalization was 22 days.

Seven patients (6 with large abscesses and 1 with a medium abscess) underwent primary surgical intervention, 33 were treated with percutaneous drainage (15 large, 13 medium, and 5 small abscesses), and 12 were observed during a 6-week or longer course of IV antibiotics (3 large, 3 medium, and 6 small abscesses). Three patients treated with antibiotics alone had refused surgical intervention and died of complications of sepsis. The 3 treatment modalities did not yield significantly different rates of resolution or reduction in hospital days. All small abscesses treated with antibiotics were resolved in immunocompetent patients; 92% of medium abscesses were successfully treated with percutaneous drainage. Approximately one third of large abscesses treated with percutaneous drainage needed additional drainage procedures or adjunct open surgical intervention.

Conclusion.—Percutaneous drainage can be as effective as open surgery for medium and large renal abscesses. Small abscesses are resolved with a course of IV antibiotics. Percutaneous drainage is cost-effective, avoids the risk of general anesthesia, and reduces morbidity, while not precluding open surgical intervention.

▶ These 2 papers present experience with percutaneous drainage of genitourinary abscesses and advocate this approach as the optimal treatment in many instances. At present, that approach is widely accepted. These experiences certainly support the conclusions of the authors. We usually use similar therapy. In regard to prostatic abscess, the authors used a Single-J drain in 5 of their 6 patients. The approach has advantages over the previous standard transurethral resection technique, in that it requires less anesthesia and should have fewer complications. The paper on renal abscesses presents an algorithm that includes medical treatment for small lesions, percutaneous therapy with antibiotics for medium lesions, and open surgical drainage for large abscesses. This plan worked in the authors' hands. We would support the editorial comments of Dr. Jackson Fowler, however, who pointed out that a 6-week course of IV medication, even on an outpatient basis, may not be cost-effective or practical, and that multiloculated lesions should be surgically drained. Finally, as with any less aggressive approach, it is essential that the physician monitor the patient carefully and be prepared to change strategy when the initial approach is not working.

S.S. Howards, M.D.

Rufloxacin Once Daily Versus Ciprofloxacin Twice Daily in the Treatment of Patients With Acute Uncomplicated Pyelonephritis
Bach D, van den Berg-Segers A, Hübner A, van Breukelen G, Cesana M, Plétan Y (St Agnes Hosp, Bocholt, Germany; Univ Hosp, Rostock, Germany; Univ of Limburg, Maastricht, The Netherlands; et al)
J Urol 154:19–24, 1995   4–5

Background.—Acute uncomplicated pyelonephritis, which typically affects women, is characterized by fever, flank pain, and costovertebral angle tenderness. It is also often accompanied by symptoms of lower urinary tract inflammation. The bacteriologic and clinical efficacy of rufloxacin and ciprofloxacin was compared in patients who had this clinical syndrome.

Methods and Findings.—One hundred ten outpatients were enrolled in a randomized, double-blind, multicenter trial. The patients received either 10 days of treatment with 200 mg rufloxacin daily, after a loading dose of 400 mg on the first day, or 500 mg ciprofloxacin twice a day. Outcomes were determined at the completion of treatment and at 2 and 4–6 weeks. The bacteriologic efficacy of rufloxacin was 55.6%, and the efficacy of ciprofloxacin was 58.8%. The success rates of rufloxacin and ciprofloxacin were 74% and 71%, respectively. Both drugs were tolerated well. Five adverse events occurred in the 53 patients who received rufloxacin, and 2 occurred in the 57 who received ciprofloxacin. This difference was not significant.

Conclusions.—Rufloxacin and ciprofloxacin are equally effective bacteriologically and clinically in patients who have acute uncomplicated pyelonephritis. Rufloxacin once daily appears to be a good alternative regimen for the outpatient antibiotic treatment of this syndrome.

▶ The results of this well-described study support the authors' conclusion that rufloxacin once daily is a good alternative to ciprofloxacin twice a day for the outpatient treatment of pyelonephritis. However, because a twice-a-day regimen is not unduly demanding, the choice probably should be based on cost. The authors did not provide that information. It may be significant that 8 of 53 patients (15%) had organisms that were resistant to rufloxacin, whereas only 3 of 57 (5%) had bacteria that were resistant to ciprofloxacin. Also, it is difficult to understand the low success rate with either drug in this series. In our experience, when a patient is treated with an antibiotic to which the bacteria are sensitive, the success rate is much higher.

S.S. Howards, M.D.

Binding of Type 1–piliated *Escherichia coli* to Vaginal Mucus
Venegas MF, Navas EL, Gaffney RA, Duncan JL, Anderson BE, Schaeffer AJ (Northwestern Univ, Chicago)
Infect Immun 63:416–422, 1995

4–6

Background.—*Escherichia coli* is responsible for most urinary tract infections (UTIs) in women. Before many UTIs, colonization of the vagina by bacteria occurs. Women who have certain blood types or the nonsecretor phenotype have an increased risk for the development of a UTI. Adhesion of some bacteria to uroepithelial cells has been shown to be mediated by proteins of the type 1 bacterial pilus. This adhesion is inhibited by mannose. An assay to examine how glycoproteins in vaginal mucus promote bacterial adhesion was developed.

Methods.—Vaginal mucus specimens were obtained from 28 women. Fourteen of the women had a history of UTIs, and 14 did not. Thirteen women were nonsecretors, and 15 were secretors. *Escherichia coli* HB101 transformed with the pW51-17, a recombinant plasmid that encodes for type 1 pili, were grown. As a control, those transformed with the vector only were also grown. *Escherichia coli* HB101 with and without pili were [3H]-labeled. Bovine submaxillary mucin (BSM) was used as a positive control for the type-1 piliated bacteria. The ascites fluid (AI) of a patient with cancer was used as a negative control. The labeled *E. coli* were incubated with mannose before being added to BSM or AI wells. Mannose antibody was added to all the wells. An enzyme-linked fluorogenic immunoassay was used to determine the secretor status of each patient.

Results.—A linear logarithmic response to binding was demonstrated in the BSM wells. Markedly less binding was seen in the AI wells, and no binding occurred with unpiliated bacteria. Binding of HB101/pWR51-17 to the 28 mucus specimens was 0.15–2.20 times that seen with the BSM control. Again, there was no binding of the unpiliated bacteria to the vaginal specimens. Mannose dependence of this binding was demonstrated by decreased binding when bacteria were preincubated with this sugar. Mannose receptors were shown with immunochemical binding by the mannose antibody. No inhibition occurred when the bacteria were preincubated with either glucose or galactose. Analysis of the samples collected during a 5-day and then a 12-week period demonstrated that any variation observed among specimens was caused by differences in the individual binding capacities to vaginal mucus, BSM, and AI.

Discussion.—Although many in vitro assays to assess bacterial adhesion exist, in vivo systems are limited. These results indicate that the type-1 piliated strain of HB101/pWR51-17 *E. coli* binds to vaginal mucus and is dependent on the number of bacteria present and the concentration of mucus in the wells. Finally, no difference was found in the bacterial binding to mucus or antimannose activity for either the secretors or the nonsecretors or for patients with and without UTI histories. The number of mannose terminal residues may actually determine the degree of bacterial binding and may be an important factor in colonization of the mucus and in assessment of a woman's susceptibility to UTIs.

Effect of Vaginal Fluid on Adherence of Type 1 Piliated *Escherichia coli* to Epithelial Cells
Gaffney RA, Venegas MF, Kanerva C, Navas EL, Anderson BE, Duncan JL, Schaeffer AJ (Northwestern Univ, Chicago)
J Infect Dis 172:1528–1535, 1995   4–7

Introduction.—Asymptomatic bacteriuria, kidney infection, or, occasionally, renal failure can result from the common bacterial urinary tract infection (UTI). A critical step is colonization of the vaginal mucosa by *Escherichia coli*, which is normally present in the bowel. How the bacteria migrates across the vaginal introitus is not well understood. Numerous factors, including bacterial characteristics, the genetic factors of the mucosal epithelial cell surface, the microenvironment of the vaginal fluid, age, menopausal status, and pH of the mucosa, have been cited. For example, the risk of UTI is reduced in postmenopausal women who take estrogen, because the pH of the vagina is lowered and colonization of bacteria is reduced. The presence of fluid on the epithelial cells at the opening of the vagina can influence a woman's chances of having a UTI by either adding a barrier to colonization or offering a receptor site for colonization. The effect of vaginal fluid on the adherence of *E. coli* to type 1 piliated epithelial cells was investigated.

Methods.—Vaginal fluid specimens were collected from 21 women, aged 23–79 years. Seven had recent UTI, and 4 had *E. coli* infections. The samples were cultured for bacteria, and pH and concentrations of protein were determined. *Escherichia coli* that encoded type 1 pili were used. *Escherichia coli* that did not encode type 1 pili were used as a negative control. Adherence and agglutination assays to the A431 cell line were determined, as was the bacterial binding to the fluid.

Results.—Low concentrations of protein enhanced bacterial binding in all specimens. At higher concentrations, binding was enhanced in some specimens but diminished in others. The increase in adherence was related to an increase in pH and in an increase in the binding of *E. coli* to the vaginal fluid.

Conclusion.—In an in vitro setting, the adherence of type 1 piliated *E. coli* to the A431 epithelial cell line is altered by the presence of vaginal fluid. The hypothesis of an effect of vaginal fluid in a required step for UTI is supported. Confirmation in a larger trial is necessary before considering the quality of the vaginal fluid as a possible factor in the in vivo development of UTI.

▶ These 2 papers are the latest work from Dr. Schaeffer and associates. This group does excellent research and has had a long-standing interest in UTI and, more specifically, in the mechanism of vaginal precolonization that leads to cystitis in women. Presumably, women who have frequent UTIs have differences in their vaginal defense mechanisms. Recent work by this group has further suggested that, at the molecular level, there are constant alterations in the ability of the vagina to resist adhesion of bacterial pathogens. These fluctuations make it even more difficult to define the specific mechanism involved. These papers add to the basic information generated by this group. The urologic community should be both proud of and grateful to the investigators at the Department of Urology at Northwestern for the excellent scientific contributions they are making. Eventually, this work will hopefully lead to therapeutic protocols for women who have recurrent UTIs.

S.S. Howards, M.D.

Relation of p53 Tumor Suppressor Protein Expression to Human Papillomavirus (HPV) DNA and to Cellular Atypia in Male Genital Warts and in Premalignant Lesions

Ranki A, Lassus J, Niemi K-M (Univ of Helsinki; Univ of Tampere, Finland)
Acta Derm Venereol 75:180–186, 1995   4–8

Purpose.—Current knowledge suggests that uncontrolled cell growth can result from functional disturbance of p53 tumor suppressor protein. Binding of human papillomavirus (HPV) E6 oncoproteins to wild-type p53 leads to loss of the negative growth control exerted by the p53 protein.

The link between aberrant p53 protein expression and HPV DNA and cellular atypia in male genital warts and premalignant lesions was determined.

Methods.—Seventy biopsy specimens of macroscopic genital warts, bowenoid papulosis (BP), or acetowhite lesions from 46 men were studied. Thirty-five lesions were histologically confirmed condylomata acuminata, 25 had BP histology, and 10 were noncondyloma lesions. Immunostaining was performed with 3 established antibodies, which recognized full-length wild-type accumulated p53 protein or its conformational mutants. In situ hybridization or polymerase chain reaction–based amplification was used to identify HPV DNA specific for HPV 6/11, 16/18, or 31/33/25.

Results.—Forty-one percent of condylomata with no keratinocyte atypia and 42% of those with slight nuclear atypia or BP histology showed both nuclear and cytoplasmic keratinocyte immunostaining. There was no apparent link between aberrant p53 expression and any specific HPV type or HPV DNA. Immunostaining for p53 was negative in normal skin and in some other penile dermatoses. After laser treatment, follow-up biopsy specimens obtained from 16 patients who had BP showed recurrent atypia only in lesions that were initially positive for both HPV DNA and p53 protein.

Conclusions.—Abnormally sequestered or loss-of-function p53 protein may be expressed by a few cells in male genital warts, even in the absence of cellular atypia. The presence of any type of HPV DNA at the same time is associated with recurrence or progression of premalignant changes. Clonal cell transformation probably involves some additional, as yet unidentified factors.

Suggested Reading

Krieger JN: New sexually transmitted diseases treatment guidelines. *J Urol* 154:209–213, 1995.

5 Renal and Urethral Injuries

Radiographic Assessment of Renal Trauma: Our 15-Year Experience
Miller KS, McAninch JW (Univ of California, San Francisco)
J Urol 154:352–355, 1995   5-1

Background.—Significant renal injury, which is staged thoroughly, represents only 10% of all renal injuries and less than 5% of all blunt renal injuries. Authorities disagree on how to identify patients who have a greater likelihood of significant renal injury, so that most patients who do not have significant injury can be spared the discomfort, possible allergic reaction, exposure to radiation, and expense of excretory urography. Criteria for radiographic imaging of renal injuries include penetrating flank or abdominal trauma, blunt trauma with gross hematuria or microscopic hematuria and shock, deceleration or major related abdominal injury, and pediatric renal trauma. The validity of these criteria was investigated.

Methods and Findings.—The medical records of 2,254 patients treated for suspected renal trauma between 1977 and 1992 were reviewed. A total of 1,588 patients had blunt trauma with microscopic hematuria and no shock. Of these patients, 1,004 did not undergo radiographic imaging, according to the above criteria. All had renal contusions. Overall, 3 patients had significant injury. These injuries, however, were identified during imaging or exploratory laparotomy for associated injuries. The status of 515 patients who did not undergo initial imaging was followed, and none of the patients had significant complications.

Conclusions.—Radiographic imaging is not required in adults who have blunt renal trauma or microscopic hematuria but no shock or major related intra-abdominal injuries. In the current series, this policy was found to be safe.

▶ This paper reconfirms a principle that, by now, has been well documented in the medical literature: Adult patients with nonpenetrating renal injuries who do not have gross hematuria or shock do not require imaging unless there are additional indications for so doing. Cass et al.,[1] Hardeman et al.,[2] Eastham et al.,[3] and the authors themselves[4] have already confirmed this. The combined series, as the authors point out, describes 2,873 patients who met the criteria. Among these patients, there were 10 significant injuries, only 1 of which was not detected with radiographic or exploratory staging procedures for additional intra-abdominal trauma.

S.S. Howards, M.D.

References

1. Cass AS, Luxenberg M, Gleich P, et al: Clinical indications for radiographic evaluation of blunt renal trauma. *J Urol* 136:370, 1986.
2. Hardeman SW, Husmann DA, Chinn HHW, et al: Blunt urinary tract trauma: Identifying those patients who require radiological diagnostic studies. *J Urol* 138:99, 1987.
3. Eastham JA, Wilson TG, Ahlering TE: Radiographic evaluation of adult patients with blunt renal trauma. *J Urol* 148:266, 1992.
4. Mee SL, McAninch JW, Robinson AL, et al: Radiographic assessment of renal trauma: A 10-year prospective study of patient selection. *J Urol* 141:1095, 1989.

Morbidity Associated With Nonoperative Management of Extraperitoneal Bladder Injuries

Kotkin L, Koch MO (Vanderbilt Univ Med Center, Nashville, Tenn)
J Trauma: Injury Infect Crit Care 38:895–898, 1995   5–2

Background.—Bladder injuries are common in trauma patients. Intraperitoneal bladder injuries are managed surgically, but extraperitoneal injuries are usually managed with Foley catheter drainage. The morbidity associated with nonsurgical management of extraperitoneal bladder ruptures was reported.

Methods.—Seventy patients who had extraperitoneal rupture caused by trauma were treated during a 10-year period. These patients were usually treated with Foley catheters alone, unless a laparotomy was indicated for another reason. All patients underwent a cystogram 10–14 days after their injury, at which time the catheter was removed unless extravasation was observed. If it was observed, then the cystogram was repeated every 5–7 days until the bladder was healed.

Results.—Of the 70 patients who had injury to the bladder, only 29 were treated with urethral catheters alone. Two of these patients died of causes unrelated to the bladder injury. Within 2 weeks, 74% of the remaining 27 individuals had a completely healed bladder. The other 26% had complications, including sepsis, vesicocutaneous fistula, and bladder calculi. These patients, when compared with those who did not have complications, had more severe injuries and lower blood pressure and required more blood transfusions. There was also an increased likelihood that these patients had functional problems with the catheter itself.

Discussion.—These results generally concur with those of previously published literature, in which nonexplorative management of extraperitoneal bladder rupture was usually appropriate. Treatment of these patients should include the use of large bore urethral catheters to maintain good drainage and a broad spectrum antibiotic regimen. In some instances, however, this management alone is not sufficient. For example, if a laparectomy is necessary for another reason, then surgical repair should be done at that time. The factors most likely to predispose an individual to an increased risk of morbidity could not be isolated.

▶ The consensus of urologists is that intraperitoneal bladder lacerations should be surgically repaired and that extraperitoneal lacerations can be managed with a catheter. Some surgeons believe that all lacerations should be repaired, whereas a few treat even intra-abdominal injuries nonoperatively. We concur with the consensus. In this retrospective study, there was a significant complication rate from nonoperative management of extraperitoneal bladder lacerations. These results are different from those reported by Corriere and Sandler,[1] who found that 87% of 39 such patients healed promptly and all did well in the long term. The take-home message from the Kotkin and Koch paper is that surgeons must be flexible both initially and subsequently, if their routine approach either seems inappropriate because of special circumstances or fails.

S.S. Howards, M.D.

Reference

1. Corriere JN Jr, Sandler CM: Management of the ruptured bladder: Seven years of experience in 111 cases. *J Trauma* 26:836, 1986.

Changing Trends in the Management of Iatrogenic Ureteral Injuries
Lask D, Abarbanel J, Luttwak Z, Manes A, Mukamel E (Hasharon Hosp, Petah Tiqva, Israel)
J Urol 154:1693–1695, 1995   5–3

Objective.—With acceptance of the percutaneous nephrostomy tube for management of late diagnosed iatrogenic ureteral injuries, the reoperation and reconstructive surgery rate decreased significantly. The outcome of management of ureteral injury before and after the introduction of the percutaneous nephrostomy tube was evaluated.

Methods.—Thirty-eight women and 6 men who had iatrogenic ureteral injuries between 1979 and 1984 were included. Six patients had immediate ureteroneocystostomy, 18 had immediate end-to-end ureteroureteral anastomosis, and 20 had percutaneous nephrostomy.

Results.—Eighty-two percent of injuries occurred during gynecologic surgery. Complications included flank pain in 82% of patients, fever in 34%, and ureterovaginal fistula in 34.5%. Patients who underwent surgery had hospital stays ranging from 14 to 35 days. Eighteen had urinary tract infections, and 8 had prolonged urinary leakage. Two patients showed mild to moderate unilateral hydronephrosis 3–6 months later. A percutaneous nephrostomy tube was used to treat 12 patients who had complete ureteral obstruction, 4 who had ureterovaginal fistula, 3 who had retroperitoneal extravasation of urine, and 1 who had a ureterosigmoid fistula. The 16 patients who recovered completely had hospital stays of 3–5 days. Four had urinary tract infections, 2 required replacement of blocked tubes, and 1 had moderate hydronephrosis at follow-up. Three of the remaining 4 patients required ureteroneocystostomy, and 1 required ureteroureteral anastomosis. The results of follow-up excretory urography were normal.

Conclusion.—Patients who have iatrogenic ureteral injuries and are treated by insertion of a percutaneous nephrostomy tube had significantly lower reoperation and morbidity rates. Most of these patients had spontaneous recoveries.

▶ There is no doubt that many ureteral injuries can and should be managed with a percutaneous nephrostomy, with or without a double J ureteral stent. There are situations, however, in which this approach is unlikely to succeed, and, particularly after iatrogenic injury, prompt surgical resolution of the situation is indicated.

S.S. Howards, M.D.

Suggested Reading

Conlin MJ, Skoog SJ, Tank ED: Current management of ureteroceles. *Urology* 45:357–362, 1995.

6 Hydronephrosis

Percutaneous Antegrade Endoscopic Pyelotomy: Review of 50 Consecutive Cases
Kletscher BA, Segura JW, LeRoy AJ, Patterson DE (Mayo Clinic and Found, Rochester, Minn)
J Urol 153:701–703, 1995
6–1

Background.—The current technique of percutaneous endoscopic pyelotomy, which is used to treat obstruction of the ureteropelvic junction, is based on the performance of intubated ureterotomies. After Wickham and Kellet, intubated ureterotomies were performed via a percutaneous nephrostomy tract. Since then, further refinements in the technique have been made. The results of 50 consecutive percutaneous antegrade endoscopic pyelotomies were analyzed retrospectively.

Methods.—Percutaneous antegrade endoscopic pyelotomy was performed in 50 patients, aged 4–87 years, who had ureteropelvic junction obstruction. Diagnosis was based on symptomatology and radiologic findings.

Results.—The overall success rate was 88%. The success rate in patients who had previous, failed renal procedures was 82%. The success rate when endoscopic pyelotomy was used as initial treatment was 90%. Follow-up was 4–74 months. Endoscopic pyelotomy failed in 6 patients. Four of these 6 patients had recurrent pain, and 2 had no pain; all had radiologic evidence of obstruction. There were 3 operative complications.

Conclusions.—Endoscopic pyelotomy as first line therapy for most adults who have obstruction of the ureteropelvic junction is supported. Excretory urography is the initial test of choice; retrograde pyelography is the initial test of choice if the patient has either an allergy to contrast medium or renal insufficiency.

▶ The authors' results in these 50 cases are very good. It should be emphasized, however, that they are very experienced and skilled. Therefore, casual use of this approach might not be successful. The authors' diagnostic approach of using excretory urography and percutaneous antegrade studies is, in our view, imprecise; we favor the direct renogram. Further, we suspect, but certainly cannot prove, that some of their patients did not need surgery.

The success rate for open pyeloplasty is 95%, compared with 85% to 90% for the percutaneous procedure. We so inform our patients and let them select the therapy. We do not perform percutaneous procedures in small children who have primary ureteropelvic junction obstruction.

S.S. Howards, M.D.

7 Calculus

Comparative Costs of the Various Strategies of Urinary Stone Disease Management
Jewett MAS, Bombardier C, Menchions CWB (Univ of Toronto; Wellesley Hosp Research Inst, Toronto)
Urology 46:S15–S22, 1995   7–1

Objective.—A cost-effectiveness study was carried out to compare 2 alternative methods of treating renal stone disease: extracorporeal shock wave lithotripsy (ESWL) and percutaneous nephrostolithotomy (PCNL).

Study Population.—An earlier cohort of 133 patients undergoing PCNL was compared with 1,000 later patients treated by ESWL. Each group consisted of consecutive adult patients with renal stones no larger than 2 cm in diameter.

Efficacy.—Ninety percent of patients with renal stones and 92% of those with ureteral stones were stone free after PCNL. The overall success rate at 3 months was 95%, and the results did not change appreciably up to 1 year after treatment. Extracorporeal shock wave lithotripsy using the Lithostar yielded a stone-free rate of 56% and a 3-month success rate of 74%. Retreatment was necessary in 19% of the first thousand patients treated. The effectiveness of ESWL using the Dornier MFL 5000 is not yet clear.

Costs.—Hospital costs per treatment and per case were substantially lower for ESWL than for PCNL (Table IV). Total fees averaged $615 for ESWL and $1,197 for PCNL. Professional fees remained the single largest

---

TABLE IV.—Hospital Costs for PCNL and ESWL

133 PCNL patients (136 treatments)	
136 treatments/year	$1,678.00/treatment
133 cases/year	$1,716.00/case
1,000 Lithostar* patients (1247 treatments)	
Inpatient	$ 764.00/treatment
Outpatient	$ 85.00/treatment
1% admission rate prorated	
$92.00/treatment	$ 115.00/case

*Similar for Dornier patients but no longer applicable as less than 0.5% admitted at present.
Abbreviations: PCNL, percutaneous nephrostolithotomy; *ESWL*, extracorporeal shock wave lithotripsy.
(Reprinted by permission of the publisher from Jewett MAS, Bombardier C, Menchions CWB: Comparative costs of the various strategies of urinary stone disease management. *Urology* 46:S15–S22, 1995. Copyright 1995 by Elsevier Science, Inc.)

component of cost, but capital costs per year and operating costs declined with increasing case volume, as did the costs of service. The cost per case increased as the annual volume decreased.

Conclusions.—Extracorporeal shock wave lithotripsy is less expensive than PCNL but less consistently renders patients free of renal stones. Total costs may be reduced by identifying, at an early stage, those patients who will require retreatment or other more expensive forms of treatment.

▶ It is not surprising that the authors found that ESWL was less expensive than PCNL. A more interesting study would be to observe these patients for a few years and examine the need for additional therapy. The rate of recurrent stone formation will be higher in the ESWL group, and the need for additional treatment will offset the savings initially achieved with ESWL.

Alan D. Jenkins, M.D.

Economic Impact of Urolithiasis in the United States

Clark JY, Thompson IM, Optenberg SA (Brooke Army Med Ctr, San Antonio, Tex)
J Urol 154:2020–2024, 1995
7–2

Objective.—Little is known about the economic impact of urolithiasis in the United States. A previous study estimated the direct and indirect costs of urolithiasis in 1984 as $898 million. Data from various sources were used to estimate the total cost treatment for upper urinary tract stones in the United States.

Methods.—Hospital discharge statistics were obtained from the Agency for Health Care Policy and Research. This provided information on the costs of evaluating and treating upper urinary tract calculi. Prevalence data for urolithiasis were assessed as well. Data on the frequency of surgical treatment were obtained from the Civilian Health and Medical Program of the Uniformed Services claims. Direct inpatient costs and direct and indirect outpatient costs were estimated.

Results.—The estimated total charges for evaluation, hospitalization, and treatment of urolithiasis in the United States were $1.23 billion per year. Estimated professional charges to hospitalized patients were $183 million. Expected costs for outpatient evaluation of urolithiasis were $278 million, and $139 million in indirect costs was attributed to lost wages. Total direct and indirect costs for urolithiasis in the United States in 1993 were estimated at $1,834 million.

Discussion.—The annual total cost of urolithiasis in the United States is about $1.83 billion, by a conservative estimate. Efforts to prevent urinary stones or manage them more effectively could yield significant cost savings to society. Although the number of office visits to urologists has not increased during the last 2 decades, the number of patients with upper urinary tract stones has increased substantially. This probably reflects the trend toward outpatient evaluation and treatment.

▶ Studies such as this can be used to compare the economic impact of urolithiasis with that of other diseases. Data such as this will be used to allocate health care dollars in the future. A more interesting finding was that professional charges accounted for only 10% of the total annual cost of urolithiasis. The vast bulk of charges were for evaulation, hospitalization, and treatment. Professional charges are an easy target for cost-cutting measures, but data such as these show that this approach will have little impact on total expenditures.

Alan D. Jenkins, M.D.

Effect of Urinary Intestinal Diversion on Urinary Risk Factors for Urolithiasis

Terai A, Arai Y, Kawakita M, Okada Y, Yoshida O (Kyoto Univ, Japan)
J Urol 153:37–41, 1995   7–3

Introduction.—Patients with urinary intestinal diversions are susceptible to many metabolic complications caused by resorption of urinary solutes across the bowel segment. Serum electrolyte abnormalities, bony demineralization, and calculus formation may occur in patients who have had bowel segments incorporated into the urinary tract. The effect of urinary intestinal diversion on risk factors for calcium urolithiasis was investigated in this report.

Methods.—Ninety-six patients were divided into 3 groups according to the type of urinary diversion they received: Kock pouch, Indiana pouch, and ileal conduit. Urine samples were collected from all patients and tested for volume, creatinine and creatinine clearance, calcium, phosphate, magnesium, uric acid, oxalate, and citrate. Data were analyzed using the unpaired generalized Wilcoxin test.

Results.—Although urinary volumes were about the same for all 3 groups, calcium, phosphate, and magnesium excretions were much higher in the continent reservoir group then in the ileal conduit group, whereas Kock pouch and Indiana pouch groups showed little difference. Hypocitraturia of less than 100 mg per day was found in 22 of 58 Kock pouch samples (38%), 14 of 25 Indiana pouch samples (56%), and 12 of 31 ileal conduit samples (39%). The mean urinary calcium, phosphate, and magnesium levels, along with other urinary risk factors, could not be correlated with the duration of diversion in any of the groups.

Conclusions.—The data indicate that the continent urinary reservoir causes long-term increases in excretions of calcium, phosphate, and magnesium that may promote the development of calcium urolithiasis and infectious stones. The results also suggest that the degree of metabolic change may be higher with a continent reservoir than with an ileal conduit.

▶ It is not surprising that the authors found an increase in urinary excretion of calcium, phosphate, and magnesium in patients with continent urinary diversion. This presumably is secondary to the hyperchloremic metabolic acidosis that occurs in these patients. Unfortunately, the authors did not evaluate systemic acid–base status. What is surprising is that the authors found that urinary citrate excretion was normal in all groups. Although more than one third of patients in each group were hypocitraturic, there were no differences between the 3 groups. If patients with continent urinary diversions had a more profound metabolic acidosis, then one would have expected urinary citrate excretion to have been uniformly low.

Alan D. Jenkins, M.D.

Genetic Factors in Calcium Oxalate Stone Disease
Goodman HO, Holmes RP, Assimos DG (Bowman Gray School of Medicine, Winston-Salem, NC)
J Urol 153:301–307, 1995   7–4

Purpose.—The development of idiopathic calcium oxalate nephrolithiasis is a complex process resulting from interaction between environmental and genetic factors. Many different urinary characteristics have been proposed to play a role, and each may be affected by environmental and genetic influences. Although the genetic contributions are difficult to extract, it can be done through careful control or assessment of the environmental factors. The literature on genetic factors contributing to susceptibility to calcium oxalate stone disease is reviewed.

Discussion.—Like other diseases with a large genetic component, calcium oxalate stone disease tends to cluster in families. The main contributing factors to this observed heritability are probably a small number—no more than 3–4—of leading gene loci. Individuals vary considerably in the excretion of certain analytes, namely calcium, oxalate, and citrate. Based on this finding and on the high prevalence of hypercalciuria, hyperoxaluria, and hypocitrauria among patients with stones, a hypothesis that alleles at 3 gene loci may be involved in determining the individual's levels of calcium, oxalate, and citrate excretion was suggested. These susceptibility genes must be reasonably frequent (i.e., affecting 20% to 60% of the population) to explain the high prevalence of calcium oxalate stone disease. People with intermediate calcium excretion appear to be more susceptible to stone disease than those with low calcium excretion. By extension, the same may be true for individuals with differing levels of oxalate or citrate excretion. With further study, it may be possible to design beneficial treatments for patients with intermediate levels of excretion. Also, efforts to identify the susceptibility genes will be aided by accurate phenotypic classification of individuals. One day, molecular biological techniques may make it possible to classify individuals through DNA testing of blood samples. The ability to obtain such an accurate genetic classification would help in making valid assessments of the relative risks associated with the susceptibility genes and in studying the effects of dietary and other factors.

Summary.—Calcium oxalate stone disease appears to be heritable, and the evidence suggests that a limited number of genetic foci are involved.

The proposed susceptibility genes affect the individual's level of calcium, oxalate, and citrate excretion in urine. Further research is needed to identify the specific genes. Once this is done, it will provide valuable insight into how calcium oxalate stone disease develops and aid in the development of effective new treatment strategies.

▶ This is an excellent review of the genetics of calcium oxalate stone disease. The mapping and sequencing of the human genome will eventually lead to the identification of the specific genes responsible for the increased risk of stone formation in some families. Traditional predictors of recurrent stone formation, such as supersaturation of crystal growth inhibition, are not very reliable. More vigorous preventive measures could be instituted in individuals who have a greater genetic predisposition.

Alan D. Jenkins, M.D.

Results of Long-Term Treatment With Orthophosphate and Pyridoxine in Patients With Primary Hyperoxaluria
Milliner DS, Eickholt JT, Bergstralh EJ, Wilson DM, Smith LH (Mayo Clinic, Rochester, Minn)
N Engl J Med 331:1553–1558, 1994   7–5

Objective.—Because patients with primary hyperoxaluria have a poor outlook without treatment, the long-term value of orthophosphate and pyridoxine therapy was studied in 25 such patients who were treated for 10 years on average, starting at a mean age of 12 years. Type I primary hyperoxaluria was confirmed in 9 patients, and type II disease was confirmed in 5. Most of the patients had symptoms of urolithiasis.

Results.—In 2 patients, urinary oxalate excretion became normal, or nearly so, shortly after the start of treatment. In 7 other cases the urinary oxalate level decreased gradually over a period of years. Calcium oxalate supersaturation and crystal formation decreased, and inhibition of calcium oxalate formation increased during treatment. No patient had evidence of metabolic bone disease. Urinary phosphorus excretion nearly doubled during treatment. Eight of 23 assessable patients had new stones or exhibited the growth of preexisting stones during long-term follow-up. Nine patients had a decrease in stone mass. Five patients progressed to end-stage renal disease after 7–23 years of treatment. Four of them underwent renal transplantation. Two transplant procedures were initially successful, and 1 patient did well after retransplantation.

Conclusion.—Combined treatment of primary hyperoxaluria with orthophosphate and pyridoxine at an early stage effectively reduces calcium oxalate crystallization in the urine and seemingly preserves renal function.

▶ Primary hyperoxaluria can be a devastating and life-threatening disease. Dr. Smith and his colleagues at the Mayo Clinic have one of the largest groups of patients with primary hyperoxaluria. They have used a combination of orthophosphate and pyridoxine for many years to treat these patients.

The last few years have seen great advances in the treatment and understanding of this disease. Liver transplantation will correct the metabolic abnormality in these patients, and concurrent renal transplantation can restore normal renal function. The biochemistry of the disorder also has been more accurately elucidated. Identification of the specific genetic defect may ultimately lead to a more elegant cure.

Alan D. Jenkins, M.D.

Urinary Calcium and Oxalate Excretion in Children
Reusz GS, Dobos M, Byrd D, Sallay P, Miltényi M, Tulassay T (Semmelweis Univ, Budapest, Hungary; Med School, Hannover, Germany)
Pediatr Nephrol 9:39–44, 1995   7–6

Background.—Most cases of nephrolithiasis in children are caused by calcium oxalate stones, and hypercalciuria is believed to be a major contributor to the development of calcium-containing renal stones. Although normative data on calcium excretion in children have been published, there are few data on urinary oxalate excretion in this age group. Levels of urinary calcium and oxalate excretion were measured in normal, healthy children as well as in children with relevant pathologic conditions.

Methods.—The normative sample consisted of 25 healthy, term newborns during the first week of life and 391 children aged 1 month to 14.5 years. Twenty-four-hour or first-morning urine samples from these children were analyzed to determine normal values for calcium/creatinine (Ca/Cr) and oxalate/creatinine (Ox/Cr) ratios. Also studied were 137 children with postglomerular hematuria and 27 children with nephrolithiasis. Ion chromatography was used to measure oxalate, and the nomograms of Marshall and Robertson were used to calculate urine saturation to calcium oxalate.

Results.—Distribution was normal for the Ca/Cr ratio and log-normal for the Ox/Cr ratio. The molar Ca/Cr ratio reached its lowest point during the first few days of life. It peaked at a mean of 0.39 mmol/mmol at 7–18 months of age then, after a slight dip, stabilized at 0.34 mmol/mmol by 6 years of age. Peak Ox/Cr values occurred during the first months of life; the geometric mean was 133 µmol/mmol. This ratio then declined gradually until the age of 11 years, reaching a mean of 24 µmol/mmol.

Of the 137 children with postglomerular hematuria, 36 had hypercalciuria: 23 absorptive calciuria and 13 renal type. The mean oxalate excretion was 38 µmol/mol in the children with absorptive hypercalciuria who were following a calcium-restricted diet compared with 22 and 23 µmol/mol, respectively, for the children with renal hypercalciuria and the normal children. Children with nephrolithiasis had a calcium oxalate urine saturation of 1.18 compared with 1.06 in the children with hematuria and

0.84 in the normal children. There was fairly good correlation between the measurements made in 24-hour and first-morning samples, but the scatter was relatively wide.

Conclusions.—Screening for hypercalciuria and hyperoxaluria in children can be performed by measuring the Ca/Cr and Ox/Cr ratios in first-morning urine samples. Age-specific reference values are needed to interpret the results, however. For children with hematuria, hypercalciuria, or nephrolithiasis, urinary calcium and oxalate excretion should both be measured. Even if the child has 1 "normal" excretion value, the clinician must persist in efforts to identify abnormal mineral excretion.

▶ The authors found that the calcium-to-creatinine ratio stabilizes after the first few days of age. This is in contrast to the oxalate-to-creatinine ratio, which is very high during the first year of life and gradually falls to a stable value during the next 4–5 years. This is illustrated in Table 1 of the original article.

Alan D. Jenkins, M.D.

Reduction of Vitamin D Induced Stone Formation by Calcium
Strohmaier WL, Seeger RD, Osswald H, Bichler KH (Eberhard-Karls Univ, Tübingen, Germany)
Urol Res 22:301–303, 1994   7–7

Introduction.—The pathogenesis of calcium-containing urinary tract stones involves 1,25-dihydroxycholecalciferol (DHCC), which is the active metabolite of vitamin D. The precise mechanism is unclear, but up to 30% of those who form calcium oxalate stones show increased vitamin D levels. The cellular processes involved in the pathogenesis of vitamin D-induced nephrolithiasis were studied in rats.

Methods.—Male Wistar rats were randomized to receive 6 days of treatment with 1,25-DHCC—alone or with the new 1,4-dihydronaphthyridine Goe 6070, a calcium antagonist—or they were randomized to a control group. The 1,25-DHCC was given subcutaneously in a dose of 120 pmol every 24 hours, whereas Goe 6070 was given by gavage, 1 mg/kg every 24 hours. After 6 days of treatment, clearance studies were performed. The kidneys were examined histologically, and their calcium tissue content was analyzed.

Results.—The rats in the 1,25-DHCC group showed substantial concretionary formation, which was significantly limited by Goe 6070 treatment. Calcium tissue content was 0.17 vs. 0.04 mg/100 mg dry weight in the 1,25-DHCC group vs. the Goe 6070 group. The glomerular filtration rate fell by nearly 4 mL/min/kg in the 1,25-DHCC group; Goe 6070 inhibited this reduction almost completely.

Conclusions.—The new calcium inhibitor Goe 6070 appears to have a protective effect against vitamin D-induced nephrolithiasis. In this rat study, 1,25-DHCC treatment is associated with both intracellular and membrane-bound concretions, which are inhibited by Goe 6070 with no significant change in biochemical parameters. These findings suggest that cellular processes play an important role in the pathogenesis of 1,25-DHCC-induced nephrolithiasis.

▶ The title of this paper is somewhat misleading because the authors actually found that vitamin D-induced stone formation was reduced by the administration of a calcium-channel blocker. Their hypothesis is that elevated vitamin D levels can lead to hypercalcemia and an increase in the influx of calcium into renal tubular epithelial cells. This leads to accumulation of calcium in mitochondria and to intracellular crystallization. The administration of a calcium-channel blocker might prevent this intracellular calcification. This is an interesting hypothesis that merits further study.

Alan D. Jenkins, M.D.

Clinical and Biochemical Features of Uric Acid Nephrolithiasis
Ito H, Kotake T, Nomura K, Masai M (Teikyo Univ, Japan)
Eur Urol 27:324–328, 1995   7–8

Objective.—The prevalence of uric acid stones varies by country, by region, by ethnicity, and over time. Questions remain about the pathogenesis of these stones, which are 1 of the 2 major noncalcium stones. Blood and urine biochemical studies were performed as part of an investigation of the frequency of uric acid stones at 1 Japanese institution.

Patients.—The study included 652 patients with upper urinary tract stones in whom the stone composition was assessable. The frequency of uric acid stones in this population was 5.5%. The patients were 33 men and 3 women, most of whom were in their forties and fifties. Hypouricemia was noted in 2 of the women. Seventy-two percent of patients had pure uric acid stones, 17% had mixed uric acid and calcium oxalate stones, and 8% had both pure and mixed stones. One patient had a mixed uric acid and sodium acid urate stone.

Biochemical Findings.—Biochemical studies were performed in male patients and controls. Men with uric acid stones had a significantly higher blood uric acid level than those with calcium stones. The blood uric acid level in the men with pure uric acid stones was no different from that in the uric acid stone group as a whole. The uric acid stone group had significantly lower urine calcium excretion than the control group. Calcium excretion also tended to be lower in men with uric acid stones and pure uric acid stones than in men with calcium stones. Oxalic acid excretion was lower in the uric acid stone group than in the calcium stone group but no different from the control group. Uric acid excretion was no different in these groups. The morning urinary pH was 5.24 in the pure uric acid stone group vs. 6.07 in the calcium stone group. In the patients with pure uric acid stones, 24-hour uric acid excretion was inversely correlated with the pH of early morning urine. Fractional excretion of urate was not significantly different between patients with uric acid stones, pure uric acid stones, and calcium stones.

Conclusions.—A clinical and biochemical investigation of uric acid nephrolithiasis is reported. The formation of these stones relies on 3 factors—acidic urine, decreased urine volume, and hyperuricosuria—of which urinary pH is the most important. The new results suggest that uric acid stones do not form until the patient excretes a large amount of uric acid with no significant decrease in urinary pH. Urinary pH is inversely related to urinary uric acid level, which points to the importance of relative hyperuricosuria in the formation of uric acid stones.

▶ These investigators found that acidic urine, decreased urine volume, and hyperuricosuria were the 3 causative factors in uric acid stone formation. Of these, urinary pH was the most important. This emphasizes that the primary treatment of uric acid stone formation is urinary alkalinization. Reduction of hyperuricosuria with allopurinol can help, but elevation of the urinary pH is far more beneficial.

Alan D. Jenkins, M.D.

A Study of Recurrent Stone Formers With Special Reference to Renal Tubular Acidosis

Singh PP, Pendse AK, Ahmed A, Ramavataram DVSS, Rajpurohit SK (Ravindra Nath Tagore Med College, Udaipur, Rajasthan, India)
Urol Res 23:201–203, 1995   7–9

Background.—In the authors' Indian state, recurrent idiopathic urinary tract calcium stones represent a major health problem. In some patients, these recurrent stones result from a distal renal tubular acidification (dRTA) defect. The reported percentage of dRTA cases among those having recurrent stones varies widely. The presence of dRTA was evaluated in selected patients with recurrent renal tract stones.

Methods.—The study included 45 patients with radiologic proof of recurrent renal stones who were seen in the surgical wards or outpatient clinic of an Indian medical college. All underwent an acid challenge test, in which they received 150 mg of ammonium chloride per kilogram of body weight, to assess the presence of dRTA. Creatinine, calcium, oxalic acid, inorganic phosphorus, uric acid, magnesium, and citric acid were analyzed in 24-hour urine samples. The patients also gave 1-hour urine samples before the acid challenge test and hourly samples for the 7 hours after the acid challenge. Creatinine, calcium, citric acid, inorganic phosphorus, titratable acidity, and ammonium were analyzed in these samples.

Results.—Twenty-two percent of the patients had a dRTA defect. Compared with the patients without dRTA defects, these patients had a significantly lower citric acid excretion and a significantly higher urinary pH. Calcium excretion was similar in the 2 groups. The patients with dRTA tended to have lower titratable acidity and ammonium excretion. After the acid challenge was given, the patients without a dRTA defect had an adequate reduction in pH; in patients with a defect, pH remained high.

Conclusions.—Those with and without dRTA defects who form recurrent stones show certain differences in their urine excretory parameters. Citric acid excretion is lower in the patients with dRTA defects, but there is no difference in calcium excretion. Urinary pH is significantly higher in the patients with dRTA defects and remains so after acid challenge. There are no previously reported data with which to compare the new findings.

▶ This paper confirms previous studies that have examined the incidence of dRTA defects in patients with calcium urolithiasis. Distal renal tubular acidification defects can be manifested completely or partially. Patients with classic dRTA have metabolic acidosis. Patients with the incomplete form do not have metabolic acidosis, but they fail to acidify their urine systemically. Both types of patients have low urinary citrate levels.

Although the authors did not examine systemic acid–base status, I presume that this was normal in their study patients. Their patients probably had incomplete dRTA. These patients usually are identified by the presence of hypocitraturia. The administration of alkali (as in bicarbonate or citrate) will correct the disorder, normalize urinary citrate levels, and halt subsequent stone formation.

Alan D. Jenkins, M.D.

Nephrolithiasis Clinical Guidelines Panel Summary Report on the Management of Staghorn Calculi
Segura JW, Preminger GM, Assimos DG, Dretler SP, Kahn RI, Lingeman JE, Macaluso JN Jr, McCullough DL (Mayo Clinic, Rochester, Minn)
J Urol 151:1648–1651, 1994   7–10

Introduction.—Struvite staghorn calculi are relatively uncommon stones that can pose serious problems. Patients with staghorn calculi often have urinary tract infections, and the stones themselves can be infected. A number of different treatments for these stones are available, each of which has its advantages and disadvantages. Evidence-based recommendations for the treatment of struvite staghorn calculi are presented.

Methods.—The recommendations were developed by the Nephrolithiasis Clinical Guidelines Panel of the American Urological Association. An explicit approach was used to develop the guidelines, based on a comprehensive literature review. Outcomes data from 110 articles that contained viable, unduplicated data on the treatment of struvite staghorn calculi were subjected to meta-analysis. Three outcomes were defined as being most important: being stone free; needing a secondary, unplanned procedure; and having treatment complications.

Results.—Two treatment standards were developed. First, active intervention was recommended as the standard for patients with newly diagnosed struvite staghorn calculi, based on the expert opinion that observation was not in the best interest of the typical patient with this type of stone. Second, patients with newly diagnosed staghorn calculi should be advised of the 4 accepted treatment modalities: open surgery, percutaneous nephrolithotomy, extracorporeal shock wave lithotripsy (ESWL), and a combination of percutaneous nephrolithotomy and ESWL.

Three guidelines were developed as well. The first was that, for the standard patient, percutaneous stone removal should be performed first, followed by ESWL repeat percutaneous treatment or both, if necessary. Treatment with ESWL alone was not viewed as a good initial choice for most patients nor was open surgery. Finally, 3 options were described. Monotherapy with ESWL and percutaneous lithotripsy were viewed as equally effective treatments for small-volume staghorn calculi in collecting systems with normal or near-normal anatomy. Open surgery was deemed appropriate for unusual patients in whom the other accepted approaches seemed unlikely to succeed. Nephrectomy was viewed as an option for patients in whom the stone-bearing kidney was poorly functional.

Summary.—Standards, guidelines, and options for the treatment of struvite staghorn calculi are described. For most standard patients, the best choice for first-line treatment is a combination of percutaneous stone removal and shock wave lithotripsy, not ESWL or open surgery alone. The article includes a discussion of the limitations of the guideline development process and outlines the basic research needs for the future.

▶ All urologists who treat patients with large kidney stones should be familiar with the recommendations in this article. Large struvite staghorn calculi should be treated initially with percutaneous lithotripsy. Extracorporeal shock wave lithotripsy and secondary percutaneous procedures can be done as needed. Primary ESWL treatment should be limited to small volume stones in patients with normal collecting system anatomy. There is no place for multiple ESWL treatments in the management of a large struvite stone.

Alan D. Jenkins, M.D.

Suggested Reading

Renal Morphology and Urodynamic Factors for Renal Stone Formation
Ishikawa Y (Kinki Univ School of Med, Osaka, Japan)
Nipon Hinyokika Gakkai Zasshi 86:263–272, 1995

▶ Studies on the pathogenesis of urolithiasis have mainly focused on metabolic disorders. However, metabolic disorders alone are not sufficient to explain the problem. In the present study, morphological and urodynamic differences of the upper urinary tract on both the stone and normal side were examined. There were 35 cases of those who had experienced unilateral, recurrent, and/or multiple stone formation.

1. Morphologic study. Study of the pelvic-caliceal system (PCS) revealed significant differences in the following parameters on the stone side as compared with the normal side. The findings were: (1) the number of minor

calices (papillaes), Np, was higher; (2) the number of major calices, Nm, was higher; (3) the number of branches, Nb, was higher; (4) the lower calyx radius, l_2, was longer; (5) the total calyx area, Ac, was larger; (6) the renal pelvic area, Ar, was larger; (7) and the total area, At, was larger.

2. Urodynamic study. Additional study of the urodynamic factors revealed significant differences in the following parameters on the stone side as compared with the normal side. These findings include: (1) the peristaltic frequency in the upper third of the ureter was less; (2) the difference in peristaltic interval was longer and the rhythm of the peristaltic discharge was irregular. However, no significant difference in the contraction pressure was found except in the pelviureteral junction. After furosemide had been administered, the contraction pressure decreased while the peristaltic frequency increased on both sides. Futhermore, it was found that on the stone side the peristaltic interval decreased significantly as well as the rhythm of the peristaltic discharge becoming regular.

The results of the two studies indicate that in the same individual the urine flow in the stone side as compared to that of the normal side is either stagnant or inconstant, thereby creating conditions conducive to the formation and growth of stones that become difficult to discharge owing to these same conditions. Therefore, morphologic and urodynamic disorders of the upper urinary tract may be considered factors contributing to stone formation. It appears that the diuretic action is an effective method for preventing stone recurrence and facilitating stone passage.

G.J. Fuchs, M.D.

8 Adrenals

Clinical, Hormonal and Pathological Findings in a Comparative Study of Adrenocortical Neoplasms in Childhood and Adulthood
Mendonca BB, Lucon AM, Menezes CAV, Saldanha LB, Latronico AC, Zerbini C, Madureira G, Domenice S, Albergaria MAP, Camargo MHA, Halpern A, Liberman B, Arnhold IJP, Bloise W, Andriolo A, Nicolau W, Silva FAQ, Wroclaski E, Arap S, Wajchenberg BL (Univ of São Paulo, Brazil)
J Urol 154:2004–2009, 1995   8–1

Introduction.—Adrenocortical neoplasms are rare but can occur at any age in both genders. The clinical, hormonal, and pathologic findings in children and adults who had functional adrenocortical neoplasms were studied, and potential prognostic factors were explored in both age groups.

Methods.—Eighteen children, aged 7 months to 14 years, and 20 adults, aged 18–57 years, in whom adrenocortical neoplasm was diagnosed between 1980 and 1992 were included. Thirteen children had signs of virilization, 1 had Cushing's syndrome, and 4 had both. Of the 20 adults, 8 had signs of virilization, 10 had Cushing's syndrome, and 2 had both. Blood specimens were obtained after fasting and analyzed for hormone concentrations. All neoplasms were completely resected. Each tumor was graded and analyzed histologically according to Weiss criteria. Clinical, hormonal, and pathologic findings, as well as survival, were compared in the adult and pediatric groups.

Results.—There was a distinct female predominance. Virilization was the predominant manifestation in children, whereas Cushing's syndrome was predominant in adults. All children but 1 had a high level of testosterone (including all children who had virilization), 17 had elevated levels of dehydroepiandrosterone sulfate, 13 had elevated levels of dehydroepiandrosterone, 17 had elevated levels of androstenedione, and 12 had elevated levels of 11-deoxycortisol. Among the adults, 10 of the 18 women had elevated levels of testosterone (including 8 who had signs of virilization), 9 of 17 had elevated levels of dehydroepiandrosterone sulfate, 10 of 17 had elevated levels of androstenedione, and 6 of 14 had elevated levels of 11-deoxycortisol. Elevated levels of cortisol were found in patients who had Cushing's syndrome, with or without virilization, in both groups. Sixteen children had localized disease, and 2 had distant disease. Nineteen adults had localized disease, and 1 had regional disease. During follow-up, 16 children remained disease-free 24–114 months after surgery, as did 16 adults 18–132 months after surgery. The 2 adults and 4 children who had both virilization and Cushing's disease had metastases; 5 of these patients died. Metastases were also associated with an elevated level of 11-deoxycortisol. Patients with isolated Cushing's disease had the longest survival rates. Prognosis was not significantly related to tumor weight and size or Weiss histologic evaluation in either age group.

Conclusions.—Children and adults are likely to have differing manifestations of adrenocortical neoplasms; virilization predominates in children, and Cushing's syndrome predominates in adults. Better prognoses were associated with young age and isolated Cushing's syndrome. High levels of 11-deoxycortisol were predictive of neoplasm recurrence in both children and adults. The poorest prognosis was associated with mixed clinical features of both Cushing's syndrome and virilization.

▶ This paper, which presents a large experience with adrenal tumors, probably reflects the high incidence of adrenal neoplasms in Brazil.[1] Most of the findings reported by the authors are typical of those noted in previous papers. The literature, however, documents rather poor results in pediatric cases. These authors reported a surprising number of pediatric cases and had a more favorable outcome. Humphrey et al.[2] recorded a 53% 5-year survival rate for children younger than 7 years of age and 17% for those older than age 7. It is difficult to explain the much better results in this series. Perhaps the results are related to the high incidence in Brazil and a different genetic disease spectrum.

S.S. Howards, M.D.

References

1. Ribero RC, Sandrini Neto RS, Schell MJ, et al: Adrenocortical carcinoma in children: A study of 40 cases. *J Clin Oncol* 8:67, 1990.
2. Humphrey GB, Physer T, Holcombe J: Overview on the management of adrenocortical carcinoma (ACC). *Cancer Treat Res* 17:349, 1983.

Therapeutic Outcome of Primary Aldosteronism: Adrenalectomy Versus Enucleation of Aldosterone-producing Adenoma
Nakada T, Kubota Y, Sasagawa I, Yagisawa T, Watanabe M, Ishigooka M
(Yamagata Univ, Japan)
J Urol 153:1775–1780, 1995   8–2

Background.—The prognosis of adrenocortical insufficiency is dismal. The removal of an aldosterone-producing adenoma, without excising the prominent part of the tumor-uninvolved glandular tissue, is therefore preferable, provided hypertension or metabolic alkalosis will respond to such a procedure. The long-term outcomes of adrenalectomy and enucleation of aldosterone-producing adenoma were compared.

Methods.—Forty-eight patients who had primary aldosteronism were treated with 1 of the 2 techniques, and their status was followed for 5 years. After unilateral solitary tumors were localized preoperatively, 22 patients underwent unilateral adrenalectomy, and 26 underwent enucleation of aldosterone-producing adenoma.

Findings.—Both procedures similarly improved hypertension, hypokalemia, the low urinary sodium-to-potassium ratio, suppressed plasma renin activity, high plasma levels of aldosterone, high urinary excretion of aldosterone, and high urinary excretion of kallikrein for 5 years. Plasma levels of cortisol and adrenocorticotropic hormone were also identical after both operations. Ambulation and administration of furosemide, combined with low sodium diet stimuli, at 5 years markedly increased plasma renin activity and plasma levels of aldosterone in the patients who underwent aldosterone-producing adenoma enucleation to levels almost similar to normal values. In the patients who underwent adrenalectomy, increment magnitudes were slight. Before surgery, infusion of angiotensin II did not increase plasma levels of aldosterone in patients who had primary aldosteronism. After surgery, plasma aldosterone responses to infusion of angiotensin II and plasma cortisol responses to administration of adrenocorticotropic hormone in the patients who underwent aldosterone-producing adenoma enucleation were more sensitive than those in the patients who underwent adrenalectomy. Recurrent hyperaldosteronism was not observed in either group throughout the study.

Conclusions.—Angiotensin II induces release of aldosterone by activating tumor-uninvolved cortical cells. The enucleation of aldosterone-producing adenoma is preferable to unilateral adrenalectomy.

▶ This important paper documents that the results achieved with enucleation of aldosterone-producing adenomas are equal to those achieved with adrenalectomy. Just as partial nephrectomy has become the treatment of choice for small renal carcinomas, partial adrenalectomy may become the option of choice for aldosterone-producing adenoma, if these findings are confirmed. We disagree, however, with the authors' assertion that adrenal failure has a dismal prognosis.

S.S. Howards, M.D.

Adrenalectomy via the Dorsal Approach: A Benchmark for Laparoscopic Adrenalectomy

Nash PA, Leibovitch I, Donohue JP (Indiana Univ, Indianapolis)
J Urol 154:1652–1654, 1995   8–3

Background.—The number of laparoscopic adrenalectomies continues to increase. More and more small adrenal tumors are discovered because of improved imaging, and it is becoming more difficult to choose between open excision or laparoscopic removal. The advantages of laparoscopic surgery in other organ systems have not been proved in laparoscopic adrenalectomy. The results of open surgical excision of aldosteronomas were reported.

Methods.—The medical records of 40 patients (mean age, 46 years) who underwent open adrenalectomy for hyperaldosteronism secondary to a unilateral solitary adenoma were reviewed. A sigmoid incision was made through the bed of the 12th rib. The costovertebral ligament was divided, and the rib was retracted inferiorly. In a transthoracic approach, a linear incision was made through the diaphragm. The peritoneal cavity was avoided in all patients.

Results.—Mean operative time was 200 minutes, and mean blood loss was 232 cc. Mean time to unassisted ambulation was 2.2 days, and mean time to return to a normal diet was 2.5 days. Mean hospital stay was 4.3 days. No intraoperative complications occurred, and there was no peri-operative mortality. No blood transfusions were required. Postoperative complications included urinary retention, prolonged ileus, urinary tract infection, wound infection, and prolonged nausea. Less narcotic was required by patients who used controlled analgesia.

Conclusions.—In these patients, open surgical excision of aldosteronomas with the use of a dorsal approach was safe and well tolerated. Morbidity was acceptable. If the pleural cavity is not entered, operative time is shorter. Morbidity is reduced if rib resection is avoided and if intrathecal narcotic and patient controlled analgesia are used. These data are offered as a standard with which results of laparoscopic adrenalectomy can be compared.

▶ Laparoscopic adrenalectomy is becoming more popular and acceptable. In the past 2 years, we have featured 3 articles that described experience with laparoscopic adrenalectomy.[1, 2] The above abstract is useful in that, as the authors point out, it provides a basis for comparison. We believe that an open surgical procedure is still the standard; in skillful hands, however, laparoscopic excision is certainly reasonable. The cost-effectiveness of a laparoscopic procedure must be evaluated. It certainly requires a longer operating time but should allow a more rapid functional recovery.

S.S. Howards, M.D.

References

1. 1994 YEAR BOOK OF UROLOGY, pp 40–41.
2. 1995 YEAR BOOK OF UROLOGY, p 28.

9 Renal Diseases

Renin Secreting Tumors: Diagnosis, Conservative Surgical Approach and Long-term Results
Haab F, Duclos JM, Guyenne T, Plouin PF, Corvol P (Saint Joseph Hosp, Paris; Broussais Hosp, Paris)
J Urol 153:1781–1784, 1995
9–1

Introduction.—Tumors of the juxtaglomerular apparatus of the kidney are rare; only about 40 cases have been described. These tumors, however, are a surgically correctable form of hypertension. The cases of 8 patients, seen during a 15-year period, who had a renin-secreting renal juxtaglomerular cell tumor were described. The mean follow-up was 98 months.

Diagnosis.—Before 1986, plasma renin activity was estimated by its enzymatic activity. At present, however, it is measured by direct radioimmunoassay. A renal venous renin ratio of 1.5 was considered clinically significant. The most recent patients have had abdominal CT scanning with contrast enhancement.

Findings.—All 8 patients had marked systolic and diastolic hypertension; mean pressures were 207 and 134 mm Hg, respectively. Hypertension had been present 7.6 years before diagnosis. The mean patient age at diagnosis was 22 years. Hypokalemia was a constant finding, and all patients had secondary hyperaldosteronism. Five of 8 tumors were localized by renal venous renin assay. Three tumors were visualized on angiography as an avascular region. Computed tomographic imaging demonstrated all reninomas.

The mean tumor size was 24 mm. All patients underwent conservative resection. It was not necessary to control the renal pedicle. Three intraparenchymal tumors were located by perioperative echography. There were no complications. Hypertension and hypokalemia resolved within a week of tumor removal, and plasma renin activity became normal within 2 days. Most elements of the tumors stained with antirenin antibody. All but 1 patient remained normotensive during follow-up. The patient who had hypertension continued to have normal plasma renin activity and a normal level of aldosterone. One of 2 women had mild hypertension during pregnancy.

Conclusions.—In a patient with hypertension who has secondary aldosteronism and no other apparent cause, renin-secreting tumor should be suspected. Exploration is indicated if renal angiography or abdominal CT demonstrates a renal tumor. Most reninomas are adequately treated by resection or partial nephrectomy.

▶ As I mentioned in my editorial comment concerning this paper,[1] the critical issue is simply to think about these rare tumors when a patient has the constellation of hypertension, hypokalemia, and a solid small renal mass. The critical test is obviously plasma renin activity, which is usually extremely high. The authors show the hypodense nature of these tumors, which previously had been shown to be hypovascular. The bottom line is that the patient should be treated with nephron-sparing surgery, i.e., partial nephrectomy, because these tumors are benign in nature.

E.D. Vaughan, Jr., M.D.

Reference

1. Vaughan ED Jr: Renal and adrenal sparing surgery for patients with primary aldosteronism and primary reninoma (editorial). *J Urol* 153:1785–1786, 1995.

Three-dimensional Analysis of Glomerular Morphology in Patients With Subtotal Nephrectomy
Remuzzi A, Mazerska M, Gephardt GN, Novick AC, Brenner BM, Remuzzi G (Mario Negri Inst for Pharmacological Research, Bergamo, Italy; Cleveland Clinic Found, Ohio; Harvard Medical School, Boston)
Kidney Int 48:155–162, 1995
9–2

Background.—Single-section assessment of kidney tissue has been found to underestimate the incidence of glomerulosclerosis. Three-dimensional evaluation of glomerular morphology improves the recognition of the incidence and distribution of sclerotic changes in the glomerular capillary tuft. This technique was used to determine the true frequency and spatial extent of glomerulosclerosis in patients undergoing extensive renal mass reduction.

Methods.—Four kidney biopsy specimens of patients with 1 kidney who had undergone partial nephrectomy for renal cell carcinoma were reevaluated. Histopathologic evaluation to detect glomerular sclerotic lesions was done on serial sections, along with 3-dimensional morphometric analysis of glomerular tuft and sclerotic regions with the use of a computer-based image processing system (Fig 1). The findings of these evaluations were compared with those of more conventional single-section examination of the same biopsy specimens.

Findings.—Only 8% of 65 glomeruli assessed by 3-dimensional morphometric analysis were normal. Forty-two percent showed segmental sclerosis, and 51% showed global sclerosis. On single-section examination, 37% of glomeruli appeared normal. The 3-dimensional distribution of sclerosis was characterized by the appearance of multifocal regions that affected a small capillary tuft volume, which eventually propagated to the whole capillary tuft.

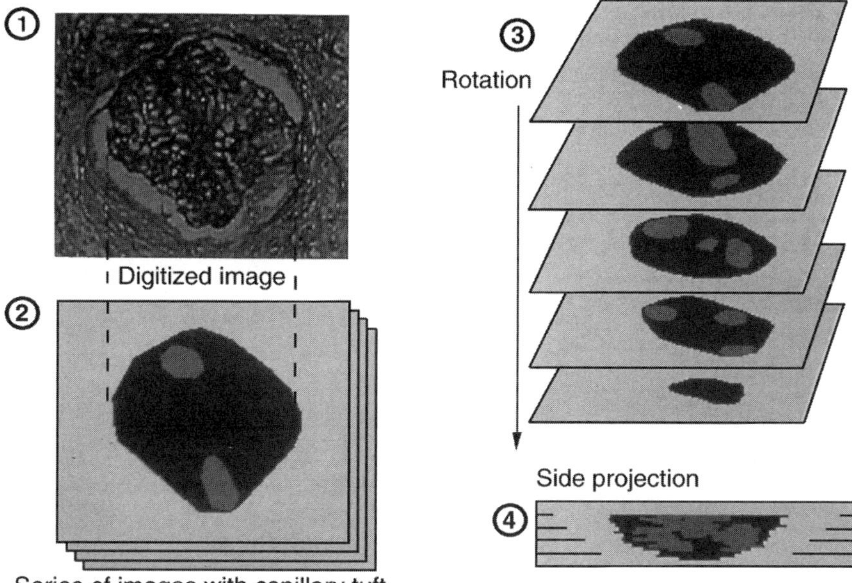

FIGURE 1.—Schematic representation of the technique used for 3-dimensional reconstruction of glomerular tufts. Digitized images from the microscope (1) were used to outline the glomerular capillary tuft and areas of sclerosis if present (2). A side view (parallel to the section plane) of the capillary tuft was then created by the projection function of Image 1.55 using all the sections of each glomerulus. The projection function represents the capillary tuft volume as transparent surface with internal localization of the sclerosis areas. (Courtesy of Remuzzi A, Mazerska M, Gephardt GN, et al: Three-dimensional analysis of glomerular morphology in patients with subtotal nephrectomy. *Kidney Int* 48:155-162, 1995.)

Conclusions.—Even when renal function is maintained, glomerulosclerosis at the time of biopsy in patients who have extensive ablation of renal mass affects nearly all of the glomerular population. Sclerotic lesions may therefore appear initially as multifocal lesions in the capillary tuft and subsequently propagate to global sclerosis.

▶ The debate continues as to how important hyperfiltration injury is, particularly in patients who have a normal contralateral kidney. This analysis is an extension of a previous paper,[1] which was an elegant study of glomerular change in these patients that revealed multifocal lesions in the glomerular tuft. Remuzzi et al. give further information concerning the progression of glomerular changes in these patients. It would be interesting to see whether early changes can be demonstrated in the contralateral kidney of patients with normal renal function who are undergoing unilateral nephrectomy.

E.D. Vaughan, Jr., M.D.

Reference

1. Novick AC, Gephardt G, Guz B, et al: Long-term follow-up after partial removal of a solitary kidney. *N Engl J Med* 325:1058–1062, 1991.

10 Renal Neoplasms

Treatment of Renal Cell Carcinoma in von Hippel-Lindau Disease: A Multicenter Study
Steinbach F, Novick AC, Zincke H, Miller DP, Williams RD, Lund G, Skinner DG, Esrig D, Richie JP, DeKernion JB, Marshall F, Marsh CL (Cleveland Clinic Found, Ohio; Mayo Clinic, Rochester, Minn; Univ of Iowa, Iowa City; et al)
J Urol 153:1812–1816, 1995   10–1

Introduction.—There is a strong predisposition for tumor development in the rate autosomal dominant disorder von Hippel-Lindau disease. Tumors may develop in the retina, cerebellum, spinal cord, pancreas, adrenal glands, and kidneys. In approximately 45% of patients who have this disorder, multicentric and bilateral carcinoma of the kidney cells develops. These cancers can metastasize and are a main cause of death in these patients. The surgical options include bilateral nephrectomy or a nephron-sparing procedure to prevent end-stage renal failure. Previous work has suggested that the nephron-sparing procedure is associated with local recurrence of the cancer. The outcome for patients who had renal replacement after bilateral nephrectomy was assessed.

Methods.—From 8 medical centers, 65 patients who had von Hippel-Lindau disease underwent surgery for treatment of renal cell carcinoma. The disease was bilateral in 54 patients and unilateral in 11. Radical nephrectomy was performed in 16 patients (8 unilateral and 8 bilateral), and nephron-sparing surgery was performed on 49 patients (8 unilateral, 19 bilateral, and 22 unilateral with contralateral nephrectomy). All tumors were staged according to established procedures. Large or suspicious lymph nodes were removed. The most common neurologic manifestations were cerebellar hemangioblastoma (69% of patients) and retinal angioma (51%). The mean follow-up was 68 months.

Results.—Stage I tumors were found in 75% of patients. Ninety percent of tumors were clear cell carcinomas. Five or more tumors were removed from 51 kidneys. There were no operative deaths or serious complications. The 5-year cancer-specific survival rate for all patients was 95%, and the 10-year survival rate was 77%. For the renal-sparing surgery patients, the 5- and 10-year survival rates were 100% and 81%, respectively. Half the patients in the latter group had a local recurrence, and 2 had metastatic disease. At 5 years, 71% were free of local recurrence, but only 15% were free of local recurrence at 10 years. Fifteen patients had end-stage renal disease. The 6 who underwent transplantation required no dialysis. One of these patients died of metastatic disease, and the other 5 were alive an average of 28 months after transplantation.

Conclusion.—Although nephron-sparing surgery is an effective initial treatment for patients who have von Hippel-Lindau disease, many patients will have local recurrence. Renal transplantation can be effective therapy for end-stage renal disease.

▶ This review of the experience of investigators at 8 institutions with surgical management of von Hippel-Lindau disease provides the best long-term data available regarding outcomes with this disease. Our experience would also suggest that long-term freedom from tumor recurrence occurs in only a distinct minority of patients who undergo nephron-sparing surgery (15% in this series). The fact that patients who have multiple foci of disease (see Abstract 10–3) do well in the short-term is based on the natural history of this disease. Further, when end-stage renal disease occurs in these patients, renal transplantation provides a feasible management strategy. In this series, only 1 of 6 patients so treated had metastatic disease while receiving the immunosuppression required to prevent rejection. It would seem reasonable, therefore, that one should not be reluctant to proceed to bilateral nephrectomy and renal transplantation (after an interval of 1–2 years) in selected patients in whom nephron-sparing surgery is impractical given the extent of their lesions on initial examination.

R. Flanagan, M.D.

Nephron Sparing Surgery for Renal Cell Carcinoma in von Hippel-Lindau Disease
Shinohara N, Nonomura K, Harabayashi T, Togashi M, Nagamori S, Koyanagi T (Hokkaido Univ, Sapporo, Japan)
J Urol 154:2016–2019, 1995   10–2

Introduction.—Both renal-cell carcinoma and cystic renal disease are part of the phakomatosis designated von Hippel-Lindau disease. From 25% to 45% of those affected have renal-cell carcinoma. Nephron-sparing surgery has been proposed because of the youth of the patients and the frequent presence of multicentric and bilateral tumors, but these cancers may metastasize and cause death.

Series.—The results of nephron-sparing surgery were reviewed in 5 patients with von Hippel-Lindau disease and non-advanced renal-cell carcinoma. Four women and 1 man with a median age of 36 years received operations. Four of them had bilateral synchronous renal-cell carcinomas, and 1 had multicentric cancer in one kidney.

Treatment.—The patient with unilateral tumors underwent extracorporeal partial nephrectomy and autotransplantation of the renal remnant. The other 4 patients had bilateral renal surgery. Three of them had in situ partial nephrectomy and/or enucleation of one kidney and extracorporeal partial removal of the other kidney with autotransplantation of the remnant. Thirty-three tumors in all were resected. One patient had microscopic invasion of the perinephric fat.

Results.—Nephron-sparing surgery succeeded in all cases. The median follow-up was approximately 5 years. All but one of the renal lesions were resected in the 9 initial procedures. Postoperative CT monitoring disclosed 35 lesions, 8 of which had enlarged. The 4 patients who initially had bilateral surgery underwent secondary renal surgery and retained adequate renal function.

Conclusion.—Nephron-sparing surgery is appropriate for patients with von Hippel-Lindau disease who have localized, low-stage renal-cell carcinomas.

▶ This paper highlights the early success that can be achieved with an aggressive approach to nephron-sparing surgery in patients who have von Hippel-Lindau disease. More importantly, it defines the growth rate of recurrent solid lesions in this group of patients (mean, 0.5 cm/yr). As such, the authors provide an algorithm (with which I would agree) that suggests that the status of such patients be followed with yearly CT scanning and that solid lesions be removed at or before the time they reach 3 cm in diameter. The results described in this paper (4 of 5 patients underwent reoperation for recurrent lesions within 77 months) would agree with those of Steinbach et al. (Abstract 10–1) that recurrent disease is highly likely with long-term follow-up.

R. Flanagan, M.D.

Prevalence of Microscopic Lesions in Grossly Normal Renal Parenchyma From Patients With von Hippel-Lindau Disease, Sporadic Renal Cell Carcinoma and No Renal Disease: Clinical Implications
Walther MM, Lubensky IA, Venzon D, Zbar B, Linehan WM (National Cancer Inst, Bethesda, Md; NCI-Frederick Cancer Research and Development Ctr, Md)
J Urol 154:2010–2015, 1995   10–3

Introduction.—Patients who have von Hippel-Lindau (VHL) disease are disposed to have multiple renal tumors and remain at risk of new tumors throughout their lives. Several cytologic and architectural tumor types have been described, but the microscopic forms of these neoplasms are unknown. The earliest renal lesions in patients who had von Hippel-Lindau disease were described.

Method.—Microscopic precursor lesions were sought by examining grossly normal renal tissue from 16 patients who had VHL disease and renal carcinomas. The patients underwent a total of 25 operations on 23 kidneys. Nephron-sparing procedures, such as partial nephrectomy and enucleation, were performed. Grossly normal tissue samples also were available from 56 patients who had sporadic renal cell carcinoma and from 19 randomly selected autopsy specimens of individuals not known to have had renal disease.

Findings.—Ten percent of samples from patients who had VHL disease exhibited microscopic lesions, including a single focus of solid renal cell tumor, a simple cystic renal cell neoplasm, and 2 complex cystic renal cell tumors. Eight atypical cysts and 13 benign cysts were also discovered. All renal cell neoplasms and atypical cysts had clear cell features. Benign cysts lined by cuboidal cells that had eosinophilic cytoplasm (resembling renal tubular cells) were found only in patients who had renal cancer. An average kidney from a patient who had VHL disease appeared to contain 1,100 benign or atypical cysts and 600 clear cell neoplasms.

Conclusions.—Clear cell renal carcinoma is the initial manifestation of cellular transformation in patients who have VHL disease. A genetic abnormality may also contribute to the development of renal cysts in these patients. The findings warrant ongoing surveillance of these patients after nephron-sparing surgery.

▶ These authors have significantly enhanced our understanding of the evolution of renal cancer in patients who have VHL disease. They first identified the *VHL* gene on chromosome 3p and have now conducted a careful investigation and provided a histologic description of the presence of large numbers of focal clear cell lesions (both cystic and neoplastic) within the grossly normal renal parenchyma of these patients. Their finding that "normal" tissue from VHL kidneys displays mutation of only 1 copy of the *VHL* gene and that the wild type (normal copy) is lost in VHL renal cancers is very important.[1] Further, although sporadic, nonfamilial renal cancers often show mutation of both copies of the *VHL* gene, normal renal parenchyma in these patients shows no VHL abnormality.[2]

R. Flanagan, M.D.

References

1. Knudson AG: Antioncogenes and human cancer. *Proc Natl Acad Sci USA* 90:10914, 1993.
2. Shuin T, Kondo K, Torigoe S, et al: Frequent somatic mutations and loss of heterozygosity of the von Hippel-Lindau tumor suppressor gene in primary human renal cell carcinomas. *Cancer Res* 54:2852, 1994.

Multicentricity in Renal Cell Carcinoma
Nissenkorn I, Bernheim J (Meir Gen Hosp, Kfar Saba, Tel Aviv, Israel)
J Urol 153:620–622, 1995   10–4

Background.—Partial nephrectomy is common in patients who have either 1 kidney and impaired renal function or bilateral renal cell carcinoma. Radical nephrectomy, however, is standard treatment for patients who have renal cell carcinoma and a normal contralateral kidney, despite dramatic changes in clinical findings of patients who have kidney tumors. Renal-sparing surgery is supported by advances in renal imaging, increased incidence of small, low-stage tumors detected incidentally, and long-term survival of patients who have partial nephrectomy. The use of partial nephrectomy decreased after reports of multicentricity of renal cell carcinoma. The presence of multicentric neoplasms in kidneys was investigated.

Methods.—The presence of multicentric neoplasms was assessed in 27 kidneys with renal cell carcinoma and 23 control kidneys from autopsies. There was no kidney tumor, renal disease, or other malignancy in the kidneys from autopsy.

Results.—Tumor size was between 2 and 9 cm. In kidneys with a tumor, the incidence of small renal cell carcinoma nodules was 11.1%. In kidneys from autopsy, the incidence of small nodules was 13%. In kidneys with a tumor 3 cm or smaller, the incidence of satellite malignant nodules was 3.7% in this series.

Conclusions.—On the basis of these findings, retroperitoneal partial nephrectomy is recommended in patients who have peripheral renal cell carcinoma smaller than 3 cm and in those who have a normal contralateral kidney.

Intrarenal Satellites of Renal Cell Carcinoma: Histopathologic Manifestation and Clinical Implication

Oya M, Nakamura K, Baba S, Hata J-I, Tazaki H (Keio Univ, Tokyo)
Urology 46:161–164, 1995   10–5

Objective.—Satellite cancers that accompany the primary lesion have been described in as many as 1 in 5 cases of renal cell carcinoma. The incidence of satellite carcinoma was determined by step-sectioning 108 nephrectomy specimens of renal cell carcinoma at 3-mm intervals. Seventy-nine tumors were found incidentally; only 29 patients were symptomatic.

Findings.—Satellite carcinomas were found in 7 specimens (6.5%); 17% were from symptomatic patients. The incidence was 7% in pathologic stage 1 cases, 3% in stage 2, and 14% in stage 3 (Table 2). Twenty-five percent of patients who had N1 disease and 5% of those who did not have nodal involvement had satellite carcinoma. Tumor grade could not be related to the presence or absence of satellite lesions.

Implications.—Satellite lesions of renal cell carcinoma are most prevalent in patients who have high-stage primary lesions but are also found in low-stage cases. Intraoperative ultrasonography may help locate a satellite cancer in patients who have low-stage primary lesions and undergo nephron-sparing surgery.

TABLE 2.—Pathologic Classification and the Incidence of Satellite Carcinoma

	Total Cases	Cases with Satellite Carcinoma	Incidence (%)	P Value
T factor				
pT1	14	1	7.10	
pT2	66	2	3	
pT1 + pT2	80	3	3.75	0.0726
pT3a	20	3	15	
pT3b	8	1	12.50	
pT3a+pT3b	28	4	14.30	
N factor				
No	100	5	5	0.238
N1	8	2	25	
M factor				
Mo	104	6	5.77	0.084
M1	4	1	25	
Tumor grade				
1	39	4	10.25	0.291
2	63	3	4.76	
3	6	0	0	0.423

(Reprinted with permission of the publisher from Oya M, Nakamura K, Baba S, et al: Intrarenal satellites of renal cell carcinoma: Histopathologic manifestation and clinical implication. *Urology* 46:161–164, copyright 1995 by Elsevier Science, Inc.)

The Incidence of Multifocal Renal Cell Carcinoma in Patients Who Are Candidates for Partial Nephrectomy

Whang M, O'Toole K, Bixon R, Brunetti J, Ikeguchi E, Olsson CA, Sawczuk TS, Benson MC (Columbia Univ, New York)
J Urol 154:968–971, 1995 10–6

Background.—Renal neoplasms discovered incidentally present a management dilemma. Partial nephrectomy has been considered in patients who have such neoplasms, because these tumors are often small, peripheral, and of a low stage. A high incidence of multifocality, however, has been reported among tumors found incidentally. The incidence of multifocal renal cell carcinoma in patients who would otherwise be candidates for partial nephrectomy was investigated.

Methods.—Thirty-one men and 13 women, aged 43–89 years, were included. All patients were suitable for partial nephrectomy but underwent radical nephrectomy. Preoperative imaging studies and surgical specimens were reviewed prospectively.

Findings.—Twenty-five percent of renal cell cancers showed pathologic multifocality. Ninety-one percent of these multifocal tumors occurred in the presence of a primary tumor 5 cm or smaller. Tumor multifocality was independent of the primary renal tumor size but occurred with a slightly greater frequency in tumors of stage T3A or higher, even when the primary tumor was small.

Conclusions.—The incidence of unsuspected multifocal renal cell cancer was high in patients who would otherwise have been considered good candidates for partial nephrectomy. This high incidence was independent of tumor size but seemed to occur with increased frequency in tumors of advanced stage. Partial nephrectomy should be reserved for patients who need nephron preservation. It should not be performed simply because it is technically feasible.

Prospective Analysis of Multifocality in Renal Cell Carcinoma: Influence of Histological Pattern, Grade, Number, Size, Volume and Deoxyribonucleic Acid Ploidy

Kletscher BA, Qian J, Bostwick DG, Andrews PE, Zincke H (Mayo Clinic and Found, Rochester, Minn)
J Urol 153:904–906, 1995

10–7

Background.—Simple or partial nephrectomy, rather than radical nephrectomy, may be considered in patients who have bilateral tumors, a tumor in a solitary kidney, or a contralateral kidney that functions poorly. More routine use of nephron-sparing surgery in patients who have renal cell carcinoma is controversial, however, because of the threat of multifocal disease. Retrospective studies have found a 7% to 19.7% incidence of multifocal disease in patients who have renal cell carcinoma. Specimens obtained from patients undergoing radical nephrectomies were studied prospectively to clarify the incidence of multifocality and the factors that predict this occurrence.

Methods.—During a 1-year period, surgical specimens obtained from 100 consecutive patients who underwent radical nephrectomies for the treatment of stage pT1N0M0 to stage pT3bN0M0 renal cell carcinoma were studied with either preoperative CT or MRI and pathologic analysis.

Results.—Sixteen specimens revealed multifocal disease. There were 1–50 lesions per specimen, with a mean of 5 and a median of 2 lesions per specimen. The secondary lesions had identical histologic patterns to the primary lesion in all but 1 specimen (6%) and identical histologic grades in all but 5 (31%). Multifocal renal cell carcinoma was suggested by the preoperative imaging findings in 7 patients (44%) and was confirmed by standard pathologic sectioning techniques in 10 specimens (62%). When tumor characteristics of those specimens with multifocal disease and those without were compared, neither diameter, volume, histologic stage or grade, nor DNA ploidy differentiated between groups. There were, however, significantly greater rates of mixed and papillary histologic patterns in the patients who had multifocal renal cell carcinoma.

Conclusions.—The incidence of unknown multifocality was 6%, which corresponds to the local recurrence rate reported in other studies. Although the papillary and mixed cell histologic patterns are associated with a greater incidence of multifocal disease, multifocality cannot be reliably predicted in patients who have renal cell carcinoma.

▶ The preceding 4 articles all involve the issue of multifocality in renal cell carcinoma. They relate the incidence of multifocality to histologic pattern, size, grade, stage, and ploidy. The incidence of 6% observed by Kletscher et al. is similar to that observed by Oya et al. Nissenkorn et al. similarly show a low incidence (3.7% in small tumors 3 cm or less). In all these studies, incidence seems to be related to the size, stage, and, to some extent, pattern of the tumor. Whang et al., however, report a much higher overall incidence of multifocality. Although the numbers are small, the data are not in significant disagreement with other data, i.e., the incidence is much less in patients who have small tumors. The Mayo Clinic group suggests a greater risk of multifocality in patients who have papillary tumors; this has been suggested in the past by others.

The underlying problem in all such studies is the definition of "malignancy." It seems clear that because local recurrence after partial nephrectomy is only in the range of 3% to 5%, many of these small tumors never become problematic. Although this finding may be the result of insufficient follow-up, and such tumors may take many years to manifest, it is also possible that they are not true malignancies and will never be a threat to the patient.

The debate regarding partial nephrectomy in the presence of a normal contralateral kidney continues. Many investigators now believe, however, that it is appropriate to perform partial nephrectomy in patients who have small tumors (3–4 cm or less) that are located in positions that allow safe removal with a reasonable amount of normal, adjacent tissue. Although radical nephrectomy may indeed remain the gold standard, most urologists believe that, in spite of the specter of multifocality and recurrence, judicious partial nephrectomy is appropriate in selected patients.

J.B. DeKernion, M.D.

Is Ipsilateral Adrenalectomy a Necessary Component of Radical Nephrectomy?
Shalev M, Cipolla B, Guille F, Staerman F, Lobel B (Hopital Pontchaillou, Rennes, France)
J Urol 153:1415–1417, 1995   10–8

Introduction.—The inclusion of ipsilateral adrenalectomy with radical nephrectomy is no longer universally recommended for all patients who have renal cell carcinoma. Some urologists still recommend adrenalectomy for patients undergoing radical nephrectomy. Ipsilateral adrenal involvement was assessed in patients who had renal cell carcinoma to ascertain whether routine ipsilateral adrenalectomy during radical nephrectomy is actually required.

Methods.—Two hundred ninety-nine patients who had renal cell carcinoma underwent radical nephrectomies. Two hundred eighty-five of these patients also underwent removal of ipsilateral adrenal glands. The patients were divided into 2 groups according to stage: Group 1 included patients who had stage T1 or T2 disease, and group 2 included those who had stage T3 or T4. Patients were further categorized according to positive or negative lymph node involvement. The likelihood ratio for adrenal involvement in relation to metastatic regional lymph node disease was calculated.

Results.—Ipsilateral adrenal gland involvement of renal cell carcinoma was found in 11 of 285 patients (3.8%). No incidental tumors were detected in this series. The tumor invaded the gland by direct extension from the upper pole in 7 of the patients who had adrenal involvement. The renal tumor was in the middle or lower portion of the kidney, and extension to the adrenal gland was by distant metastasis in the remaining 4 patients. All 11 patients had lymph node metastases. Distant metastases were found in the lung of 2 patients. Adrenal metastases were observed by CT in 2 patients before surgery. In 274 patients (96.2%), the excised ipsilateral adrenal glands were free of disease; 98 of these patients (35.7%) had stage pT3 carcinoma, and 4 (1.4%) had stage pT4. Lymph node involvement was detected in 52 (18.9%). The likelihood ratio for adrenal involvement was 2.7 in relation to T stage; it was 5.2 in relation to lymph node involvement (N stage).

Conclusion.—The likelihood of adrenal involvement was high with nodal metastases. Nodal involvement was far more predictive of adrenal involvement than was local tumor spread. Adrenalectomy during radical nephrectomy should be restricted to suspected direct extension of the tumor from the kidney into the gland. It should also be performed when an adrenal gland is the site of a single metastasis.

▶ Whether to take out the adrenal gland during radical nephrectomy for renal cancer has become controversial. The data provided by the authors certainly support their conclusion that adrenalectomy is necessary only when there is suspicion of direct extension into the gland or there is a solitary adrenal metastasis. On the other hand one usually knows from a CT scan whether there is a normal contralateral adrenal gland that would maintain normal physiologic function. This issue came up recently at our institution and was discussed by a distinguished visiting urologic oncologist who believed that, because of instances of local recurrence, the gland should be removed. This has been our practice.

S.S. Howards, M.D.

Frequent Somatic Mutations and Loss of Heterozygosity of the von Hippel-Lindau Tumor Suppressor Gene in Primary Human Renal Cell Carcinomas

Shuin T, Kondon K, Torigoe S, Kishida T, Kubota Y, Hosaka M, Nagashima Y, Kitamura H, Latif F, Zbar B, Lerman MI, Yao M (Yokohama City Univ, Japan; Yokohama City Univ Hosp, Japan; Natl Cancer Inst–Frederick Cancer Research and Development Ctr, Md)
Cancer Res 54:2852–2855, 1994
10–9

Background.—A number of genetic changes that activate proto-oncogenes and inactivate tumor suppressor genes appear to have a role in the development of human renal cell carcinoma (RCC). These changes include mutations of the von Hippel-Lindau (VHL) tumor suppressor gene, *VHL*. Mutations of *VHL* have been observed in patients who have VHL and in cell lines from sporadic RCCs. Mutations of *VHL* were determined with use of the polymerase chain reaction and single-strand conformational polymorphism (SSCP) analysis of DNA.

Methods.—Forty-seven primary sporadic RCCs, 39 clear cell tumors, and 8 non–clear cell lesions were examined. Tumors that were SSCP-positive were subjected to direct sequencing.

Results.—Somatic mutations of *VHL* were documented in 56% of clear cell RCCs. Deletions were most frequent, but insertions, missense mutations, and a nonsense mutation were also observed. Nineteen of the 22 mutations were predicted to truncate the VHL protein. They were found mainly in the last one-third region of exons 1, 2, and 3. Loss of heterozygosity of *VHL* was observed in 84% of 19 informative clear cell tumors but not in any of the non–clear cell carcinomas.

Conclusion.—Inactivation of *VHL* appears to be a major molecular mechanism in the development of human RCCs, especially clear cell carcinomas.

▶ This paper confirms the pioneering work, initiated approximately 10 years ago at the National Cancer Institute, by Drs. Linehan and Zbar that resulted in their classic paper (*Science* 260:1307–1320, 1993, and recently reviewed in *JAMA* 273:564–570, 1995) in which the *VHL* tumor suppressor gene was identified. These important studies will eventually enable us to design a molecular, rather than pathologic, classification of RCC, thereby opening the field to new molecular tumor markers that will help the clinician predict better the biological behavior of the different variants of RCC.

A.S. Belldegrun, M.D.

International Renal-cell Cancer Study: I. Tobacco Use
McLaughlin JK, Lindblad P, Mellemgaard A, McCredie M, Mandel JS, Schle-
hofer B, Pommer W, Adami H-O (Natl Cancer Inst, Bethesda, Md; Univ Hosp,
Uppsala, Sweden; Danish Cancer Society, Copenhagen; et al)
Int J Cancer 60:194–198, 1995   10–10

Background.—The relative risk between use of tobacco and development of renal cell carcinoma (RCC) is considered moderate. To verify this
finding, the relationship between tobacco use and RCC was examined in
a large-scale, population-based international study.

Method.—A total of 1,732 individuals, aged 20–79 years, were included
in the study group. A control group of 2,309 individuals was matched by
gender and 5-year age groups. Data concerning tobacco use in its many
forms, drug and alcohol use, and medical history were obtained during
personal interviews. The odds ratio was used to measure the relationship
between use of tobacco and risk of RCC. Logistic regression methods
determined the adjusted relative risk.

Results.—Men and women in the study group (81% and 44%,
respectively) were more likely to use tobacco, particularly cigarettes, than
were men and women in the control group (77% and 41%, respectively).
There was a significant increase in risk for exclusive cigarette smokers and
users of mixed products. Current tobacco users had a higher excess risk
than ever-smokers, and former smokers had the lowest excess risk. Renal
cell cancer was attributed to smoking in 16% of patients: 24% of men and
9% of women had RCC directly related to smoking. No increase in risk
occurred for users of cigars, pipes, or smokeless tobacco. Age at which
smoking began was inversely related to risk.

Discussion.—Smoking is a causal risk factor for RCC. A cessation effect
occurred that reduced the risk of long-term smokers to 75% to 80% of
current smokers. Elimination of the smoking habit would reduce the
number of new cases of RCC.

▶ This international, multicenter, population-based pooled analysis, which
represents the largest study to date, adds convincing evidence to a growing
body of literature relating cigarette smoking as a causal risk factor for RCC
(1:4 for men, 1:10 for women). Importantly, a cessation effect was noted,
which indicates that an elimination of smoking would contribute to a reduction in the number of RCC cases worldwide.

A.S. Belldegrun, M.D.

Nuclear Morphometry in Differential Diagnosis of Renal Oncocytoma and Renal Cell Carcinoma

Castrén JP, Kuopio T, Nurmi MJ, Collan YU (Univ of Turku, Finland)
J Urol 154:1302–1306, 1995   10–11

Introduction.—Approximately 4% of all kidney neoplasms are renal oncocytomas, which are benign, nonmetastasizing tumors. Ultrasound, CT, MRI, and angiography have been unreliable methods for detecting renal oncocytomas. The applicability of nuclear morphometry in diagnosing renal oncocytoma was studied.

Methods.—Specimens from 16 oncocytomas and 16 renal cell carcinomas, grade 1 or 2 and stage T1 to 2N0M0, were reviewed with the use of nuclear morphometric measurements. Statistic analyses were conducted.

Results.—In more than 80% of specimens, oncocytomas could be distinguished from carcinomas on the basis of nuclear morphometry (Fig 1). The shape descriptors form AR, form PE, form NCI, contour ratio, and nuclear roundness helped distinguish oncocytoma from carcinoma. With form AR, there was a 93.8% sensitivity in detecting oncocytoma; forms PE, NCI, contour ratio, and nuclear roundness each had a 81.3% sensitivity.

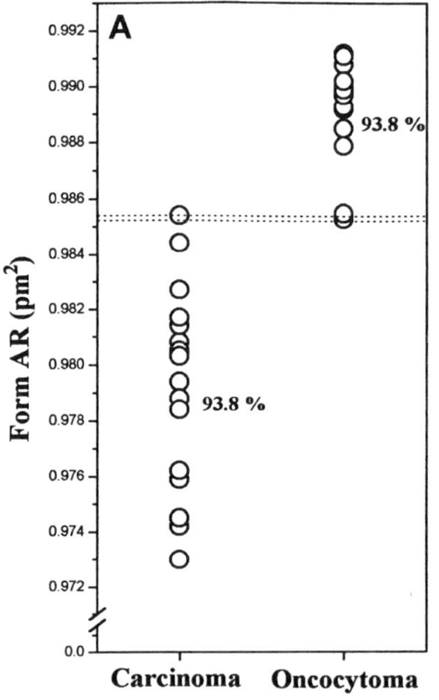

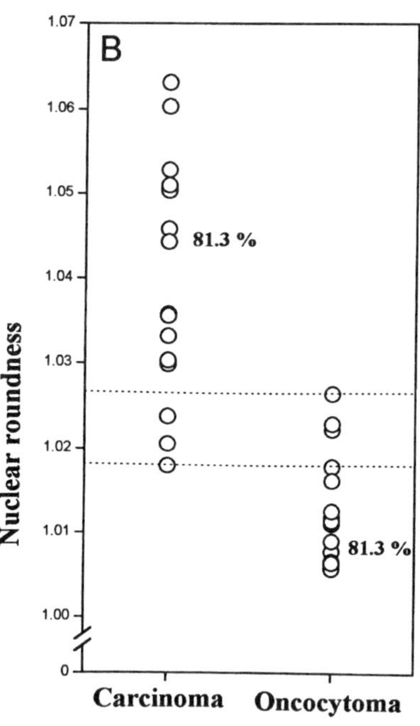

FIGURE 1.—Values of shape descriptors form AR (**A**) and nuclear roundness (**B**) in carcinomas and oncocytomas. *Dashed lines* show borders of undetermined regions. Reliable distinction of carcinoma and oncocytoma is possible beyond these lines. (Courtesy of Castrén JP, Kuopio T, Nurmi MJ, et al: Nuclear morphometry in differential diagnosis of renal oncocytoma and renal cell carcinoma. *J Urol* 154:1302–1306, 1995.)

Conclusion.—To support diagnostic decisions in problematic cases, morphometrically determined nuclear shape descriptors can be used. In the first of 2 diagnostic phases for renal tumors, attention should be given to shape descriptors. In the second diagnostic phase, grading of renal cell carcinoma can be based on morphometry.

▶ Preoperative differentiation between oncocytoma and renal cell carcinoma remains a diagnostic challenge. Molecular markers will, in the near future, be available to assist the clinician in making the differential diagnosis. Nuclear morphometric measurements were suggested to predict prognosis accurately, specifically tumor recurrence, in patients with renal cell carcinoma.

The specimens analyzed in this study were obtained from paraffin sections (frozen sections will alter nuclear size). Further studies are therefore needed to assess the value of nuclear morphometry data obtained preoperatively from needle biopsy specimens.

A.S. Belldegrun, M.D.

A New Protocol for the Followup of Renal Cell Carcinoma Based on Pathological Stage

Sandock DS, Seftel AD, Resnick MI (Case Western Reserve Univ, Cleveland, Ohio)

J Urol 154:28–31, 1995

10–12

Background.—There is no consensus on which laboratory and imaging studies are needed to follow the status of patients who undergo radical nephrectomy for renal cell carcinoma. A protocol to detect recurrences that may be amenable to treatment is needed. One experience was reviewed to define better which patients require more or less intensive follow-up.

Methods and Findings.—The records of 158 patients who underwent radical nephrectomy were reviewed retrospectively. All patients had a final diagnosis of renal cell carcinoma. Twenty-one patients had node-positive or metastatic disease, and 137 had no evidence of metastases at diagnosis. In this latter group, 19 patients had pathologic stage T1N0M0, 82 had T2N0M0, and 36 had T3N0M0 tumors. Recurrences were documented in 0%, 14.6%, and 52.8%, respectively. The mean interval to recurrence was 29.5 months for patients who had stage T2 carcinoma and 22 months for those who had stage T3 tumors. Useful follow-up information was obtained from a symptom history, serum liver function tests, and chest radiographs at defined intervals.

Conclusions.—Patients who have stages T2N0M0 and T3N0M0 disease should provide a thorough symptom history and undergo physical examination, serum liver function tests, and a posteroanterior and lateral chest radiograph every 6 months for 3 years and annually thereafter. Only symptom history is needed for patients who have stage T1 disease, as their prognosis is excellent. Only symptomatic patients or those who have increased liver function tests need to undergo abdominopelvic CT. In addition, bone plain films, radionuclide bone scans, and head CT scans are required only for symptomatic patients.

▶ The use of standard guidelines for postoperative follow-up of patients who have renal cell carcinoma is timely and important in the era of cost-effective medicine. Abdominal CT scans and/or ultrasound for postoperative monitoring still are widely used in many institutions, including ours. Once tumor recurrence is recognized, patients are immediately involved in an immunotherapy protocol. Additional such studies are therefore needed to define better safe guidelines for the follow-up of patients who have large or locally extensive tumors.

A.S. Belldegrun, M.D.

Interleukin-2 Based Home Therapy of Metastatic Renal Cell Carcinoma: Risks and Benefits in 215 Consecutive Single Institution Patients
Hänninen EL, Kirchner H, Atzpodien J (Medizinische Hochschule–Hannover Univ, Germany)
J Urol 155:19–25, 1996   10–13

Objective.—Although recombinant interleukin-2 (IL-2) and interferon-α2 (INF-α2) therapy for metastatic renal cell carcinoma have shown promising results, administration of IL-2 is expensive and is associated with significant side effects. Subcutaneous administration of recombinant IL-2 with or without concomitant administration of INF-α2, at doses much lower than maximum tolerable doses has shown good therapeutic effects. The results of the risks and benefits of at-home subcutaneous recombinant IL-2 treatment, alone or in combination with subcutaneous recombinant INF-α2 and/or IV 5-fluorouracil, in 215 consecutive patients who had metastatic renal carcinoma were reported.

Methods.—Therapy was administered to 215 patients, aged 18–75 years, who had renal cell carcinoma and no other health problems. The patients had received no other therapy during the previous 4 weeks. Therapeutic responses were evaluated between each cycle using World Health Organization (WHO) criteria of complete response, partial response (50% or more reduction in size of lesions and no new lesions or increase in size of lesions), and progressive disease. Toxicity grade and survival were recorded.

Results.—Median survival was 20.2 months in patients at low risk, with significant survival differences between each category of low (39.4 months), medium (15 months), and high (6.2 months) risk. Tumor response rate was 33%, with 9% complete remissions and 24% partial remissions. In 16 patients who received recombinant IL-2, the tumor response rate was 6%. In 5 patients, the cancer stabilized. Six of 79 patients who received subcutaneous recombinant IL-2 and INF-α2 had complete remission for 10–55 plus months, 16 had partial remission for 2–11 months, and 38 had stable disease. Of the 120 patients who received both recombinant cytokine plus IV 5-fluorouracil, 13 had complete remission for 8 plus to 47 plus months, and 34 had partial remission for 2–31 plus months. Five percent of all patients remain disease free. Most patients experienced local tissue hardening and transient inflammation from recombinant IL-2, and most had WHO grade 1 or 2 side effects consisting of fever, malaise, and chills in all 3 treatment cycles. Mild anorexia, nausea, vomiting, and/or diarrhea also occurred in most treatment cycles. No patients had grade 4 toxicity.

Conclusion.—The 3-drug combination outpatient treatment was as effective as the high-dose bolus or IV treatments but less expensive than inpatient treatment. Most patients experience low to moderate side effects of WHO grade 1 or 2.

▶ This retrospective, single institution experience with subcutaneous IL-2–based immunotherapy clearly demonstrated that some patients (5%) who have advanced renal cell carcinoma can achieve long-lasting remission and remain disease free after completing therapy. This regimen is safe and is associated with relatively low toxicity. Whether chemoimmunotherapy with 5-fluorouracil adds to the combination of IL-2 and INF-α alone remains unclear and requires prospective randomized studies.

A.S. Belldegrun, M.D.

Dynamic MRI of Small Renal Cell Carcinoma

Yamashita Y, Miyazaki T, Hatanaka Y, Takahashi M (Kumamoto Univ, Japan)
J Comput Assist Tomogr 19:759–765, 1995   10–14

Background.—Detecting small renal cell carcinomas (RCCs) can be difficult. Although contrast-enhanced CT is the standard method for detection, MRI has some advantages. Administration of a paramagnetic contrast agent has been shown to improve tumor detection. On dynamic studies, early enhancing tumors can be clearly detected because of tumor hypervascularity. In the current study, the efficacy of contrast-enhanced dynamic MRI for the diagnosis of small RCCs was compared with that of conventional spin-echo techniques.

Methods.—Twenty-seven patients with 28 small RCCs underwent conventional spin-echo and contrast-enhanced dynamic MRI to detect and characterize their tumors. In all patients, tumors were detected by contrast-enhanced CT and confirmed surgically. Dynamic MRI was performed after rapid injection of gadolinium-diethylenetriamine pentaacetic acid (Gd-DTPA). A breath-hold fast low-angle shot method was used. Renal masses were characterized by visual analysis of tumor vascularity and by quantitative assessment of the contrast-noise ratio (CNR) and degree of enhancement.

Findings.—Conventional spin-echo MRI detected 18 of the 28 small RCCs, and dynamic MRI detected 26. The tumor–renal medulla contrast was marked at 90–120 sec after Gd-DTPA administration in the dynamic studies. The tumor–renal medulla contrast was more pronounced in the dynamic study than in postcontrast T1-weighted imaging, T2-weighted imaging, and T1-weighted imaging.

Conclusions.—Dynamic imaging may be valuable for detecting small RCCs, especially in patients who are allergic to iodine contrast agents, patients with indeterminate or calcified renal masses, or patients with renal failure. Further research is needed to better define the role of dynamic MRI in the detection and characterization of small RCCs.

▶ Magnetic resonance imaging is continuously evolving. In this paper the authors have detected 93% of small renal neoplasms by using directed dynamic MRI after IV injection of a paramagnetic contrast agent. In the same series conventional MRI detected only 64%. Dynamic MRI is nothing else but frequent (every 20 sec) acquisition of the same image before and after an IV bolus of contrast agent while the breath is held. A neoplasm will enhance and will stand out clearly in contrast compared with normal renal parenchyma. This is great news for patients who are allergic to iodinated contrast material (used in CT) and for those with renal failure (paramagnetic contrasts are not nephrotoxic).

Z.L. Barbaric, M.D.

Intraoperative Sonography for the Evaluation and Management of Renal Tumors: Experience With 100 Patients
Polascik TJ, Meng MV, Epstein JI, Marshall FF (Johns Hopkins Med Inst, Baltimore, Md)
J Urol 154:1676–1680, 1995   10–15

Introduction.—Partial nephrectomy can be an alternative to radical nephrectomy in selected patients, especially those with small, incidentally detected tumors and a normal, contralateral kidney. Real-time intraoperative sonography was evaluated prospectively for its capability to determine the extent and location of the tumor and to aid in obtaining a tumor-free margin in patients undergoing radical nephrectomy or nephron-sparing surgery.

Patients and Methods.—Intraoperative sonography was used for 100 patients who underwent surgery between September 1988 and August 1994. A single surgeon performed all procedures and evaluated the kidneys with an ultrasound unit equipped with a triple-head sector transducer and duplex Doppler imaging capability. Data recorded included the size, number, echo texture, and location of suspected lesions, as well as their relationship to the collecting system, vasculature, and renal capsule. Ab-

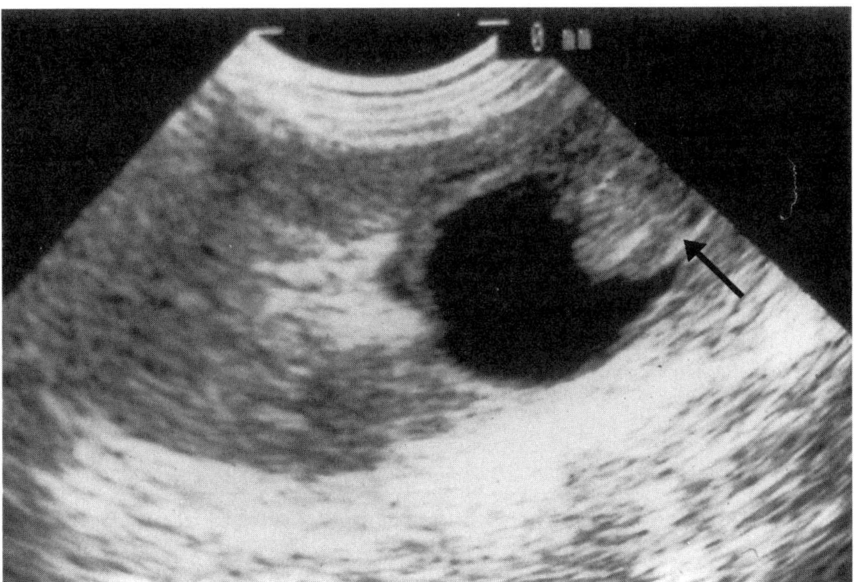

FIGURE 2.—Transverse intraoperative sonogram shows renal tumor (*arrow*) within renal cyst. (Courtesy of Polascik TJ, Meng MV, Epstein JI, et al: Intraoperative sonography for the evaluation and management of renal tumors: Experience with 100 patients. *J Urol* 154:1676–1680, 1995.)

dominal CT was used to evaluate all patients preoperatively; excretory urography, MRI, renal angiography, and transabdominal renal sonography were performed selectively.

Results.—Radical nephrectomy was performed in 56 patients, and partial nephrectomy was performed in 40; 3 patients underwent unroofing of renal cysts, and 1 had a renal biopsy. Among patients treated by radical nephrectomy, 46 had renal cell carcinoma, 2 had collecting duct carcinoma, and 8 had benign disease. Except for 2 patients with angiomyolipomas, malignant disease was suspected preoperatively in all cases. In 8 cases the surgical approach was preoperatively unclear. Nephrectomy was performed in all 8 cases when intraoperative sonography showed the lesion to be more extensive than anticipated. Except for the 3 patients with angiomyolipomas, all 40 patients who underwent partial nephrectomy were thought to have a malignancy. Three patients were spared nephrectomy when intraoperative sonography and frozen section confirmed benign multilocular cysts. In 1 case, sonography identified a tumor located at the base of a cyst (Fig 2). Intraoperative sonography also identified an unsuspected adrenal mass that proved to be metastatic renal cell carcinoma. All surgical margins were negative in patients undergoing partial nephrectomy.

Conclusion.—Intraoperative sonography is particularly useful as an adjunct to partial nephrectomy and may help to obtain a tumor-free margin.

The technique is also valuable for further radiographic assessment of preoperatively indeterminate lesions and for additional imaging of extra-renal anatomy.

▶ This is a follow-up on an earlier study of the use of intraoperative sonography of renal tumors. It confirms the usefulness of such an approach whenever a partial resection is contemplated and whenever preoperative diagnostic uncertainty exists. The high prevalence of small satellite neoplasms in the ipsilateral kidney is frightening. It is disconcerting that such lesions are too often unrecognized despite excellent surgical exposure, high-frequency transducers, and real-time duplex Doppler imaging. Finally, it is not ultrasound alone that provides the wonderfully useful information presented in this paper. It is the accomplished user who makes the difference.

Z.L. Barbaric, M.D.

Renal Arteriovenous Malformations Masquerading as Renal Cell Carcinoma

Vasavada SP, Manion S, Flanigan RC, Novick AC (Cleveland Clinic Found, Ohio; Loyola Univ, Maywood, Ill)
Urology 46:716–721, 1995   10–16

Background.—The diagnosis of arteriovenous malformations is sometimes difficult to establish with standard uroradiographic imaging procedures. The clinical presentation and management of 6 patients with renal arteriovenous malformations that masqueraded as renal cell carcinomas are presented

Patients.—The 6 patients, aged 29–57 years, were initially seen for gross or microscopic hematuria, flank or abdominal pain, and/or hypertension. Physical examination revealed flank or abdominal bruits in 3 of the patients and hypertension in 2 of the patients. In the 4 patients who had the procedure, IV urography revealed markedly delayed nephrograms with a suggestion of a renal mass. Although CT scan findings were helpful, discerning the exact nature and extent of the presumed renal vascular malformation was often difficult. In all 6 patients, angiography proved the diagnosis of an arteriovenous malformation. Two patients with small malformations were successfully treated with vascular embolization. Three patients had successful nephron-sparing surgery, and 1 patient had a nephrectomy.

Discussion.—A renal arteriovenous malformation should be considered in a young or middle-aged patient with significant hematuria. About 70% of patients are reported to have flank or abdominal bruits, and about 50% are reported to have hypertension. Although cardiomegaly and symptoms of congestive heart failure are reported to be present in about 50% of patients, none of the patients in this series had apparent heart problems. Although routine diagnostic imaging studies and CT scans are helpful in establishing the diagnosis, angiography remains the gold standard. Renal angiography confirms the diagnosis, helps differentiate benign from malignant lesions, and provides a vascular "roadmap" for surgical management or embolization therapy.

Conclusions.—Renal arteriovenous malformations are sometimes difficult to differentiate from renal cell carcinomas. A younger patient with hematuria is particularly at risk for a renal vascular malformation. Angiography should be done in patients with suggestive findings, because it is the gold standard for diagnosis and for providing a roadmap for decisions about treatment.

▶ This is a great discussion about arteriovenous malformation; however, looking at the CT images, there is no problem regarding diagnosis, except, perhaps, in case 2. Between modern CT and color Doppler imaging there should be very few undiagnosed cases before angiography. A selective renal angiogram will still be needed to evaluate whether a selective embolization is feasible or to provide a preoperative map.

Z.L. Barbaric, M.D.

11 Laparoscopy and Endourology

Gasless Laparoscopy-Assisted Nephrectomy Without Tissue Morcellation for Renal Carcinoma
Suzuki K, Masuda H, Ushiyama T, Hata M, Fujita K, Kawabe K (Hamamatsu Univ, Japan; Univ of Tokyo)
J Urol 154:1685–1687, 1995   11–1

Background.—Laparoscopic nephrectomy has been a common surgical procedure since 1991. It is still difficult, however to retrieve a kidney and tumor from the abdominal cavity. The results of gasless laparoscopy–assisted nephrectomy without tissue morcellation were reported and compared with those of open nephrectomy.

Method.—Seven patients, aged 44–83 years, who had renal tumors were included. Two specially designed lifting retractors were attached to either side of the incision, and another specially designed retractor was inserted into the abdomen. The retractors were suspended from a frame, and the abdominal wall was raised. Sufficient working space was created with this technique, and a pneumoperitoneum was not required. The tissue was removed en bloc from the abdominal cavity with or without a laparoscopy sac.

Results.—Mean surgical time was 260 minutes, which was longer than the time required for open radical nephrectomy. An epidural catheter in situ was required for an average of 1.7 days after the new technique and 3.4 days after open nephrectomy. Patients who underwent gasless laparoscopy–assisted nephrectomy did not require postoperative pain medication and reported full recovery after 5.4 weeks.

Discussion.—Because this method uses the same forceps, scissors, and retractors used in open surgery, it was easier than standard laparoscopic surgery. Recovery time was significantly shorter with gasless laparoscopy–assisted nephrectomy. Preoperative renal artery embolization is recommended in patients who have advanced renal cell carcinoma. Long-term follow-up will confirm the prognosis of renal cancer after this procedure.

▶ Gasless laparoscopy offers several advantages. First, the risks of the pneumoperitoneum (i.e., arrhythmia, pulmonary embolism, acidosis, and postoperative diaphragmatic irritation) are avoided. Moreover, the potential exists to perform procedures using a local or regional anesthetic. Finally, this technique permits the use of standard open instrumentation through small skin incisions.

Although this technique is promising, there are also disadvantages that hinder its widespread application. A major limitation is that the space obtained with the current gasless methods is not as large or as uniform as that obtained with the pneumoperitoneum. Further, the pneumoperitoneum tamponades capillary bleeding, thereby resulting in a drier operative field. As gasless techniques evolve and standardize, these approaches may become a routine part of laparoscopic procedures.

L. Kavoussi, M.D.

Percutaneous Management of Transitional Cell Carcinoma of the Renal Collecting System: 9-Year Experience
Jarrett TW, Sweetser PM, Weiss GH, Smith AD (Long Island Jewish Med Ctr, New Hyde Park, NY)
J Urol 154:1629–1635, 1995   11–2

Introduction.—Although radical nephroureterectomy remains the definitive treatment for transitional cell carcinoma of the renal collecting system, certain patients are better treated with parenchymal-sparing surgery. The results of endoscopic resection of these relatively uncommon tumors were reported.

Patients and Methods.—Eleven women and 23 men (36 kidneys) who met the criteria for percutaneous management were included. Selection criteria included a solitary kidney in 11 patients, bilateral disease in 3, significant medical risk for a major operation in 8, chronic renal insufficiency in 5, patient choice in 6, and an incidental finding at nephroscopy for calculus in 3. The patients underwent percutaneous resection between March 1984 and June 1993. All cases incorporated the principles of complete resection, second-look nephroscopy, and a third look to confirm the absence of tumor (Fig 1). Location of the tumor determines approach, and more than 1 access may be required. Adjunctive therapy with bacillus Calmette-Guérin was administered in 19 patients after the second-look nephroscopy. Patients were evaluated every 3 months during the first year, every 6 months for 4 years, then yearly.

Results.—Six of 36 kidneys were treated with immediate nephroureterectomy for aggressive disease; 3 were grade 2, and 3 were grade 3 tumors. Nine patients (11 kidneys) had superficial, grade 1 tumors with an average size of 1.55 cm. Seven of these patients were alive a mean of 54.9 months after endoscopic resection; the 2 deaths were not cancer related. Two patients (18%) had superficial recurrences; 1 patient underwent repeat endoscopic resection, and the other underwent nephroureterectomy because of large volume disease. Twelve patients had grade 2 tumors, all but 2 of which were superficial. During a mean follow-up of 42 months, the

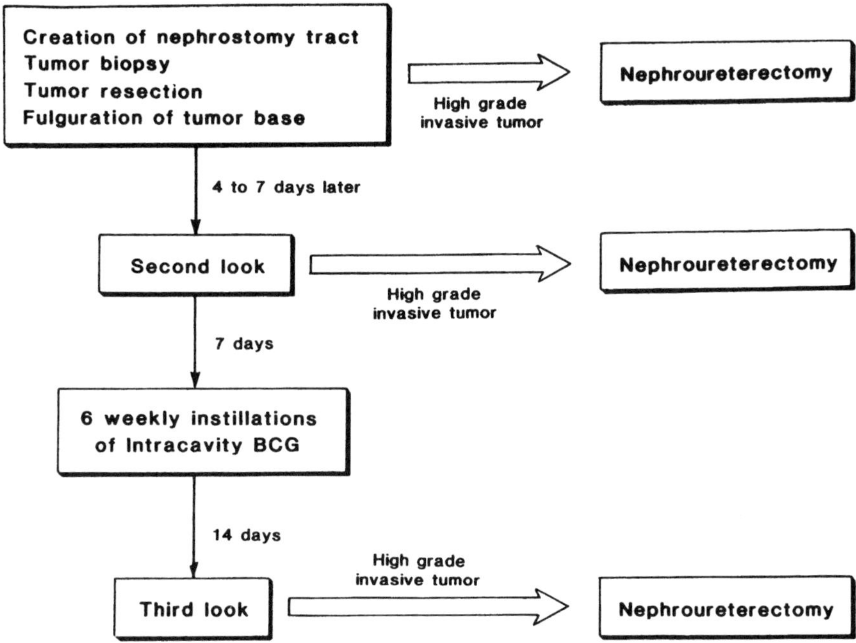

FIGURE 1.—Percutaneous approach to transitional cell carcinoma of upper urinary tract. (Courtesy of Jarrett TW, Sweetser PM, Weiss GH, et al: Percutaneous management of transitional cell carcinoma of the renal collecting system: 9-year experience. *J Urol* 154:1629–1635, 1995.)

recurrence rate for grade 2 tumors was 33%. Thirteen patients had grade 3 tumors, only 3 of which were superficial. Five of 10 patients who had grade 3 tumors and received a full course of endoscopic treatment underwent delayed nephroureterectomy for recurrent disease 2–17 months after the initial therapy. Six patients, all with grade 3 tumors, died of disease progression.

Conclusion.—Radical nephroureterectomy may be associated with a significant rate of morbidity and mortality and/or lifetime hemodialysis. Because endoscopic local tumor resection carries the risk of recurrence, however, the consequences of suboptimal surgery must be weighed against the hazards of major surgery. With vigilant follow-up, patients who have grade 1 transitional cell carcinoma of the renal collecting system and selected patients who have grade 2 disease may benefit from percutaneous management.

Definitive Tumor Resection and Percutaneous Bacille Calmette-Guérin for Management of Renal Pelvic Transitional Cell Carcinoma in Solitary Kidneys

Vasavada SP, Streem SB, Novick AC (The Cleveland Clinic Foundation, Ohio)
Urology 45:381–386, 1995   11–3

Background.—Because of the high risk of ipsilateral recurrences with conservative surgery in patients who have upper tract transitional cell carcinoma (TCC), nephroureterectomy is the standard management. A nephron-sparing approach obviously should be considered for patients who have anatomically or functionally solitary kidneys in whom nephrectomy would lead to dialysis dependence or renal transplantation. The safety and initial efficacy of definitive tumor resection combined with percutaneous bacille Calmette-Guérin (BCG) for the treatment of renal pelvic TCC in patients who have solitary kidneys were investigated.

Methods and Findings.—Eight patients who had anatomically solitary kidneys and a previous history of TCC elsewhere in the urinary tract were included. Two patients were treated with partial nephrectomy, and 6 with percutaneous resection. All received a 6-week course of topical percutaneous BCG. Seven patients could tolerate the entire course of BCG with no adverse effects. In 1 patient, treatment had to be stopped because of renal insufficiency, which resolved thereafter. Six patients underwent follow-up nephroscopy 3 months after initial tumor resection. The status of all patients was followed regularly at 3- to 6-month intervals after nephroscopy with radiographic, cytologic, and, in some, ureteroscopic evaluation. Follow-up ranged from 9 to 59 months (mean, 22 months). Local tumor recurrence became evident in only 1 patient, who died 20 months after treatment. In another 2 patients, distant metastatic disease developed. Both of these patients had invasive TCC elsewhere in the urinary tract

TABLE 2.—Results of Treatment

Patient	Serum Creatinine Post-treatment (mg/dL)	Follow-up (months)	Current Status
BC	1.1	9	Died with metastatic disease; no local recurrence
AZ	1.8	59	Alive; no recurrence
RB	4.4	17	Alive; no recurrence
JP	0.9	12	Alive; no recurrence
AB	1.0	14	Alive; no recurrence
MQ	1.6	17	Alive; no recurrence
FL	1.7	18	Alive with metastatic disease; receiving systemic chemo-therapy; no local recurrence
MM	2.2	20	Died with local recurrence

before their upper tract cancer was treated. One died with metastatic disease 9 months after therapy (Table 2).

Conclusions.—The combination of a 6-week course of percutaneous topical BCG and definitive tumor resection may ultimately reduce the incidence of local tumor recurrence in this high-risk patient population. This treatment is also generally well tolerated.

▶ These papers demonstrate the durability and safety of percutaneous management of transitional cell carcinoma of the upper collecting system. Success was highly dependent on appropriate patient selection and deliberate use of multiple procedures (second- and third-look nephroscopy). As is the case with open resection, low-grade and low-stage tumors respond best to this form of surgical therapy. The numbers are too small to determine whether BCG resulted in improved success; however, these authors demonstrate that when adequate precautions are taken, BCG may be safely used in the upper urinary tract.

L. Kavoussi, M.D.

Effect of Alkaline Citrate Therapy on Clearance of Residual Renal Stone Fragments After Extracorporeal Shock Wave Lithotripsy in Sterile Calcium and Infection Nephrolithiasis Patients

Cicerello E, Merlo F, Gambaro G, Maccatrozzo L, Fandella A, Baggio B, Anselmo G (Treviso Gen Hosp, Italy; Univ of Padova, Italy)
J Urol 151:5–9, 1994

11–4

Objective.—Extracorporeal shock wave lithotripsy (ESWL) is now the first treatment choice for most patients who have renal stones. What happens to the stones after ESWL, however, is not completely clear. The stone fragments may carry some risk of new stone formation and persistent urinary tract infection. The use of alkaline citrate therapy to improve the clearance of stone fragments has been considered, although this treatment has not been evaluated in patients who have infection stones. The effects of alkaline citrate therapy on stone fragment clearance in patients who have calcium oxalate and infection stones were evaluated.

Methods.—Forty consecutive patients who had sterile calcium stones and 30 who had struvite stones were included in a 12-month follow-up study. All had residual fragments of less than 5 mm after ESWL. The patients were randomly selected to receive either citrate therapy, 6–8 g/day, or hygienic measures only. All patients who had infection stones received sufficient antibiotic treatment. Plain abdominal radiography and kidney ultrasound were performed at baseline and at 6 and 12 months, and excretory urography was performed at baseline and 12 months.

Results.—Stone clearance rates at 1 year in the patients who had calcium oxalate stones were 75% with citrate treatment vs. 32% in the control group. For patients who had infection stones, 1-year clearance rates were 86% with citrate treatment vs. 40% in controls. In the citrate-treated patients who did not have stone clearance, citrate prevented the growth or reaggregation of residual fragments. Citrate treatment was associated with stone clearance by 6 months in most patients. Of the 19 control patients with sterile calcium stones who completed treatment, 13 did not have stone clearance. Six of these patients had residual fragment growth after 1 year, and 3 had stone reaggregation.

Conclusions.—In patients who have residual calcium and infection stones after ESWL, the residual stone fragments commonly persist or grow. Treatment with alkaline citrate can improve the stone clearance rate in these patients and reduce the growth or agglomeration of residual fragments. Prevention of residual stone fragment growth may be critical to their eventual passage.

▶ Recently, a number of subspecialized endourologists have embarked on a "boost therapy" of 3 months of citrate administration after treatment with SWL and percutaneous surgery for the management of residual fragments.[1] Cicerello et al. treated a cohort of patients who had residual stones, including those who had infection stones, after SWL therapy with alkaline citrate for an extended period of 1 year; a control group received hygienic treatment only. Their results corroborate the work of Streem (Abstract 11–5) and my own observations with regard to the usefulness of management of urinary infection and administration of citrate to facilitate stone passage and reduce stone recurrence and regrowth. Further investigation regarding the optimum dosage of citrate and duration of therapy is warranted.

G. Fuchs, M.D.

Reference

1. Bagley D, Clayman R, Fuchs G, et al: Personal communication, 1995.

Long-term Incidence and Risk Factors for Recurrent Stones Following Percutaneous Nephrostolithotomy or Percutaneous Nephrostolithotomy/Extracorporeal Shock Wave Lithotripsy for Infection Related Calculi
Streem SB (Cleveland Clinic Found, Ohio)
J Urol 153:584–587, 1995

11–5

Introduction.—The clinical importance of early intervention for the removal of infected renal calculi was recognized more than 20 years ago with the introduction of new surgical procedures that permitted complete stone removal without stopping renal function. Early intervention is now even more important because of the almost universal use of noninvasive technologies for stone management. Despite these advances and improved morbidity associated with stone removal, however, residual and recurrent stone and infection rates have remained about the same. The long-term incidence and causes of recurrent stones after percutaneous nephro-stolithotomy, alone or in combination with extracorporeal shock wave lithotripsy (ESWL), were examined.

Methods.—The status of 44 patients who underwent percutaneous nephrostolithotomy alone or in combination with ESWL was followed a mean of 41.7 months. All patients received antibiotics and underwent clinical, radiologic, and bacteriologic examinations at 6- to 12-month intervals. To determine the annual risk factor for stone recurrence, a Kaplan-Meier plot was developed, and data were analyzed with the use of Cox's proportional hazards model.

Results.—Recurrent stones developed in 12 patients (27%) 12–61 months (mean, 32.3 months) after treatment. With the Kaplan-Meier estimate, the risk of new stone formation at 5 years was 36.8%. Analysis of potential risk factors with Cox's proportional hazards model found that only an anatomical urinary tract abnormality caused significant risk. Eleven patients (25%) had such abnormalities, and their risk for recurrent stones was 5.7 times greater than that of patients who had normal tracts.

Conclusions.—Mandatory surveillance for recurrent stones is necessary, even in patients who are initially free of stones and in those who maintain sterile urine. Because patients who have urinary tract abnormalities are statistically much more likely to have recurrent stones, future studies on recurrence rates should stratify patients according to anatomical status.

▶ This author shakes one of the basic beliefs of the endourology subspecialty community. He postulates that removing infected stones from a patient does not significantly affect the stone recurrence and regrowth rate. The author's approach to treating patients who have infected stones, relies heavily on SWL (used in 70.5% of patients for a stone-free rate of 72.7%) as an adjunct to percutaneous endoscopic surgery. Trends in specialized endourology stone centers, however, are going toward the more aggressive use of endoscopic clearance of stone material, especially in patients at risk for recurrence, i.e., patients who have anatomical and/or functional abnormalities of the urinary tract.[1, 2] Flexible endoscopy (including the use of Holmium Laser energy for vaporization of stones that are difficult to remove) and multiple renal access (including the technically more difficult upper pole access) can increase the stone-free rate to greater than 90% without the use of the less predictable SWL technology.[1, 2] The author stresses the importance of chronic antibiotic suppression in patients who have undergone treatment for infected stones; however, he does not offer recommendations as to the choice of antibiotic, dosage, and duration of antibiotic suppression. We administer 10 days of preoperative quinolone antibiotic, given twice a day orally, and perioperative IV administration of antibiotics, followed by continuation of the preoperative dosage until removal of all drainage tubes (percutaneous nephrostomy and ureteral stent). We have found that this regimen, complemented by a 3-month course of mandellamine given daily (in case the culture remains negative 2 weeks after discontinuation of the quinolone), effectively controls recurrence of infection.

This regimen, in conjunction with the use of citrate (3 months of potassium citrate 20 mEq 3 times per day) indeed seems to be beneficial in improving stone-free rates and decreasing rates of recurrent infection, even in the presence of a small amount of residual stone material. We found it helpful to evaluate patients who had undergone treatment for struvite stones and those who had undergone treatment for stones associated with anatomical abnormalities (regardless of whether the stone was infected) twice a year with renal ultrasound (radiographs only when ultrasound indicates presence of stone in kidney or hydronephrosis), urine analysis, and urine culture. This way, recurrence of stone and/or infection can be detected early, the further follow-up interval can be individualized, and intervention can be planned as necessary.

G. Fuchs, M.D.

References

1. Fuchs GJ, Patel A, Tognoni P: Management of stones associated with anatomic abnormalities, in Coe FL, Favus MJ, Pak CYC, et al (eds): *Kidney Stones: Medical and Surgical Management.* Lippincott-Raven, Philadelphia, 1996, p 1037.
2. Pearle M, Clayman RVC: Outcomes and selection of surgical therapies of stones in the kidney and ureter, in Coe FL, Favus MJ, Pak CYC, et al (eds): *Kidney Stones: Medical and Surgical Management.* Lippincott-Raven, Philadelphia, 1996, p 709.

A Prospective Trial Comparing the Efficacy and Complications of the Modified Dornier HM3 and MFL 5000 Lithotriptors for Solitary Renal Calculi

Chan SL, Stothers L, Rowley A, Perler Z, Taylor W, Sullivan LD (Univ of British Columbia, Vancouver, Canada)
J Urol 153:1794–1797, 1995 11–6

Introduction.—One hundred and ninety-eight adult patients who had solitary stones in the upper collecting system were randomly assigned to lithotripsy with either the Dornier MFL 5000 or modified HM3 lithotriptor; 170 patients were available for follow up for 3 months. Abdominal plain films, tomograms, and ultrasound were used to evaluate patients at 1, 4, and 12 weeks after treatment. Outcomes, complication rates, and treatment times were compared between the 2 groups.

Results.—Ninety-one of the solitary calculi were located in a renal calix, 66 were located in the ureter, and 39 were in the renal pelvis. Although the average number of shocks received was similar between patient groups, the mean treatment time was 0.7 hours for the MFL 5000 device compared with 0.4 hours for the modified HM3 lithotriptor. Both units showed equivalent turnover times between treatments. The only significant difference in stone-free status at 3 months between the 2 groups was seen in patients who had lower pole caliceal stones, with a success rate of 80% in the modified HM3 group compared with 56% in the MFL 5000 group. When stratified over time, patients who had pelvic calculi (Fig 4) and

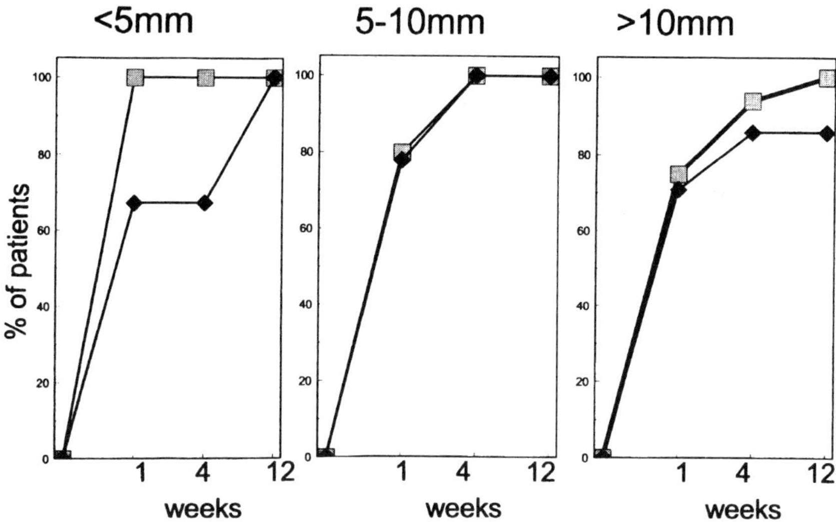

FIGURE 4.—Rate of renal pelvic stone-free status achieved 3 months after treatment with MFL 5000 (*filled squares*) and modified HM3 (*shaded squares*) lithotriptors. (Courtesy of Chan S, Stothers L, Rowley A, et al: A prospective trial comparing the efficacy and complications of the modified Dornier HM3 and MFL 5000 lithotriptors for solitary renal calculi. *J Urol* 153:1794–1797, 1994.)

caliceal calculi achieved a stone-free status sooner with the modified HM3 unit. No statistically significant difference in complication rate was observed between the 2 groups.

Discussion.—The MFL 5000 lithotriptor appears to offer no significant clinical advantage, in terms of treatment success and complication rate, compared with the modified HM3 units. Further, treatment time with the MFL 5000 device is almost twice as long.

▶ Newer is not necessarily better. This paper compares a modification of the "workhorse" HM3 Dornier lithotriptor (40-nanofarad version) with a so-called third-generation multifunctional lithotriptor, the Dornier MFL 5000. With regard to the treatment outcomes at the 3-month follow-up, few differences in terms of stone-free rates were noted. The major differences between the 2 machines were the treatment times (0.4 vs. 0.7 hours, in favor of the modified HM3 device) and the stone-free rate for stones located in lower calyces (80% vs. 56%, again in favor of the HM3).

Both machines can be used "anesthesia free" with the patient under heavy sedoanalgesia. This perceived advantage is, at the same time, 1 drawback of the newer devices, because it necessitates higher re-treatment rates. A larger shockwave aperture reduces the shock wave energy density at the skin level, thereby lowering the perception of pain and obviating the need for regional or general anesthesia. The geometric design of these anesthesia-free energy sources also results in a smaller focal area, which negatively affects the efficacy of stone comminution. As our work with ureteroscopically monitored and/or assisted shock wave lithotripsy

(SWL) (Dornier MFL 5000) has shown stone, fragmentation with this lithotriptor occurs only when the stone is located exactly in the center of the cross hairs of the fluoroscopy screens. Any deviation of the stone, such as with breathing excursion or patient movement, will result in missed shots. Therefore, in the patient under sedoanalgesia with uncontrolled breathing excursion (i.e., movement of the kidney containing the stone) most shock wave pulses are fired in vain, which reduces efficacy, prolongs treatment times, and frequently results in repeat treatment sessions. This problem occurs to a lesser degree for stone contained in the ureter (less movement with respiration). Therefore, the results for these stones more closely resemble the results of previous machine generations.

The true "selling point" for the multipurpose, third-generation machines in the era of declining SWL case loads is the ability to perform simultaneous endoscopic surgery and SWL treatment for complex stones that require, for example, repair of intrarenal strictures. The machine can also be used to treat residual stone burden up to 2.5 cm with simultaneous SWL and ureteroscopic lithotripsy. To optimize utilization of the costly unit, it can also serve as a radiologic x-ray table or endoscopic surgery table.

G. Fuchs, M.D.

Electrohydraulic Versus Pneumatic Disintegration in the Treatment of Ureteral Stones: A Randomized, Prospective Trial

Hofbauer J, Höbarth K, Marberger M (Univ of Vienna)
J Urol 153:623–625, 1995   11–7

Background.—Approximately 25% of patients who have ureteral stones are unsuitable for treatment with extracorporeal shock wave lithotripsy (ESWL). Available options for such patients include electrohydraulic and pneumatic lithotripsy. The latter, a recently developed method of intracorporeal lithotripsy, is reported to minimize tissue trauma. A consecutive series of 72 patients who could not spontaneously pass ureteral stones or undergo ESWL were randomly selected to undergo electrohydraulic or pneumatic lithotripsy.

Methods.—The 2 treatment groups were comparable in age, sex, and location and size of stone. A crossover was offered to patients who did not respond to the initial treatment. All interventions were performed in a standardized manner with the patient under general anesthesia. Before hospital discharge, patients were examined with a nephrosonogram and a plain film of the kidneys to determine the presence of 5-mm fragments pushed up into the kidney. A positive finding was followed immediately by an ESWL treatment. The patients' status was followed for residual calculi and perforations.

Results.—Stones were disintegrated into fragments of 3 mm or smaller in 89.5% of the pneumatic lithotripsy group and in 85.3% of the electrohydraulic lithotripsy group, not a significant difference. There was a significantly higher rate of perforation, however, in the electrohydraulic

TABLE 2.—Results of Electrohydraulic and Pneumatic Lithotripsy for Ureteral Stones

	Electrohydraulic Lithotripsy (34 pts.)		Pneumatic Lithotripsy (38 pts.)	
No. disintegration (%):				
Successful (fragments 3 mm. or less)	29	(85.3)	34	(89.5)
Failed	1	(2.9)*	—	
No. technical defects (%)	—		1	(2.6)*
No. crossover (%)	1	(2.9)*	1	(2.6)*
No. fragments disclosed/ESWL (%)	5	(14.7)	4	(10.5)
No. perforation (%)	6	(17.6)	1	(2.6)
No. hemorrhage (%)	1	(2.9)	0	
Anesthesia time (mins.)	74 ± 28		64 ± 31	
Mean postop. hospitalization (days)	1.1		1.1	
No. stone-free after stent removal (%)	31	(91.2)	34	(89.5)

Note: There were no late complications.
* Identical patients.
(Courtesy of Hofbauer J, Höbarth K, Marberger M: Electrohydraulic versus pneumatic disintegration in the treatment of ureteral stones: A randomized, prospective trial. *J Urol* 153:623–625, 1995.)

group (17.6% vs. 2.6%). Mean period of hospitalization and stone-free rate after calculus removal were similar for the 2 treatment groups (Table 2). One patient in each group was crossed over to the alternative treatment method and achieved complete disintegration of stones.

Conclusion.—Although electrohydraulic and pneumatic lithotripsy were equally successful in disintegrating ureteral stones, the perforation rate was significantly greater with the electrohydraulic method. Pneumatic lithotripsy has a higher initial equipment cost but is significantly easier to handle and has become the method of choice at the study institution for patients who cannot be treated with ESWL.

▶ A perforation rate of 17.6% associated with the use of electrohydraulic energy in the ureter seems to be excessively high, especially in experienced hands. When energy sources cause damage in the urinary tract, the culprit is either the technology (device) or the technique (operator). These authors and others who have experienced the same problems should really look into the possibility that this high perforation rate is a function of the lithotrite used. In our experience with electrohydraulic lithotripsy (EHL) in the ureter of more than 10 years on more than 1,000 patients, only 1 perforation occurred (a hole was "electrocuted" into the ureter by inadvertently touching the wires of a basket with the tip of the electrode). From animal experiments, it is known that EHL is potentially the most harmful of energy sources used for the fragmentation of stone when activated against tissues. When stone is encased in copious edema and full visualization is not possible (about 4% of patients at a tertiary care referral center), it is therefore prudent to pass a ureteral stent first and allow the edema to subside. This is usually accomplished in a 2-week period. Subsequent stone fragmentation with EHL and removal are then much more easily accomplished, and the risk of perforation is greatly reduced. Another possible cause for the higher perforation rate with the EHL probe is the authors' use of miniature ureteroscopes with a smaller field of view and reduced irrigation. Electrohydraulic lithotripsy always causes a minute amount of mucosal bleeding from the shock wave delivery. In view of the smaller field of view and reduced irrigation through the small ports, even minor bleeding may obscure the vision enough to cause the operator to lose control of the electrode tip and inadvertently hit the wall of the ureter. According to our animal experiments, this is the only way to cause a perforation of the ureteral wall. The only energy source we would recommend for in situ use in the setting of an impacted stone covered with copious edema is the Holmium Laser. The shallow (0.5 mm) penetration of the Holmium energy does not carry the risk of bleeding and impaired visibility.

Upward migration is one of the potential downsides for electrohydraulic and pneumatic direct contact lithotripsy of ureteral stones. Indeed, 14.7% of patients treated with EHL and 10.5% treated with pneumatic lithotriptor needed repeat treatment for stones larger than 5 mm that had migrated up into the kidney during treatment. Also, the authors elected to fragment only the stones in situ in the ureter and did not actively remove the stone debris. Prudence would dictate that if one performs an endoscopic surgical procedure for management of stones, the fragments should be removed from the ureter; the passage of debris should not be left to chance because of possible complications. Stone fragments that have migrated up into the kidney during treatment can be readily removed with flexible instrumentation under the same anesthesia, thus avoiding an extra treatment session and the added cost of SWL. In our experience, both EHL and the Swiss Lithoclast are safe energy sources in the urinary tract, and tissue damage can be avoided by cautious use, The pneumatic lithotriptor is an excellent tool for fragmentation of stones. We have found this device to be especially effective with large impacted hard stones in the ureter as well as with renal stones with poor or slow response to ultrasound or electrohydraulic energy.

We agree with the authors that, in the long run, the Lithoclast may be less expensive than EHL and certainly is less expensive than any of the laser systems.

G. Fuchs, M.D.

Suggested Reading

1. Denstedt JD: Advances in intracorporeal lithotripsy. *Curr Opin Urol* 5:212, 1995.

12 Extracorporeal Shock-Wave Lithotripsy

Extracorporeal Shock Wave Lithotripsy: Multicenter Study of Kidney and Upper Ureter Versus Middle and Lower Ureter Treatments
Ehreth JT, Drach GW, Arnett ML, Barnett RB, Govan D, Lingeman J, Loening SA, Newman DM, Tudor JM, Saada S (Univ of Arizona, Tucson; Spartanburg Regional Med Ctr, South Carolina; Stanford Univ, Calif; et al)
J Urol 152:1379–1385, 1994   12–1

Purpose.—For patients with urinary calculi measuring less than 2 cm and located in the renal calyces or pelvis or upper ureter, extracorporeal shock wave lithotripsy (ESWL) is the treatment of choice. A number of different studies have evaluated the use of ESWL to treat patients with stones of the middle and lower ureter. The results have varied, apparently depending on the device used and the characteristics of the stone. The use of ESWL to treat calculi in the kidney and upper ureter vs. the middle and lower ureter was evaluated in a multicenter study.

Methods.—All 6 U.S. institutions participating in the study used a Dornier MFL-5000 multifunctional flat table lithotriptor. The analysis included a total of 766 treatments in 658 patients with stones of the kidney and upper ureter and 391 treatments in 323 patients with stones of the middle and lower ureter. The total number of patient events was 981, including patients who received treatment for both the kidney and ureter. Eighty-one percent of patients completed follow-up. The evaluation included the safety, efficacy, and clinical use of ESWL as well as the incidence of side effects and the anesthetic requirements.

Results.—The ninety-day stone-free rate was 83% in the patients with middle and lower ureter stones vs. 67% in those with kidney and upper ureter stones. Ninety percent of the former group were treated for single stones, compared with 72% of the latter. Eighteen percent of patients with middle and lower ureter stones and 13% of those with kidney and upper ureter stones required 2 or more treatments. Twenty-seven percent of the kidney and upper ureter group received anesthesia compared with 19% of the middle and lower ureter group. Anesthesia was most often given at the request of the patient or physician or for some adjunctive procedure. There were few complications, including ureteral obstruction; the overall complication rate was about 2% in both groups. Laboratory results suggested no significant treatment effects. Six percent of the patients with kidney and upper ureteral stones and 4% of those with middle and lower ureteral stones had diastolic blood pressure increases to more than 95 mm Hg after ESWL. Another 11% of patients in both groups had resolution of hypertension after ESWL was performed.

Conclusions.—When a group of patients with specific indications is considered, ESWL may be even more effective for patients with stones in the middle and lower ureter than for those with stones in the kidney and upper ureter. In either case, the treatment has few complications or side effects. Among other factors, stone size has an impact on the need for retreatment.

▶ Evidence continues to accumulate showing that stone-free efficacy is greater in cases in which the treatment target is a small stone and/or a single stone in a nonobstructing location. A small, nonobstructing single stone in the superior calyces, renal pelvis, or ureter has the highest probability of becoming "stone free" after ESWL. Multiple stones, obstructing stones, radiographically "dense" stones, and large stones (greater than 1–1.5 cm) have a lower possibility of becoming stone free.[1]

D.P. Griffith, M.D.

Reference

1. Griffith DP, Politis G: ESWL: Stone free efficacy based upon stone size and location. *World J Urol* 5:525, 1987.

Extracorporeal Shock-Wave Lithotripsy of Middle Ureteral Stones: Are Ureteral Stents Necessary?
Nakada SY, Pearle MS, Soble JJ, Gardner SM, McClennan BL, Clayman RV (Univ of Wisconsin, Madison; Univ of Texas Southwestern, Dallas; Washington Univ, St Louis; et al)
Urology 46:649–652, 1995   12–2

Background.—Because of problems related to visibility and positioning, pretreatment with a stent is widely used in patients undergoing extracorporeal shock wave lithotripsy (ESWL) for the treatment of middle ureteral stones (i.e., those overlying the pelvic bone). This practice continues despite the lack of studies demonstrating any advantage of stent bypass over in situ ESWL. The effect of placement of a ureteral stent on the outcome of ESWL for middle ureteral stones was investigated.

Methods.—The retrospective study included 26 of 33 patients undergoing ESWL for middle ureteral stones during a 3-year period. The patients (average age, 58 years) were treated by 16 different urologists. Fourteen patients received stent bypasses, 8 received in situ treatment, and 4 had EWSL after percutaneous nephrostomy (PCN). An unmodified Dornier HM-3 lithotriptor was used for initial treatment in all patients, all but 4 of whom underwent EWSL in the prone position on a modified Stryker frame. All patients were assessed at an average follow-up of 8 weeks by telephone interview, abdominal radiography, IV urography, and sometimes retrograde urography.

Results.—The patients received an average of 2,423 shocks at an average of 22 kV. Overall, the stone-free rate after at least 1 month of follow-up was 73%, and the efficiency quotient was 69. Single-treatment stone-free rates were 71% with stent bypass, 63% with in situ ESWL, and 75% with PCN. The retreatment rate was 4%. Auxiliary treatments were required by 19% of patients, and admission for renal colic was recorded for 8%. Nine patients had stones measuring 10 mm or larger: 33% were stone free after stent bypass or in situ ESWL compared with 67% after PCN. Success rates increased to 82% for stent bypass, 80% for in situ ESWL, and 100% for PCN in patients with smaller stones.

Conclusions.—For patients undergoing ESWL for middle ureteral calculi, pretreatment with a stent appears to offer no advantage in terms of outcome. Avoidance of the use of a stent avoids transurethral and ureteral manipulation, which makes ESWL a truly noninvasive therapy. Lithotripsy is an appropriate initial treatment for patients with middle ureteral stones measuring less than 10 mm.

▶ Ureteral stents dilate the ureter, provide better fluoroscopic localization of the ureter, reduce ureteral colic, retard the passage of large stone fragments, and improve the predictability of clinical management. This manuscript demonstrates that stents confer no improvement in treatment outcome. However, the use of stents in selected patients may "smooth," or make more predictable, clinical management. One policy does not fit all patients.

D.P. Griffith, M.D.

Painless ESWL by Cutaneous Application of Vaseline
Heidenreich A, Bonfig R, Wilbert DM, Engerlmann UH (Univ of Cologne, Germany; Eberhard-Karls-Univ, Tübingen, Germany)
Scand J Urol Nephrol 29:155–160, 1995   12–3

Background.—Although newer generations of lithotriptors have facilitated anesthesia-free extracorporeal shock wave lithotripsy (ESWL) treatments, pain necessitating IV anesthesia, analgosedation, or a reduction in the number and/or power of shock waves still occurs in 30% to 50% of the patients. Most pain associated with ESWL appears to originate in the skin, which suggests that a cavitation phenomenon may be the cause. Fluids high in viscosity can inhibit the development of cavitation bubbles. Thus, it was hypothesized that the cutaneous application of Vaseline (petroleum jelly) would decrease pain during ESWL.

TABLE 2.—Requirements for Supplementary Analgesic Sedation in
Relation to Stone Location

	Group 1	Group 2	
Upper calyceal stones	0/23	4/10 (40%)	$p < 0.03$
Lower calyceal stones	4/20 (20%)	3/9 (33%)	n.s.
Renal pelvis stones	0/21	8/15 (53%)	$p < 0.001$
Mid and upper ureteral stones	0/55	3/30 (30%)	n.s.
Distal ureteral stones	6/31 (19%)	8/11 (78%)	$p < 0.001$
	10/150 (6.7%)	26/75 (35%)	$p < 0.001$

(Courtesy of Heidenreich A, Bonfig R, Wilbert DM, et al: Painless ESWL by cutaneous application of Vaseline. *Scand J Urol Nephrol* 29:155–160, 1995. Used by permission.)

Methods.—In one group of 150 patients, petroleum jelly was applied to a 10- × 20-cm area of skin corresponding to the entry site of shock waves just before ESWL was begun. In a second group of 75 patients, ESWL was done without petroleum jelly.

Findings.—Additional analgesic sedation was required in 6.7% of those treated with petroleum jelly and in 36.4% treated without it. The need for additional analgosedation was most marked for patients with lower calyceal and distal ureteral stones (Table 2). Median pain scores were 2.5 and 4.25 in patients treated with and without petroleum jelly, respectively.

Conclusions.—The local application of petroleum jelly significantly decreases pain during ESWL. The high viscosity of petroleum jelly inhibits cavitation bubble development at the surface of the skin. Cutaneous petroleum jelly application may be especially useful in outpatient ESWL procedures.

▶ This is a very scholarly, practical, and useful concept. It should become routine use in all lithotriptic centers. However, it should be used selectively and appropriately. In the cited paper the authors show that the thickness of cutaneous petroleum jelly is inversely proportional to successful stone fragmentation. Thus, a layer of cutaneous petroleum jelly less than 1 mm thick decreases pain somewhat and decreases fragmentation effectiveness minimally. Thicker layers of petroleum jelly are deleterious to effective pulverization.

D.P. Griffith, M.D.

Long-term Radiographic and Functional Outcome of Extracorporeal Shock Wave Lithotripsy Induced Perirenal Hematomas

Krishnamurthi V, Streem SB (Cleveland Clinic Found, Ohio)
J Urol 154:1673–1675, 1995

12–4

Introduction.—The preferred treatment for most renal calculi is extracorporeal shock wave lithotripsy (ESWL). Perirenal or intrarenal hematomas are a relatively frequent complication of ESWL, and there is little known about their long-term consequences. Therefore, the long-term outcome of ESWL-induced perirenal hematomas was investigated.

Methods.—Renal ultrasonography identified 21 perirenal hematomas after ESWL in 19 patients who had a minimum of 3 months of clinical and radiographic follow-up. Of the 19 patients, 14 were asymptomatic and 5 had symptoms suggestive of ESWL. The symptomatic patients were treated conservatively with supportive therapy only. The blood pressure and serum creatinine levels were measured in all patients before ESWL and at follow-up visits. Anatomical changes in the hematoma were assessed on follow-up ultrasound studies.

Results.—The ultrasound studies revealed complete radiographic resolution of 18 of the 21 hematomas (85.7%) within 3–46 months. There were no significant changes in mean blood pressure, either individually or overall. Only 1 patient, who had been azotemic before undergoing ESWL and had a persistent hematoma at 15 months, demonstrated a significant increase in serum creatinine levels.

Conclusions.—Most ESWL-induced perirenal hematomas can be expected to resolve spontaneously within 1–2 years. These hematomas are unlikely to adversely affect blood pressure or renal function. Therefore, it is suggested that patients with ESWL-induced perirenal hematomas be monitored every 6–12 months with blood pressure measurements and radiographic studies until resolution of the hematoma, and additional periodic monitoring of renal function should be done in patients with a solitary kidney or preexisting azotemia.

▶ In investigative imaging (CT and MRI) after ESWL, hematomas (mostly subcapsular) have been revealed in 20% to 25% of patients. Only a small percentage of these show clinical symptoms. This paper demonstrates that the symptomatic hematomas, which are likely to hold the greatest potential risk in terms of damaging sequelae, are not likely to impair renal function or cause hypertension in the majority of cases.

However, risk factors for hematomas—hypertension, nonsteroidal anti-inflammatory medications, and bleeding abnormalities—should be addressed and optimized before ESWL.

D.P. Griffith, M.D.

13 Transplantation

The Fate of Renal Allografts Functioning for a Minimum of 20 Years (Level 5A): Indefinite Success or Beginning of the End? A Proposed Classification of Long-term Allograft Survivals
Braun WE, Popowniak KL, Nakamoto S, Gifford RW Jr, Straffon RA
(Cleveland Clinic Found, Ohio)
Transplantation 60:784–790, 1995

13–1

Background.—When a renal allograft functions for more than 20 years, the potential for open-ended success exists. This potential and the effect of acute rejection and delayed function in patients in whom renal allografts had been functioning for 20 years or more were investigated.

Methods.—Fifty-five renal allografts that had functioned for 20.1–30.7 years were assessed. Forty-four allografts were obtained from 44 living-related donors, and 11 were obtained from cadaver donors. Patients were divided into 3 groups according to renal function. The 26 patients in group 1 had a glomerular filtration rate (GFR) of 60 mL/min/1.7 m² or greater or serum levels of creatinine of 1.4 mg/dL or lower and no proteinuria. The 9 patients in group 2 had a GFR of 60 mL/min/1.7 m² or greater or serum levels of creatinine 1.4 mg/dL or lower but had more than 150 mg proteinuria/24 hours. The 20 patients in group 3 had a GFR of less than 60 mL/min/1.73 m² and/or serum levels of creatinine greater than 1.4 mg/dL with or without proteinuria.

Findings.—Acute rejection occurred in 62% and delayed function in 55% of the cadaver grafts. These factors, however, did not preclude 20-year success or the prospect of continued survival. Acute rejection, however, occurred in a limited period in the first 3 months after transplant in all group 1 and 2 patients but in only 7 of 16 group 3 patients. Acute rejection was treated with IV methylprednisolone in 14 patients in groups 1 and 2 and in 6 patients in group 3. In 87% of these transplants, donor age was 50 years or younger and recipient age was 40 years or younger. Ninety-eight percent of living-related transplants involved 1- or 2-HLA haplotype matching. Three patients died of coronary artery disease, 1 died of malignancy, and 3 died of severe infection and hepatitis. Hypertension developed in 25 recipients, and diabetes mellitus developed in 12. Renal dysfunction in groups 2 and 3 compromised potential open-ended success. In 12 patients in group 1, however, open-ended success seemed possible.

Conclusions.—Over the years, immunosuppressed renal allograft recipients continue to be at increased risk for eventual renal allograft dysfunction and cardiovascular, neoplastic, infectious, and metabolic diseases. A simple classification system based on minimum and mean allograft survival was proposed to standardize the phrase "long-term."

► It is heartening to see that long-term renal allograft survival is attainable, even without modern immunosuppressive agents, such as cyclosporine, mycophenolate mofetil, and antilymphocyte antibodies. Increased 1-year graft survival seen with the newer agents may not translate to longer-term graft survival, however, unless the mechanisms of chronic allograft nephropathy are elucidated. Although intriguing surrogate molecular markers are being defined in rodents, none yet exists in human beings. The authors' point that long-term success, despite delayed graft function and acute rejection, is possible is not surprising; these factors are strong predictors of chronic allograft nephropathy. However, chronic allograft loss is multifactorial, and no one factor need be the "kiss of death." Nevertheless, only 50% of the episodes of acute rejection in this study were biopsy proved. Therefore, not all the group 1 patients with acute rejection may have had the condition by modern criteria. Furthermore, 80% of group 3 patients had experienced delayed graft function. Although this finding was not statistically significant, the study was probably not powered to preclude a significant difference in this factor given the small numbers.

Reduction of both acute rejection episodes and nonimmune damage (e.g., cold ischemia, hypertension, hyperfiltration injury, infection, and hyperlipidemia) currently remains the best way to improve long-term graft survival.

D.A. Shoskes, M.D.

Malignancies of the Genito-urinary System Following Renal Transplantation
Schmidt R, Stippel D, Krings F, Pollok M (Univ of Cologne, Germany)
Br J Urol 75:572–577, 1995   13–2

Background.—Organ transplant recipients have an increased risk of malignancies. Lymphomas, skin cancer, and cancer of the genitourinary system are most common. The development of genitourinary system malignancies after renal transplantation was analyzed.

Methods.—Eight hundred sixty-eight renal graft recipients were included. Mean follow up was 41.8 months. Fifteen grafts were obtained from living-related donors, and 853 were from cadavers.

Findings.—Cancer of the genitourinary system developed in 12 patients (1.4%) (Fig 3). Eleven tumors were de novo malignancies. In 1 patient, a small renal carcinoma was transplanted from a living-related donor. The incidence of genitourinary system tumors was 34 per 100,000 patient-years in patients treated with cyclosporin and 32 per 100,000 patient-

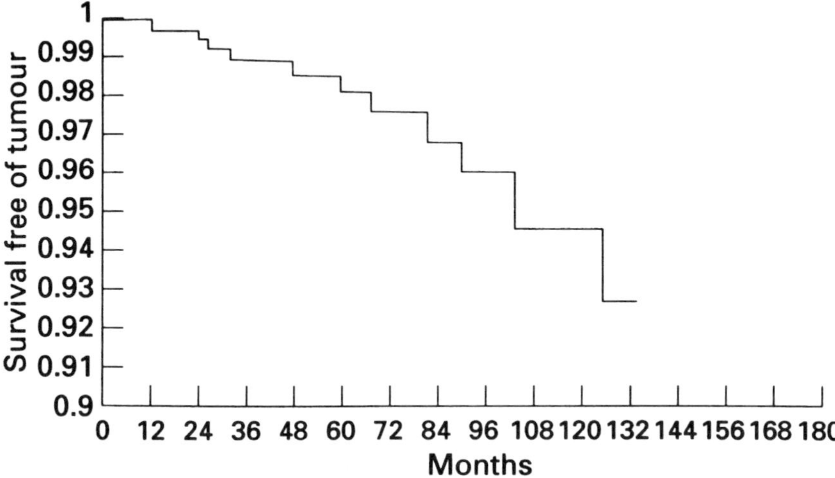

FIGURE 3.—Incidence for development of malignancies of the genitourinary system. Five-year *P* value, 0.982; 10-year *P* value, 0.947. (Courtesy of Schmidt R, Stippel D, Krings F, et al: Malignancies of the genito-urinary system following renal transplantation. *Br J Urol* 75:572–577, 1995.)

years in those treated with conventional therapy. Compared with a reference population, the incidence of malignant genitourinary system tumors was increased by a factor of 7.3 in male patients and 11.2 in female patients. Four patients died 0–48 months after the malignancies were diagnosed. Median survival time for these patients was 14.4 months.

Conclusions.—The frequency of malignancies in renal transplant recipients necessitates routine assessment in all such patients before and at regular intervals after surgery. Routine examinations should include cervical smears in female patients.

▶ Excluding skin cancers, the genitourinary system is the most frequent site of occurrence of de novo malignancy in organ transplant recipients. Genitourinary tumors currently comprise approximately one third of all noncutaneous tumors in this population. The increased incidence of renal tumors reflects not only intercurrent immunosuppressive therapy but also underlying primary renal disease.[1] Acquired renal cystic disease occurs in 30% to 95% of long-term dialysis patients and is associated with an increased risk of renal cell carcinoma. Renal transplant recipients also have a higher than expected incidence of renal pelvic transitional cell carcinoma because of the large number of patients with analgesic nephropathy. Data from the Australia and New Zealand transplant tumor registry have suggested an increased risk of transitional cell carcinoma of the bladder in transplant recipients.[2] Another recent study highlighted the increased potential for squamous cell carcinoma of the bladder in patients who have end-stage renal disease because of spina bifida or spinal cord injury.[3] Genitourinary malignancies will probably be detected more frequently in transplant recipients in the future because of the higher age and increasing longevity of these patients.

A.C. Novick, M.D.

References

1. Penn I: Primary kidney tumors before and after renal transplantation. *Transplantation* 59:480–485, 1995.
2. Sheil AGR, Disney APS, Matthew TH, et al: De novo malignancy emerges as a major cause of morbidity and late failure in renal transplantation. *Transplant Proc* 25:1383–1384, 1993.
3. Yaqoob M, McClelland P, Bell GM, et al: Bladder tumors in paraplegic patients on renal replacement therapy. *Lancet* 338:1554–1555, 1991.

Steady Improvement in Renal Allograft Survival Among North American Children: A Five Year Appraisal by the North American Pediatric Renal Transplant Cooperative Study
Tejani A, Sullivan EK, Fine RN, Harmon W, Alexander S (State Univ of New York, Brooklyn; EMMES Corp, Potomac, Md; State Univ of New York, Stony Brook; et al)
Kidney Int 48:551–553, 1995   13–3

Background.—Although renal transplantation is now viewed as the optimal replacement treatment for children who have end-stage renal disease, the results have not equalled those achieved in adults. Trends in graft survival were examined with the use of data from the North American Pediatric Renal Transplant Cooperative Study.

Methods.—From 1987 through 1994, 1,641 children who received cadaver kidneys were enrolled. The patients were from 83 participating centers in the United States and Canada. Of 1,410 cadaver kidney transplants done from 1987 to 1991, 1,258 were index transplants.

Results.—The 1987 cohort had 1- and 2-year graft survival rates of 72% and 65%, respectively, compared with 83% and 78% for the 1991 cohort. The relative risk of graft failure in the earlier cohort was 1.4. T-cell induction antibody was administered to 38% of patients in the 1987 cohort and to 67% in the latter group. Cyclosporine was used for at least 1 month after transplantation in 87% of the earlier group and in 97% of patients in the 1991 cohort. The respective average daily maintenance doses 1 year after transplantation were 6.5 and 7.5 mg/kg. Random transfusions were given less often to the 1991 cohort. The use of younger cadaver kidney donors also declined over time.

Implication.—The finding that improved survival of cadaver kidney transplants relates to advances in practice is encouraging, as identification of those factors that influence graft survival could enhance the quality of life for pediatric transplant recipients.

▶ Renal transplantation is the principle therapeutic modality for children who have end-stage renal disease, because a well-functioning graft allows for better quality of life and rehabilitation than can be achieved with dialysis. Graft survival rates in children have improved in recent years because of both the availability of cyclosporine and the preponderance of living-related donors in this population. Predialysis or preemptive renal transplantation is being increasingly performed in children to obviate dialysis-related morbidity and to optimize overall rehabilitation.[1]

Growth retardation secondary to renal failure has been an important clinical problem in children who have end-stage renal disease. Transplantation is most likely to have a positive impact on subsequent growth in children if done before the age of 7 years. Small children who weigh less that 20 kg have traditionally been considered high-risk recipients because of the technical difficulties associated with surgery and dialysis in this group. Refinements in pediatric anesthesia, intensive care practice, and surgical technique have substantially improved transplant outcome, and size alone is no longer a contraindication to transplantation. Other strategies that have been successfully and safely used to improve the growth velocity of pediatric renal allograft recipients are alternate-day steroid dosing[2] and administration of recombinant human growth hormone.[3]

A.C. Novick, M.D.

References

1. Donnelly PK, Oman P, Henderson R, et al: Predialysis living donor renal transplantation: Is it still the gold standard for cost, convenience, and graft survival? *Transplant Proc* 27:1444–1446, 1995.
2. Jabs K, Sullivan EK, Avner ED, et al: Alternate-day steroid dosing improves growth without adversely affecting graft survival or long-term graft function. *Transplantation* 61:31–36, 1996.
3. Fine RN, Yadin O, Moulten L, et al: Extended recombinant human growth hormone treatment after renal transplantation in children. *J Am Soc Nephrol* 2:274S–283S, 1992.

Cold Ischemia and Outcome in 17,937 Cadaveric Kidney Transplants
Peters TG, Shaver TR, Ames JE IV, Santiago-Delpin EA, Jones KW, Blanton JW (South-Eastern Organ Procurement Found, Richmond, Va; Univ of Florida Health Science Ctr, Jacksonville; Walter Reed Army Med Ctr, Washington, DC; et al)
Transplantation 59:191–196, 1995   13–4

Introduction.—With the increasing need for kidneys for transplantation, it is important that no available kidneys be wasted, unless sound reasons are evident. Questions remain regarding the ultimate outcome in organ transplantation and varying cold ischemic times. The presence or absence of adverse effects was analyzed in 17,937 cadaveric renal transplants performed with varying cold preservation times.

Methods.—Information regarding the organ donor, the kidney, the transplant recipient, and periodic post-transplant follow-up was gathered prospectively from 1982 to 1991. Separate analyses were performed for patients who received kidneys preserved for 1–16, 16–32, 32–48, and more than 48 hours. The University of Wisconsin solution became widespread after 1989. A separate analysis was therefore done for the 13,800 kidneys transplanted before January 1, 1990, and the 4,137 subsequent kidneys transplanted through 1991. An HLA match at 3 or more loci occurred in 6,067 transplants (34%).

Results.—Before 1990, graft functional survival was significantly better for kidneys stored for 1–16 hours than those preserved for longer periods. Graft functional survival was similar in kidneys stored 16–32, 32–48, and more than 48 hours during the years 1982–1989. There was no significant difference, however, in preservation times and allograft survival in 1990–1991. One-year actuarial graft survival rates were 74%, 83%, and 76%, respectively, for grafts transplanted from 1982–1989, 1990–1991, and overall. Before 1990, the strongest outcome factors were delayed graft function degree of match, retransplanted recipient, black race, and previous transfusion for all kidneys. During 1990–1991, the most significant outcome factors were delayed graft function and degree of match. Poorer outcomes were observed overall in older patients, regardless of the date of transplant. Delayed graft function occurred significantly more frequently in all kidneys preserved longer than 16 hours. The 1-year allograft survival rate was not related to the duration of organ preservation in the event of delayed graft function.

Conclusion.—Functional viability of kidneys preserved 48 hours or longer may be expected with current preservation methods. Prolonged cold ischemic time is no longer a major factor in discarding organs.

▶ This multicenter study is important both for what it says and for what it doesn't say. The authors show that increased cold ischemia time is 1 contributing factor for delayed graft function and that delayed graft function is a strong predictor of poor outcome but that increased cold ischemia time alone does not invariably lead to poor graft survival. They don't say that a prolonged cold ischemia time is harmless to the graft. Clearly, delayed graft function is multifactorial, and other important donor and recipient factors will define the tolerable range of cold ischemia time for the individual kidney, which may well extend longer than 48 hours.[1] Nevertheless, the nonimmune damage present in the kidney after transplantation sets the baseline function below which immune-mediated damage will harm the kidney further, thereby setting up an inflammatory injury response that can lead to chronic allograft nephropathy.[2] These data should therefore not be used as an excuse to prolong cold ischemia time unnecessarily or perform cadaveric renal transplantation only during elective surgery hours. Neither should otherwise good kidneys with prolonged cold ischemia time be needlessly discarded.

D.A. Shoskes, M.D.

References

1. Shoskes DA, Churchill BM, McLorie GA, et al: The impact of ischemic and immunologic factors on early graft function in pediatric renal transplantation. *Transplantation* 50:877–881, 1990.
2. Shoskes DA, Halloran PF: Delayed graft function in renal transplantation: Etiology, management and long-term significance. *J Urol* 155:1831–1840, 1996.

Ureteral Complications of Renal Transplant Surgery
Shah MH (Kidney Centre, Rawalpindi, Pakistan)
Transplant Proc 27:2708–2711, 1995   13–5

Introduction.—Urinary leakage is a major cause of morbidity in recipients of renal transplants. The incidence of ureteral complications was studied in the 15-year experience of renal transplants performed by a single surgeon. The influence of the type of ureterovesical (UV) anastomosis on the incidence of ureteral complications was analyzed.

Methods.—Seven hundred thirty renal transplants were performed with the use of live donors. These patients were divided into 3 groups, defined by the type of UV anastomosis used during the transplantation procedure. In the 50 patients in group 1, UV anastomosis was achieved with an anterolateral external ureteroneocystostomy. In the 435 patients in group 2, a bladder flap was created over the anterolateral bladder wall. The spatulated ureteric end was pulled through a small mucosal hole and anastomosed to the mucosa. A Ryle's tube or small lumen polythene tube was sutured within the ureter and was either removed through the bladder wall or left inside the bladder and removed with a cytoscope 2 weeks later. In the 245 patients in group 3, the preceding technique was modified by using an unsutured Double-J ureteric tube instead of Ryle's tube or polythene tube.

Results.—There were ureteral complications in 2.87% of procedures, which accounted for 33.33% of urologic complications. The incidence of ureteral complications was 26% in group 1, 1.36% in group 2, and 0.81% in group 3.

Conclusions.—The incidence of ureteral complications can be reduced by using a modification of Boari's flap technique for ureterovesical anastomosis. This approach requires a smaller length of donor's ureter.

▶ The author reports a 26% ureteral complication rate with the use of an external ureterocystostomy. When properly done, the complication rate for this technique should be no higher than 4%. There is little role for the Boari flap–type repair that the author advocates. This approach decreases the capacity of an already small bladder and increases the risk of bladder leak and hemorrhage. If a short or compromised donor ureter is encountered, the procedure of choice is native ureteropyelostomy.

D.A. Shoskes, M.D.

Flank Versus Transabdominal Living Donor Nephrectomy: A Randomized Clinical Trial

Mehraban D, Nowroozi A, Naderi GH (Tehran Univ, Iran)
Transplant Proc 27:2716–2717, 1995   13–6

Objective.—Whether the flank approach or the transabdominal transperitoneal approach yields greater benefits and fewer complications was determined in a clinical trial involving 104 live-donor nephrectomies.

Methods.—The kidney donors were randomly selected to undergo either flank or transabdominal transperitoneal nephrectomies. All procedures were performed by the same surgeon. Data were collected on nephrectomy side, number of donor arteries, family relationship of the donor and recipient, operation time, cold ischemia time, analgesic requirements, graft function, hospital stay, and complications.

Results.—The 2 kidney donor groups were similar in mean age, male-female ratio, percentage of related donors, nephrectomy side, number of donor kidney arteries, operation time, and duration of hospital stay. Cold ischemia time was significantly longer in the transabdominal approach, and mean time to oral feeding showed a statistically significant difference between the transabdominal (36 hours) and flank (20 hours) groups. There were no major complications in either group, but the rate of minor complications (Table 2) was higher in the flank group (17%) than in the transabdominal group (11%). Most donors who underwent the transabdominal approach were unhappy with their abdominal scar at 6-month follow-up.

Conclusion.—Because of the lack of important differences in outcome between the flank approach and the transabdominal approach to live-donor nephrectomies, the study was terminated and the flank technique was selected as the preferred method. Donor satisfaction was not a variable, but the young donors had a clear preference for the flank approach.

▶ The advantages of a flank approach for living-donor nephrectomy have long been established. This study shows essentially no difference between the 2 approaches, apart from resumption of oral feeding half a day sooner in

TABLE 2.—Types and Numbers of Complications in Each Group

	Flank	Transabdominal
Pleural injury	6	0
Lumbar artery injury	0	1
Lumbar vein injury	1	0
Mesocolon hematoma	0	1
Injury to colonic serosa	1	0
Major bleeding	0	3
Mild, transient ATN	1	0
Sinus tachycardia	1	0
Bladder injury	1	0

the flank group. If the surgeon is more comfortable with a transperitoneal approach, I would favor a subcostal or modified chevron incision over the long midline that the authors used. Whether laparoscopic-assisted donor nephrectomy will establish a routine role in transplantation awaits more widespread use.[1]

D.A. Shoskes, M.D.

Reference

1. Ratner LE, Ciseck LJ, Moore RG, et al: Laparoscopic live donor nephrectomy. *Transplantation* 60:1047–1049, 1995.

Influence of End-stage Renal Disease and Renal Transplantation on Serum Prostate-specific Antigen

Morton JJ, Howe SF, Lowell JA, Stratta RJ, Taylor RJ (Univ of Nebraska Med Ctr, Omaha)
Br J Urol 75:498–501, 1995   13–7

Background.—Kidney transplant recipients and patients on dialysis who are awaiting transplantation have increased risk of de novo malignancy, compared with the general population. There has been an upward trend in the age of transplant recipients, and more men in their fifth to seventh decades have required dialysis and eventual transplantation. Clinically significant prostate cancer will undoubtedly develop in some of these men, either before or after transplant. The effects of end-stage renal disease and transplantation on serum levels of prostate-specific antigen (PSA), and the ability of PSA to detect prostate cancer in patients on dialysis and after kidney transplantation, were studied.

Study Design.—All men in a kidney transplant program who were older than 40 years of age and had received a kidney transplant between 1974 and 1992 or were currently on dialytic therapy awaiting transplantation were included in an ongoing prospective longitudinal study. Serum levels of PSA were determined and digital rectal examinations (DREs) were performed yearly. Twelve patients were evaluated before transplant and 70 were evaluated after transplant, for a total of 136 PSA levels determined for 42 months (mean, 1.7). The results were compared with those of age-matched controls who did not have known prostate cancer.

Results.—Mean levels of PSA were not affected by either dialysis or transplantation, irrespective of age, when compared with controls. Further, mean levels in the 12 patients who were evaluated while on dialysis and who subsequently underwent transplantation did not differ significantly before and after transplantation. In 3 patients, the results of DRE and the serum level of PSA were used to diagnose localized prostate cancer after transplant, for an incidence of 3.7%. Two patients who had undergone radical prostatectomy and were free of disease at 24 and 36 months after surgery with no change in renal function. Immunosuppression was not modified.

Conclusion.—Transplantation and dialysis do not appear to affect clinical serum levels of PSA. Serum levels of PSA and DRE appear to be equally applicable as screening modalities for detection of prostate cancer in patients on dialysis and after transplant, when compared with the general population. Radical surgery is a feasible treatment option for localized prostate cancer in this group of patients.

▶ Patients who have end-stage renal disease are twice as likely to be men than women. They also include a higher proportion of blacks and Hispanics, who are known to have an increased risk for prostate cancer. Therefore, screening of male transplant candidates or recipients who are older than 40 years of age is likely to identify patients who have localized disease that can be treated. The prevalence of prostate cancer in solid organ transplant recipients is currently not known. The Urologic Society for Transplantation and Vascular Surgery recently completed a prospective multicenter study to evaluate the problem of prostate cancer in renal transplant recipients.[1] Three hundred eighty-nine men, aged 40 years or older, were screened with serum levels of PSA and DRE 1–6 years after successful renal transplantation. Thirty-three patients (8.5%) had abnormalities of either DRE or PSA or both; 20 of these patients underwent transrectal ultrasound–guided prostate biopsies. Prostate cancer was detected in 7 patients, for an overall incidence of 1.8%. All these patients underwent radical prostatectomy with no adverse sequelae. These data emphasize that there is a high prevalence of clinically significant prostate cancer in renal transplant recipients and that these patients can undergo radical prostatectomy safely. The study by Morton and associates underscores the utility of screening for prostate cancer in this population with serum levels of PSA and DRE.

A.C. Novick, M.D.

Reference

1. Khauli RB: Genitourinary malignancies in organ transplant recipients. *Semin Urol* 12:224–232, 1994.

Suggested Reading

Transplantation of Pediatric Cadaver Kidneys Into Adult Recipients
Gourlay W, Stothers L, McLoughlin MG, Manson AD, Keown P (Univ of British Columbia, Canada)
J Urol 153:322-325, 1995

▶ The continued cadaveric organ shortage mandates exploration of donor sources at the extremes of age and organ function. Pediatric donors, especially those younger than 4 years of age, have been used reluctantly because of higher rates of technical complications, acute rejection, and the concern of transplanting an insufficient nephron mass. This retrospective review of pediatric kidneys into adult recipients confirms the higher rate of vascular complications and episodes of acute rejection, although the serum level of creatinine at 1 year was equivalent to that seen with adult donors. Parenthetically, transplanting pediatric kidneys into pediatric recipients yields uniformly abysmal results and should be avoided. Of note, the pediatric donor group in this study had a significantly higher cold ischemic time (although rates of delayed graft function were not quoted), and kidneys were flushed with Collin's solution, which may have contributed to the inferior results.

I continue to use pediatric kidneys in adults but attempt to select recipients with an improved chance for success. If the donor weighs less than 25 kg or if the kidneys are less than 7 cm long, I transplant both kidneys en bloc. I exclude recipients who are very large, are highly sensitized, or have extensive atherosclerotic disease or in whom the cold ischemia time is expected to be longer than 36 hours.

Intraoperatively, I stent all pediatric ureters, ensure a sufficiently large retroperitoneal pocket to place en bloc kidneys without angulation, and use antilymphocytic induction therapy. If these precautions are needed, results with pediatric donors should approach those seen with adults.

D.A. Shoskes, M.D.

14 Voiding Dysfunction and Neurogenic Bladder

Sacral Anterior Root Stimulation for Bladder Control in Patients With a Complete Lesion of the Spinal Cord
van der AaHE, Hermens H, Alleman E, Vorsteveld H (Rehabcentre't Roessingh Enschede, The Netherlands)
Acta Neurochir (Wien) 134:88–92, 1995   14–1

Background.—Neurostimulation with the Finetech-Brindley bladder controller is very effective in the management of neurogenic bladders in patients who have spinal cord lesions. The results of this system in selected patients who had a complete spinal cord lesion were reported.

Methods.—A Finetech-Brindley bladder controller was implanted in 17 patients who had a complete lesion of the spinal cord. The sacral roots were identified during a microscopic procedure in the cauda equina, and the posterior components of the S2, S3, and S4 roots were cut. Stimulators were intradurally placed around the anterior components of the S2, S3, and S4 roots and around the S5 root. The patients' status was followed 1–6 years.

Findings.—Bladder capacity was increased in all 17 patients. At the most recent assessment, 16 patients had a residual volume of less than 30 mL. Urinary tract infection occurred rarely. Full continence was achieved in 12 patients. All men could sustain a full erection with the implant. Thirteen patients used the implant for bowel function. There were no significant complications.

Conclusions.—Sacral anterior root stimulation is effective in the treatment of neurogenic bladder in patients who have a complete spinal cord lesion. With this procedure, bladder capacity is improved, and the residual volume is reduced. Almost all patients become continent. Urinary tract infections occur rarely, and defecation is facilitated. The risk of renal damage is also reduced. Socially and psychologically, the patients' condition is much improved.

▶ This report presents the largest review to date of anterior sacral root stimulators combined with posterior sacral rhizotomy to achieve micturition and defecation. Through a series of empirical observations, investigators have found that intradural stimulators combined with posterior rhizotomy produced most effective evacuation. Posterior rhizotomy improves continence by limiting afferent input from the bladder and pelvic structures, which can elicit involuntary bladder contractions. Rhizotomy also increases bladder compliance. The price of rhizotomy, however, is the loss of sacral sensation and impotence in some patients.

It is important to remember that these patients are highly selected at their respective centers. Preoperative or intraoperative evoked testing is used to determine whether stimulation of a special nerve root results in an effective detrusor contraction. Obviously, patients who have cauda equina lesions or poor detrusor contractility are not candidates for such a device. Stimulation parameters are chosen that elicit bladder contraction yet do not stimulate the external urethral sphincter. Most of the 500 patients who underwent implantation are still using the device. So what is the catch? Should all patients who have spinal cord injury be given an opportunity to use such a device? These challenging questions involve risk-benefit and cost-benefit ratios. It is unclear whether many patients would have benefited from rhizotomy alone. As for emptying the bladder, the greatest challenge is to show that this device is as effective and safe as alternative therapy, namely intermittent self-catheterization. No data are presented in this report of residual urines, continence, urodynamics, or prevalence of autonomic dysreflexia. The obvious costs include surgery and possible reoperation. Long-term data appear encouraging, but some dark clouds may be on the horizon. Rhizotomies initiate changes in the bladder that cannot be predicted and do not become apparent for many years. Reimbursement for such devices is also an issue. Sacral anterior root stimulators are no longer merely experimental, and the decision whether to be part of the very time-consuming and challenging program is difficult for both the patient and urologist. The costs and potential for adverse effects theoretically exceed those of intermittent self-catheterization.

W.D. Steers, M.D.

The First 500 Patients With Sacral Anterior Root Stimulator Implants: General Description
Brindley GS (Royal Natl Orthopaedic Hosp, Stanmore, England)
Paraplegia 32:795–805, 1994   14–2

Introduction.—Between 1976 and 1992, sacral anterior root stimulators for bladder control were implanted in 500 patients. The results of this procedure were determined during a total follow-up time of 2,033.5 years. Excluding periods of non-use, the total time of use was 1,897.1 years.

Method.—Posterior rhizotomy (within the range S2-5) was complete near root exits in 251 patients. In 405 patients, an intrathecal, 30-channel stimulator was used. In 477 patients, the electrodes were implanted intrathecally at the level of the fifth lumbar vertebra and last intervertebral disc. In 12 patients whose primary deafferent was at the conus and in 11 other patients, the electrodes were implanted extradurally in the sacrum.

Results.—Of the 479 survivors, 424 were using their stimulators between 3 months and 16.1 years (mean, 4 years) after implantation. In 45 patients, the implants were intact but not used, mainly because of inadequate implant-driven micturition. Other reasons for non-use included pain when using the stimulator and autonomic dysreflexia. For bladder management, 15 of these patients used intermittent self-catheterization. One percent of stimulators were lost because of infection. Upper urinary tract function deteriorated in 12 patients, including 10 who had incomplete deafferentation or none. One patient died of renal failure, another had grade 1 ureteral reflux, and 10 had radiologic signs of upper tract deterioration (9 were in good health, except for 1 who had kidney stones). Ninety-five operations were performed to remedy faults in implants, including 75 for replacing blocks or rejoining broken cables and 20 for implanting new extradural stimulators. Among 143 patients who had nondeafferentation or incomplete deafferentation, 25 subsequently underwent a secondary deafferentation at the conus medullaris. Seven of the 251 patients in whom complete deafferentation was attempted underwent a secondary deafferentation.

Summary.—Sacral anterior root stimulators provide bladder control in most patients who have spinal cord injury. It is usual to cut the posterior roots at the time of implantation of the electrodes, and the results of the implantation of a stimulator are much less successful without than with posterior rhizotomy. Detrusor areflexia after S2-5 posterior rhizotomy is permanent if it is achieved. The use of extradural electrodes are justified only in the presence of severe arachnoiditis.

▶ As with the multicenter report previously discussed, herein are presented the results of combined S2-S4 posterior sacral rhizotomy with implantation of the Finetech-Brindley intradural anterior sacral root stimulator. Again, improved continence and increased bladder compliance result from rhizotomy alone. The author presents a more detailed account of residual urines, which are surprisingly low (30 cc) in these highly selected patients. Selection is based in part on the response to sacral root stimulation. It is unclear how many of these patients had undergone previous manipulations, such as sphincterotomy, or had received drugs that affected the outlet; these approaches could also partially facilitate low residuals after neurostimulation. The author states that erections persisted. But more precisely, erections were induced by the stimulator. In general, reflex erections are lost. Stimulation of nerves does much more than cause contraction. In experimental models, mast cell degranulation, changes in immune response, and vascular permeability also occur. Do these events occur in the bladder? It may take years to discover. Call me a doubting Thomas, but the results are more favorable than anecdotal reports. As an aside, some investigators have abandoned neuromodulation because of the time, expense, and recurring problems seen with any prostatic device. We may be witnessing results in patients so highly selected over many years as to be inappropriate for a large population. Alternatively, if results continue to improve, we may find ourselves adopting this methodology for many more patients who have spinal cord injury. Even assuming marked reductions in morbidity, however, such devices have to compete with intermittent self-catheterization, especially in this cost-conscious health environment. Although some patients want to avoid self-catheterization, the trade-off must be carefully weighed and explained to the patient. It is important to remember that a rhizotomy is permanent and self-catheterization is not. Despite skepticism, this evolving technology may eventually result in changes in routine patient care.

W.D. Steers, M.D.

Sacral (S3) Segmental Nerve Stimulation as a Treatment for Urge Incontinence in Patients With Detrusor Instability: Results of Chronic Electrical Stimulation Using an Implantable Neural Prosthesis

Bosch JLHR, Groen J (Erasmus Univ, Rotterdam, The Netherlands)
J Urol 154:504–507, 1995   14–3

Objective.—In patients who have urge incontinence and whose conditions are resistant to conservative treatment, unilateral sacral segmental nerve stimulation by a permanent foramen S3 electrode provides a nondestructive alternative. The effectiveness of this treatment in patients who had urge incontinence caused by bladder instability was determined.

Methods.—A foramen electrode connected to a subcutaneously placed pulse generator was implanted into 15 women and 3 men, (average age, 46 years). Patients and voiding-incontinence diaries were examined at 1, 3, 6, 9, 12, 15, 18, and 24 months.

Results.—Voiding frequency, average voided volume, number of incontinence episodes, and number of pads used were significantly improved in all patients (Table 3). Partial or excellent results were achieved in 83% of patients. Symptomatic and urodynamic changes were not completely correlated, because 9 patients who were dry at last follow-up still had bladder instability, whereas 2 patients who were not dry had stable bladders. One

TABLE 3.—Results of Neuromodulation According to Predefined Criteria in 18 Patients

	More Than 90% Decrease (excellent)	No. Pts. 50 to 90% Decrease (partial)	Less Than 50% Decrease (failed)
Pad use	11	3	4
Incontinence episodes	10	5	3
Pad use and/or incontinence episodes	11	4	3

(Courtesy of Bosch JLHR, Groen J: Sacral (S3) segmental nerve stimulation as a treatment for urge incontinence in patients with detrusor instability: Results of chronic electrical stimulation using an implantable neural prosthesis. *J Urol* 154:504–507, 1995.)

patient required repositioning of the electrode, 2 patients required repositioning of the lead, and 1 patient required repositioning of the pulse generator.

Conclusion.—Sacral segmental nerve stimulation is an effective treatment for refractory urge incontinence in patients who have detrusor instability.

▶ Stimulation of sacral roots excites both afferents and efferents that supply the urinary bladder. Efferent stimulation causes contraction of the bladder and pelvic floor. Afferent stimulation causes striated muscle contraction, which in turn generates an afferent volley. Afferent volleys reflexively inhibit the bladder and form the basis of anal and vaginal stimulators. Stimulation of nonbladder sacral afferents inhibits micturition and involuntary bladder contractions through complex mechanisms within the sacral spinal cord. In highly selected patients, S3 root stimulation inhibits urge incontinence. The direct stimulation of S3 is probably more effective than diffuse stimulation of the anus, vagina, or posterior tibial region with implanted stimulators. Biofeedback may also work by the same mechanism. As with all treatments for urinary incontinence, however, outcome measurements are crucial. In this difficult population of patients, success is defined by a 50% to 90% decrease in pad usage. What was the dry rate? Were patients prospectively given pads to count or merely retrospectively asked about pad usage? As with outcome for surgery for stress urinary incontinence, the survey instrument and method of verification can dramatically influence the results by as much as 30% to 40%. The lack of correlation between the urodynamic parameters and symptomatic changes in this report may be partially explained by the methods used to evaluate incontinence. The authors, however, are bluntly honest about 2 patients who are continent even after electrostimulation was discontinued. Whether this resulted from retraining, altered nerve function, or the natural history of the disorder is unclear. Alternatively, one can argue that deterioration of nerve roots may help eliminate detrusor hyperreflexia. Cautious optimism should be reserved for implantable neuromodulation techniques. Cost and morbidity should be carefully weighed.

W.D. Steers, M.D.

Selective Sacral Rhizotomy for the Management of Neurogenic Bladders in Spina Bifida Patients: Long-term Followup
Schneidau T, Franco I, Zebold K, Kaplan W (Westchester County Med Ctr, Valhalla, NY; Children's Memorial Hosp, Chicago)
J Urol 154:766–768, 1995   14–4

Background.—Selective sacral rhizotomy was originally performed in children who had myelodysplasia to treat lower extremity spasticity. Selective sacral rhizotomy was combined with cord untethering in the management of the high pressure bladder often present in these patients.

Favorable results with selective sacral rhizotomy in 8 patients who had spina bifida were reported in 1992. Long-term results of this procedure in the same 8 patients and additional patients were reported.

Methods.—The records of the original 8 patients and 3 additional patients who underwent selective sacral rhizotomy combined with cord untethering were reviewed. At surgery, all patients were aged 3–18.5 years. Maximum follow-up was 49 months. Follow-up included cystometry and radiologic studies.

Results.—Overall, bladder volume increased by 83%; 2 of the original 8 patients had a decrease in bladder volume. Leak point pressure was not significantly changed, which indicates that there was no induced sphincteric damage. No patient had worsening of urinary or bowel control, and uninhibited bladder contractions resolved. In patients who had perineal sensation before surgery, sensation did not change after surgery. Bladder compliance increased by 139%.

Conclusions.—Selective sacral rhizotomy combined with cord untethering is superior to cord untethering alone. The effects are long lasting, and no signs of denervation supersensitivity have been noted. Because patients younger than 9 years of age had a more favorable response, early intervention is recommended.

▶ This series of 11 patients whose status was followed for up to 4 years, shows that selective sacral rhizotomy can increase bladder compliance and eliminate involuntary contractions. No mention is made, however, of associated defects, such as loss of sacral sensation, impact on future potency, or fecal incontinence. The authors point out that the results are much more favorable if rhizotomy precedes development of bladder fibrosis. Theoretical concerns can be raised. For example, myogenic changes may take years to develop after sectioning of nerves. Experimental studies have revealed that loss of direct neural contact or transmitters can lead to biochemical and structural changes in the bladder. Fibrosis may still develop late in patients who have not had rhizotomy. In experimental animals, the elimination of sacral input stimulates growth and overactivity of thoracolumbar input to the bladder. These scenarios could take longer than 4 years to develop. Finally, in this report the influence of spinal cord tethering is unclear. We generally inform our patients that sectioning the filum terminale may prevent future deterioration in lower limbs or bladder but may not restore function already lost.

W.D. Steers, M.D.

Reappraisal of Endoscopic Sphincterotomy for Post-traumatic Neurogenic Bladder: A Prospective Study

Fontaine E, Hajri M, Rhein F, Fakacs C, Le Mouel M-A, Beurton D (Univ of West Paris, Boulogne, France)
J Urol 155:277–280, 1996   14–5

Introduction.—Endoscopic sphincterotomy for rehabilitation of the neurogenic bladder is designed to facilitate bladder emptying without high intravesical pressures. The procedure has been performed for many years, yet its value remains controversial and its acceptance by patients is not clearly established. The results of endoscopic sphincterotomy in patients who had supra-sacral spinal cord injury and detrusor-sphincter dyssynergia were evaluated.

Methods.—Ninety-two men who had spinal cord injury were included. Forty-seven had quadriplegia, and 45 had paraplegia. All had detrusor-sphincter dyssynergia, as indicated by increased external urethral sphincter activity on electromyography during involuntary detrusor contraction. The mean interval between spinal cord injury and sphincterotomy was 47.5 months. The patients' status was followed a mean of 20.6 months. Postoperative evaluations included subjective patient assessment, voiding cystourethrography, and urodynamic examinations.

Results.—All but 6 patients were available for follow-up. Quality of voiding was objectively improved in 83.7% of patients, and 73% expressed subjective satisfaction with results of the procedure. Subjective autonomic dysreflexia was resolved in 41 of 44 patients. Objective improvement was similar in both patient groups, but more patients with quadriplegia reported a subjective improvement in quality of voiding. Febrile urinary tract infections disappeared in 33 of 44 patients. None of the 75 patients who had erections preoperatively experienced a deterioration in sexual function. The rate of post-sphincterotomy complications was 10.9%. Seven patients required a second procedure, but no patient with an initially satisfactory result had a deterioration in function during follow-up.

Conclusion.—Patients who have detrusor-sphincter dyssynergia after spinal cord injury in whom other methods designed to restore continence have failed can benefit from sphincterotomy. The procedure had a high degree of success, both objectively and subjectively, in this series of patients.

▶ In this study, objective improvement after sphincterotomy was defined as a reduction of voiding pressure by greater than 25 cm H_2O and maintenance of voiding pressure less than 50 cm H_2O. Indications for sphincterotomy included urinary incontinence, retention, inability or refusal to perform intermittent self-catheterization, autonomic dysreflexia, bladder calculi, or febrile urinary tract infections. Only 12% of patients had hydronephrosis or reflux. Follow-up was short at 20 months. Although mean residual urine decreased from 210 to 110 cc, inspection of some patients revealed an increase in residual urine. Febrile urinary tract infections disappeared in 77% of patients. However, the timing and frequency of infections before sphincterotomy are unclear. Over time, infection rates may be comparable.

So why has sphincterotomy been all but abandoned in many centers? The authors state that they have converted high pressure urinary incontinence to low pressure urinary incontinence, yet only 13% of patients had reflux or hydronephrosis. We reserve sphincterotomy for patients (usually those with quadriplegia) who have upper tract deterioration, inability to empty the bladder, and high detrusor leak point pressure and cannot perform self-catheterization. For many urologists, the initial enthusiasm for sphincterotomy has been dampened by return of urinary tract infections and residual urines over time. Few clinicians realize that some degree of dyssynergia may actually be beneficial and help maintain a poorly sustained detrusor contraction mediated by a spinal reflex in patients who have spinal cord injury. This is accomplished by triggering repeated afferent volleys from the bladder when the bladder is contracted against an intermittently closed outlet. Decreasing outlet resistance through sphincterotomy reduces this afferent volley, more ineffective reflex bladder contractions, and the increase in residual urine. With more conservative approaches and close follow-up, we rarely see renal problems in our patients who have not had a sphincterotomy. Most paraplegics would rather maintain periods of continence and perform intermittent self-catheterization than undergo sphincterotomy, which has gotten a bad name in the spinal cord injury community. At best, sphincterotomy still condemns the patient to a condom catheter, which results in tremendous long-term morbidity.

W.D. Steers, M.D.

Voiding Dysfunction and Urodynamic Findings in Patients With Lumbar Spinal Stenosis and the Effect of Decompressive Laminectomy
Hellström PA, Tammela TLJ, Niinimäki TJ (Oulu Univ Hosp, Finland)
Scand J Urol Nephrol 29:167–171, 1995   14–6

Background.—Patients who have spinal stenosis, in which narrowing of the spinal cord leads to lumbago, root pains, and then spinal claudication, may also have such clinical problems as impotence, incontinence, cauda equina syndrome, and bladder claudication. Few studies have examined the urodynamic findings of patients who have spinal stenosis. Bladder function was evaluated in 18 patients who had lumbar spinal stenosis, and the effects of decompressive laminectomy were investigated.

Methods.—Twelve men and 6 women (mean age, 55 years) were included. The presence of lumbar spinal stenosis was clinically and radiologically verified in every patient; the patients were not selected according to their voiding symptoms. The level of stenosis was L3-L5 or L4-L5 in 16 patients. Urodynamic examinations were performed before decompressive laminectomy in 16 patients and afterward in 15. The laminectomy procedure sought to decompress the stenotic central channel and, when appropriate, to widen the root canals.

Results.—Preoperatively, two thirds of patients had symptoms of voiding dysfunction, but only 2 had abnormal urodynamic findings (1 detrusor hyperreflexia and 1 obstruction). Three patients said that their voiding was improved after laminectomy, but 3 showed obstructive voiding. There was 1 case of detrusor areflexia with difficulties in bladder emptying after surgery. Maximum urethral pressure and urethral closure pressure increased after surgery; these were the only significant urodynamic changes. In terms of radicular symptoms and back pain, the overall outcome was judged excellent or good in 6 patients, fair in 6, and poor in 4.

Conclusions.—In patients who have lumbar spinal stenosis, decompressive laminectomy has controversial and unexpected effects on bladder and urethral dysfunction. Urodynamic testing is indicated for patients who have voiding complaints, but the laboratory setting and the patients' back pain may alter the findings and thus lead to a mistaken diagnosis. Electrophysiologic studies should be used more extensively in patients who have lumbar spinal stenosis and voiding dysfunction.

▶ Lumbar stenosis and spinal degenerative joint disease in elderly individuals may contribute to urinary incontinence. It is even unclear whether the high prevalence of urge incontinence with aging may, in part, be attributed to subclinical, nonradiographically documented impingement of nerve roots. This study revealed that surgical outcome was as reliable as a "flip of the coin" with respect to pain. Only 2 urodynamic abnormalities were discovered preoperatively in this report. This study supports the advice of our neurosurgeons that surgery may or may not help bladder symptoms. In effect, results are unpredictable. In my mind, an important question remains: Are voiding complaints in elderly patients often caused by lumbar deficits in the absence of somatic complaints? Only when somatic complaints (lower extremity pain or weakness) are present are neurosurgeons willing to correct spinal deformity. Theoretically, small diameter, unmyelinated visceral nerves may be damaged with spinal stenosis or disc disease before injury to somatic axons. Very few outcome studies of this sort have been reported.

W.D. Steers, M.D.

15 Incontinence

Modified Pereyra Bladder Neck Suspension: 10-Year Mean Followup Using Outcomes Analysis in 125 Patients
Trockman BA, Leach GE, Hamilton J, Sakamoto M, Santiago L, Zimmern PE
(Kaiser Permanente Med Ctr, Los Angeles)
J Urol 154:1841–1847, 1995
15–1

Background.—Modified Pereyra bladder neck suspension is now commonly performed in patients with stress urinary incontinence. Short-term success rates have been reported to range from 77% to 96%. However, there have been few studies of the long-term success rates associated with this surgical procedure.

Methods.—The medical records of 177 patients who had undergone modified Pereyra bladder neck suspension at 1 center more than 5 years earlier were reviewed. Attempts were made to contact the patients by telephone or mail, and the patients were asked to complete a questionnaire.

Findings.—Seventy-one percent of the patients completed the survey. Mean follow-up for these 177 patients was 9.8 years. Sixty-eight percent had had modified Pereyra bladder neck suspension alone, and 32% had related vaginal surgery also. Twenty percent of the patients reported no incontinence of any type. Fifty-one percent reported stress urinary incontinence with or without urge incontinence. Seventy-one percent said their incontinence was significantly improved, and 73% were satisfied with treatment outcomes. Accurate preoperative predictors of long-term outcome could not be identified. The method and length of follow-up significantly affected continence status after the procedure.

Conclusions.—The rate of recurrent stress incontinence after modified Pereyra bladder neck suspension is high. However, subjective improvement is maintained, and most patients continue to be satisfied with the results of the procedure.

▶ This excellent, timely, very interesting study of long-term outcome after needle bladder neck suspension shows that women so treated do not do as well as one would hope. Although only 20% reported total absence of incontinence when they were questioned, about 70% overall said they were reasonably satisfied with the operative results.

Now, why did those who failed fail, and why did those who did well not fail? The preoperative workup included all the recommended tests including "multi-channel urodynamics." We know the number of pads, and the grade of incontinence each woman had preoperatively. These patients "fit" a typical referral practice: 37% had had a prior procedure; 75% to 80% had moderate to severe incontinence; 13% had definite, urodynamic, bladder instability; and the usual 67% had both stress and urge incontinence symptoms even if the cystometrogram was negative for definite detrusor instability. Upon analysis of the data the authors found preoperative pad use weakly related to outcome, but preoperative "urge incontinence" symptoms were completely unrelated.

The obvious quick conclusion here is that the operation needs to be replaced with something better, but I think that we may have applied a single operative procedure to a large group of women and some failed. On the basis of the data available, we cannot tell why that happened. Needle suspensions do work, but we don't seem to have enough information about on whom to use them appropriately. We do know that a cystometrogram won't help to define the problem—something I think someone else said before this.

E.J. McGuire, M.D.

The Polypropylene Pubovaginal Sling for the Treatment of Recurrent Stress Urinary Incontinence

Morgan JE, Heritz DM, Stewart FE, Connolly JC, Farrow GA (Univ of Toronto)
J Urol 154:1013–1015, 1995   15–2

Objective.—The pubovaginal sling operation has proved to be an effective approach for women having recurrent incontinence secondary to a deficient sphincter (type III stress urinary incontinence). Eighty-eight consecutive women aged 32–73 years underwent a two-team procedure utilizing a polypropylene (Marlex) sling in the years 1986–1992. The women had averaged 1.6 previous failed vaginal or retropubic procedures other than hysterectomy.

> *Procedure.*—The bladder neck was released from scar tissue under direct vision and the sling was placed with minimal tension at the neck of the bladder by 2 teams, 1 operating abdominally and 1 vaginally. A suprapubic catheter drained the bladder. A urethral catheter and perioperative antibiotics were not routinely used.

Results.—The average follow-up was approximately 4 years. Eighty-five per cent of the women were cured of stress incontinence and another 9%—mainly with urge incontinence—were improved. Five operations (6%), 4 of them in women with recurrent stress incontinence, and 1 in a woman with urge incontinence, failed. Five of 6 women with preoperative detrusor instability were continent postoperatively. There were no major complications.

Conclusion.—The 2-team pubovaginal sling procedure using polypropylene mesh is an effective means of treating complicated or recurrent stress urinary incontinence.

▶ Fascial slings (rectus, or more recently, fascia lata) have been used since the turn of this century in the management of stress urinary incontinence (SUI). The sling technique has become an accepted procedure for intrinsic sphincteric deficiency (or type 3 SUI) because of its benefit: a high likelihood of being dry long term outweighs its risks, namely, obstruction resulting in bladder instability (urge and urge incontinence) and retention requiring life-long intermittent catheterization. The added risks of using a synthetic material (infection, erosion, fistulas) are a matter of personal preference. A urethrolysis is part of the procedure because the retropubic space and the periurethral tissues need to be free to position the sling adequately beneath the urethra and to anchor it suprapubically. I use a vaginal approach and a short suprapubic incision (1 team only). I transfer the ends of the autologous sling, or the sutures placed at each extremity in case of a short fascial sling, from the vaginal area to the suprapubic region with a long curved clamp or the Raz-Pereyra needle. I fix the sling beneath the urethra to keep it flat (avoid bunching). My trick to secure the sling in place with minimal tension is to visualize cystoscopically when the sling elevates the posterior wall of the proximal urethra. Support but do not occlude! Most important, all my patients learn to perform self-intermittent catheterization preoperatively. Those who are unsuccessful and those who have hypocontractile bladders on pressure-flow study are offered an artificial urinary sphincter instead.

P.E. Zimmern, M.D.

Dependence of Male Voiding Efficiency on Age, Bladder Contractility and Urethral Resistance: Development of a Voiding Efficiency Nomogram
Bosch JLHR, Kranse R, van Mastrigt R, Schröder FH (Erasmus Univ, Rotterdam, The Netherlands)
J Urol 154:190–194, 1995   15–3

Background.—Benign prostatic hyperplasia (BPH) is characterized by symptoms of prostatism, increased prostate volume, and voiding dysfunction. Quantitatively relating voiding efficiency with urodynamic parameters may predict the occurrence of acute retention in patients. The influence of age, urethral resistance, and the bladder contraction strength variable on male voiding efficiency was assessed.

Methods.—Pressure-flow studies were performed in 138 men aged 18–86 years. The urethral resistance parameter and maximum bladder contraction strength were determined. A bladder contraction strength decay factor was used to quantify premature fading of bladder contraction. Postvoid residual urine volume was used to express voiding efficiency as a percentage of the initial bladder volume.

Findings.—According to a multiple regression analysis, voiding efficiency depended significantly on urethral resistance, maximum bladder contraction strength, and bladder contraction stength decay factor, in that order of importance. Patient age was not an independent variable. There was no correlation between maximum bladder contraction strength and bladder contraction strength decay factor, indicating that maximum bladder contraction strength and its decay may represent different properties of bladder contractile function.

Conclusions.—A voiding efficiency nomogram was developed based on the values for maximum bladder contraction strength and urethral resistance in individual patients. Such a nomogram may help predict the occurrence of acute retention. A prospective longitudinal study is now needed to validate the voiding efficiency nomogram.

▶ This study examined voiding efficiency, defined as percent residual urine, using a multivariant analysis of age, bladder contractility, and urethral resistance. The urethral resistance factor (URA) has been used by the group at Rotterdam, while bladder contractions were assessed using the contractility variable W. The authors have shown that urethral resistance appears to be more important than the bladder contraction strength or detrusor decay strength in determining percent residual urine. The patient's age is not an independent factor. There is hope that through the development of such programs or nomograms one would be able to predict the surgical response to therapy after acute urinary retention. Routine pressure-flow studies have not been shown to have prognostic significance in the face of acute urinary retention. The authors postulate that slight increases in urethral resistance are most important in determining retention, especially if patients have somewhat impaired contractility or premature loss of bladder contractions. One problem acknowledged by the authors in the study is that residual urine is measured at the time of the pressure-flow study. It is our experience that patients with little or no residual urine when undergoing a pressure-flow study invariably showed increased residual urine when voiding around a urethral catheter, not to mention the potential inhibition with urodynamics. Whether these calculations are of clinical importance remains to be determined and will require prospective evaluation of large numbers of patients. Attempts to develop predictors for successful surgery after urinary retention are to be applauded.

W.D. Steers, M.D.

Urodynamic Findings in Patients With Diabetic Cystopathy

Kaplan SA, Te AE, Blaivas JG (Columbia Univ, New York)
J Urol 153:342–344, 1995   15–4

Introduction.—Diabetic cystopathy is classically characterized by decreased bladder sensation, increased bladder capacity, and impaired detrusor contractility. However, because many diabetic patients have other concomitant lesions, they may have varying symptom presentations, complicating the diagnosis. The various voiding dysfunction features in symptomatic diabetic patients were studied by retrospectively analyzing their synchronous video–pressure-flow urodynamic studies.

Methods.—The urodynamic studies of 115 men and 68 women with diabetes and persistent voiding symptoms were reviewed and analyzed. Synchronous video pressure studies were obtained while the patient was not taking any medications that affect bladder or sphincter function.

Results.—The most common symptoms were nocturia (87%) and urinary frequency (78%), followed by hesitancy (62%), decreased stream (52%), and the sensation of incomplete bladder emptying (45%). The patients had a first sensation of filling at a mean of 298 mL with a mean bladder capacity of 485 mL. Voiding dysfunction features included detrusor instability in 52%, impaired detrusor contractility in 23%, detrusor areflexia in 10%, and poor compliance in 24%. Sixty-six men had bladder outlet obstruction, and 17 patients had urinary retention. Sacral cord signs occurred in 42 patients, including 5 with detrusor instability, 21 with impaired detrusor contractility, 6 with indeterminate findings, and 10 with detrusor areflexia. Of the 33 patients with poor bladder compliance, 20 had bladder outlet obstruction and 13 had positive sacral cord signs with either detrusor areflexia or indeterminate findings.

Conclusions.—The classic features of diabetic cystopathy were not the most common urodynamic diagnoses. The majority of the men had bladder outlet obstruction, and a majority of those also had other urodynamic diagnoses. Therefore, urodynamic studies should be required to identify all voiding dysfunction features before initiating therapy in diabetic patients.

▶ This large group of well-studied diabetic patients had a wide spectrum of urodynamic findings mirroring the population as a whole. The most surprising finding is the large number of patients with outlet obstruction and poor contractility. The authors make a plea for urodynamic studies in all diabetic patients contemplating therapy. Although I would agree with their conclusion, I am still somewhat surprised at their results. Whether their data reflect the highly selective nature of referrals to their university is unclear. Most people associate the sensory neurogenic bladder with diabetes. However, when early neuropathic degeneration of small nerve fiber occurs, it could elicit detrusor hyperreflexia initially and symptoms of urgency. The most common diagnosis was impaired contractility in 50% of these patients. This finding may be more related to our inability to separate myogenic and neurogenic causes for a low amplitude detrusor contraction. Further work will be needed in this regard. The bottom line is that when faced with a diabetic patient contemplating an invasive procedure, one should perform urodynamics to exclude obstruction. Finally, there have been reports correlating decreased irritative voiding symptoms resulting from prostatism in diabetic men. One study even found that diabetic patients are less likely to undergo a transurethral prostatectomy, presumably because irritative symptom scores are less. Whether prostatic growth or prostatic, urethral sensory nerve function, and in turn "prostatism," is influenced by diabetes and/or insulin-like growth factors is an intriguing question.

W.D. Steers, M.D.

Incontinence After Radical Prostatectomy: Detrusor or Sphincter Causes

Chao R, Mayo ME (Univ of Washington, Seattle)
J Urol 154:16–18, 1995   15–5

Objective.—Incontinence after radical prostatectomy, as a result of decreased detrusor compliance, may be a temporary condition. The video urodynamic records of 74 men were reviewed retrospectively to determine the cause of incontinence.

Methods.—Urine flow rate, postvoid residual volume, filling and voiding monitoring, sphincter activity, and urine loss were assessed in 74 men aged 54–81 years, an average of 3.8 years after radical retropubic (n=64) or radical perineal (n=10) prostatectomy.

Results.—Sphincter weakness only was diagnosed in 42 men, detrusor instability and/or decreased compliance plus sphincter weakness was found in 29, and detrusor instability only in 3. Nineteen men had anastomotic strictures. There were 31 men who voided by the Valsalva maneuver.

Conclusion.—In the majority of men in this study, incontinence was the result of sphincter weakness rather than detrusor instability or decreased compliance.

▶ The lack of correlation between incontinence symptoms after radical prostatectomy and the underlying lower urinary tract dysfunction has long been recognized. Unless you decide to treat all your patients with an artificial urinary sphincter and manage their bladder dysfunction secondarily should it occur, a simple initial urodynamic testing is helpful to segregate patients with bladder dysfunction (possibly pre-existing) who might benefit from anticholinergic therapy alone, from those with sphincteric deficiency (alone or in association with bladder dysfunction). In my experience, fluoroscopic monitoring (video urodynamic) adds little to sort out between these 2 categories. A functional anastomotic stricture can be responsible for bladder instability (obstructive mechanism) and should be excluded by cystoscopy. The management of patients with mixed etiologic factors remains challenging, often requiring the placement of an artificial urinary sphincter and long-term anticholinergic therapy.

P.E. Zimmern, M.D.

Artificial Urinary Sphincter in Patients Following Major Pelvic Surgery and/or Radiotherapy: Are They Less Favorable Candidates?

Martins FE, Boyd SD (Univ of Southern California, Los Angeles)
J Urol 153:1188–1193, 1995

15–6

Background.—Patients undergoing major pelvic surgery and/or radiotherapy commonly experience severe complications resulting in urinary incontinence caused by sphincteric damage. Periurethral injections of collagen or polytetrafluoroethylene and sling cystourethropexy are the 2 established treatments of these complications. However, the AMS800 artificial urinary sphincter has been shown to be highly effective in the treatment of urethral sphincter insufficiency from a variety of causes. The role of the AMS800 artificial sphincter was investigated retrospectively in a high-risk group of patients with male urinary incontinence secondary to major pelvic operation and/or radiotherapy.

Methods.—During a 4-year period, 81 men with urinary incontinence secondary to major sphincter injury underwent placement of an AMS800 artificial sphincter. Bulbar urethral cuff placement was used in all patients with the balloon reservoir placed in a preperitoneal pouch created in the lower quadrant of the abdomen. The balloon reservoir pressure was 51–60 cm water in 18 patients and 61–70 cm water in the rest. The patients were classified into 3 groups: those who underwent major pelvic surgery without radiotherapy, those who underwent either definitive or adjuvant radiotherapy, and those with a neobladder.

Results.—Of the 81 patients, 31 (38%) required a total of 43 surgical revisions. Three of the revisions were indicated because of mechanical malfunction. The remaining 40 revisions were required because of nonmechanical complications; 50% of these occurred in the irradiated group. The revisions required in response to infection and erosion were more common in the patients in the postradiation and neobladder groups. The postradiation group also had the greatest incidence of inadequate cuff compression and urethral atrophy, which was the indication for 32 of the revisions. These were corrected by increasing the balloon reservoir pressure. Socially acceptable continence was achieved by 91% of the patients, with comparable distribution in the 3 patient groups.

Conclusions.—The AMS800 artificial sphincter has excellent mechanical reliability and durability and produces objective results that compare favorably with periurethral injection and sling cystourethropexy. Even patients treated with radiation therapy should not be excluded from placement of the AMS800 artificial sphincter.

▶ The artificial urinary sphincter has revolutionized the treatment of male incontinence. Prior pelvic surgery has no real impact on the placement of the sphincter cuff around the bulbar urethra. Patients who have received radiation constitute a high-risk group for complications such as urethral atrophy, infection, and erosion. When incontinence recurs after sphincter placement[1] and the sphincter is functioning adequately, one must remember about possible bladder wall changes, namely, reduced compliance and/or bladder instability, changes that are difficult to assess preoperatively in a bladder with limited storage capacity from a deficient sphincter. Should urodynamic testing confirm adequate bladder function, the main dilemna resides in changing the cuff to a more distal site along the urethra, which is technically difficult because the patient tends to "sit" on his sphincter afterward, or to place a higher pressure balloon, as chosen by these authors. However, because urethral atrophy is already present, this decision in the face of radiated tissues could result in urethral erosion. To minimize the long-term risk of urethral atrophy in all patients, I still continue to use a small cuff (4 or 4.5 cm) and a low pressure reservoir (51–60 cm water) and I delay activation to at least 4 weeks.

P.E. Zimmern, M.D.

Reference

1. Leach GE: Incontinence after artificial urinary sphincter placement: The role of perfusion sphincterometry. *J Urol* 138:529, 1987.

Periurethral Implantation of Glutaraldehyde Cross-Linked Collagen (Contigen) in Women With Type I or III Stress Incontinence: Quantitative Outcome Measures

Moore KN, Chetner MP, Metcalfe JB, Griffiths DJ (Univ of Alberta, Edmonton, Canada; Misericordia Hosp, Edmonton, Canada)
Br J Urol 75:359–363, 1995   15–7

Objective.—Although published reports indicate that periurethral collagen implantation with a glutaraldehyde cross-linked substance (GAX collagen) improves or cures, for up to 2 years, 75% to 94% of women with stress incontinence, attempts to quantify outcome have led to varying results. The outcome of a 10-hour pad test and home-monitoring results of 10 women with type I or III stress incontinence treated with a periurethral collagen implant were compared with both the patients' own response to treatment and the published reports.

Methods.—Twelve women aged 46–87 years received periurethral collagen implants. Eleven had previously undergone at least 1 procedure to treat incontinence. All required adult diapers during the day. Six patients had more than 1 medical problem including obesity, chronic obstructive lung disease, depression, insulin-dependent diabetes, heart disease, and smoking. One patient was withdrawn and another declined follow-up. Severity of incontinence and voiding patterns were studied by stress testing. Incontinence was defined as a weight increase of 5 g or greater in 1 or more pads. Severity of incontinence was determined by the increase in weight of the wettest diaper.

Results.—Nine patients required a second implant 3–5 months after the first procedure. Urine loss, number of wet pads, and weight of the wettest pad 7–8 weeks after the second implantation were significantly lower than the baseline value. Two patients with urine loss of 5 g or less did not consider themselves to be cured. One patient reported being cured, although she had 1 pad containing 11 g of urine. Two patients reported no change, although urine loss had decreased by more than 60%. Six patients reported improvement, although urine losses remained high. There were no significant differences in maximum single-voided volume, maximum flow rate, and residual volume from baseline to second implantation.

Conclusion.—Eight weeks after the second implantation, urine loss decreased significantly. Two (18%) patients were cured. There was no correlation between objective findings and subjective patient reports of cure or improvement. No findings of significant obstruction were present.

▶ The highlight of this small study on the outcome of collagen injection in the treatment of female incontinence lies in the demonstration of how divergent patient reports of dryness can be, compared with our objective measures. For example, consider the patient who reported subjectively that she was "cured", although objectively the pad test continued to detect leakage of urine; or the 2 patients who reported that they were treatment "failures" despite objective evidence of a decrease in grams of urine loss and in grams of their wettest pad. These examples underscore the difficulty in measuring and reporting outcomes in the treatment of stress incontinence. In this study what is the "true" success rate of collagen injection; 10% of patients according to their subjective report, 30% of patients who decreased the number of wet pads to 0–1, or 20% of patients who had less than 5 g of urine loss? Other authors have recognized such discrepancies in the interpretation of objective tests such as the International Continence Society pyridium pad test[1] or pad weighing.[2] The need for a validated, reproducible, and reliable score for the measurement of severity of urinary incontinence is clearly evident.

L. Stothers, M.D.

References

1. Wall LL, Wang K, Robson I, et al: The pyridium pad test for diagnosing urinary incontinence. A comparative study of asymptomatic and incontinent women. *J Reprod Med* 35:682–684, 1990.
2. Victor A: Pad weighing test: A simple method to quantitate urinary incontinence. *Ann Med* 22:443–447, 1990.

Collagen Injection for Intrinsic Sphincteric Deficiency in Men
Aboseif SR, O'Connell HE, Usui A, McGuire EJ (Univ of Texas, Houston; Univ of California, San Francisco)
J Urol 155:10–13, 1996   15–8

Introduction.—In 1993, the Food and Drug Administration approved the use of collagen for the treatment of intrinsic sphincteric deficiency. Glutaraldehyde cross-linked collagen is a highly purified suspension of bovine dermal collagen associated with minimal inflammatory response and no tendency to migrate. The early experience with collagen injections in the treatment of male urinary incontinence caused by intrinsic sphincteric deficiency was reported.

Patients.—Eighty-eight men aged 54–82 years (mean, 68 years) with mild-to-severe intrinsic sphincter deficiency were treated. Urinary incontinence secondary to intrinsic sphincteric deficiency was caused by prostatectomy in 85, trauma in 1, myelodysplasia in 1, and chondroma of the sacral roots in 1. All men were incontinent for 1 year and failed to respond to medical treatment.

Procedure.—All patients underwent skin testing with 0.1 mL of glutaraldehyde cross-linked collagen and were observed for 4 weeks. Except for 15 patients who required general anesthesia, all other injections were given under local anesthesia (1% lidocaine). Under direct vision, collagen was injected slowly and submucosally proximal to the external sphincter on both sides until urethral mucosa coaptation was achieved. The end point for treatment was either cure or administration of 5 injections at intervals of at least 1 month.

Outcome.—The mean follow-up was 10 months. The mean number of treatments was 3.5, and mean total volume of collagen injected was 25 mL. Patients were subdivided into 2 groups based on the response to collagen injection. Group 1 included 61 (85%) patients with normal bladder compliance who gained some benefit from collagen therapy, including 42 who became completely dry (47%) and 19 (19%) with substantial improvement but who required 1–3 pads per day. Group 2 included 27 patients with severe incontinence who required more than 4 pads per day before treatment. Of these, 14 consistently used fewer pads but still more than 3 per day after treatment, and 13 showed no improvement. Both groups were similar in age, duration of incontinence, volume of collagen used, and number of injections given. Worse response to collagen therapy was associated with more severe pretreatment incontinence, concomitant detrusor abnormalities, and etiology of the sphincteric deficiency. No significant morbidity occurred; only 11% of patients required clean intermittent catheterization for 24–48 hours.

Conclusion.—Transurethral injection of collagen is effective and safe in carefully selected patients with intrinsic sphincteric deficiency. Many patients who respond to treatment have previously undergone only uncomplicated radical retropubic prostatectomy without another procedure and have normal bladder function.

▶ When considering the effectiveness of collagen injection for the treatment of male intrinsic sphincter dysfunction, the issues of length of follow-up, severity of incontinence, and cost become imperative if this treatment is to be compared with other available treatment options such as the artificial urinary sphincter. In short-term follow-up, the authors found that the best outcome was seen in patients with very mild incontinence. By pad status, 42 of the 61 patients in group 1 used no pads or 1 pad per day. Even with such infrequent pad use, 22.7 mL of injected collagen was needed to achieve dryness or improvement in pad status. The poor outcome in group 2 with severe incontinence requiring more than 4 pads per day incurred the cost of an average of 25.5 mL of collagen without achieving substantial improvement. In such patients, the cost-effectiveness of collagen is questionable. Contrary to this case series, some authors have reported worsening continence status after collagen injection in up to 10% of patients.[1,2] This risk should be balanced against the minimal impact on continence status in patients with severe intrinsic sphincter dysfunction.

L. Stothers, M.D.

References

1. Gill HS, Payne CK: Experience with collagen injection therapy in men with urinary incontinence. *Proceedings of the American Association. J Urol Suppl* 153:277A, 1995.
2. Stothers L, Chopra A, Raz S: A cost effectiveness and utility analysis of the artificial urinary sphincter and collagen injection in the treatment of postprostatectomy incontinence. *Proceedings of the American Urological Association. J Urol Suppl* 153:278A, 1995.

16 Diversion

Subcutaneous Urinary Diversions for Palliative Treatment of Pelvic Malignancies
Desgrandchamps F, Cussenot O, Meria P, Cortesse A, Teillac P, Le Duc A
(Saint-Louis Hospital, Paris)
J Urol 154:367–370, 1995
16–1

Background.—Palliative urinary diversion for patients who have advanced pelvic malignancies poses difficult challenges in maintaining quality of life. Percutaneous nephrostomy causes problems because of the posterior location of the tube, which prevents the patient from reclining comfortably and requires assistance during dressing changes; mechanical complications are also a risk. Pyelovesical bypass and anterior cutaneous nephrostomy were developed as alternative procedures for patients undergoing permanent palliative percutaneous nephrostomy.

Methods.—Twenty-one patients who were undergoing permanent subcutaneous urinary diversion because of advanced pelvic tumors that were invading or compressing the urinary tract were included. The percutaneous nephrostomy tube was replaced by a self-retaining expanded polytetrafluoroethylene-silicone tube tunneled beneath the skin. Thirteen patients underwent a total of 19 pyelovesical bypass procedures, in which the distal extremity of the tube was introduced into the bladder (Fig 1). This procedure was always done after failure of Double-J stent diversion. Eight patients whose lower urinary tract precluded use of the bladder underwent a total of 13 anterior cutaneous nephrostomy procedures, in which the distal extremity of the tube was brought out directly through a cutaneous orifice (Fig 2).

Results.—Secondary complications occurred in 2 of 31 evaluable subcutaneous diversions; 1 patient had delayed healing with exposure of the graft, 1 had obstruction by an intrarenal nodule. One patient in each group, therefore, required removal of the prostheses and replacement with a standard nephrostomy tube. There were no instances of tube dislodgement, and none of the tubes became blocked by incrustation or angulation. All patients noted improvement in quality of life after these procedures. In addition, all could continue adjuvant therapy for their underlying disease.

Conclusions.—Pyelovesical bypass and anterior cutaneous nephrostomy are useful alternatives to a permanent palliative percutaneous nephrostomy tube. Pyelovesical bypass avoids the need for external drainage in

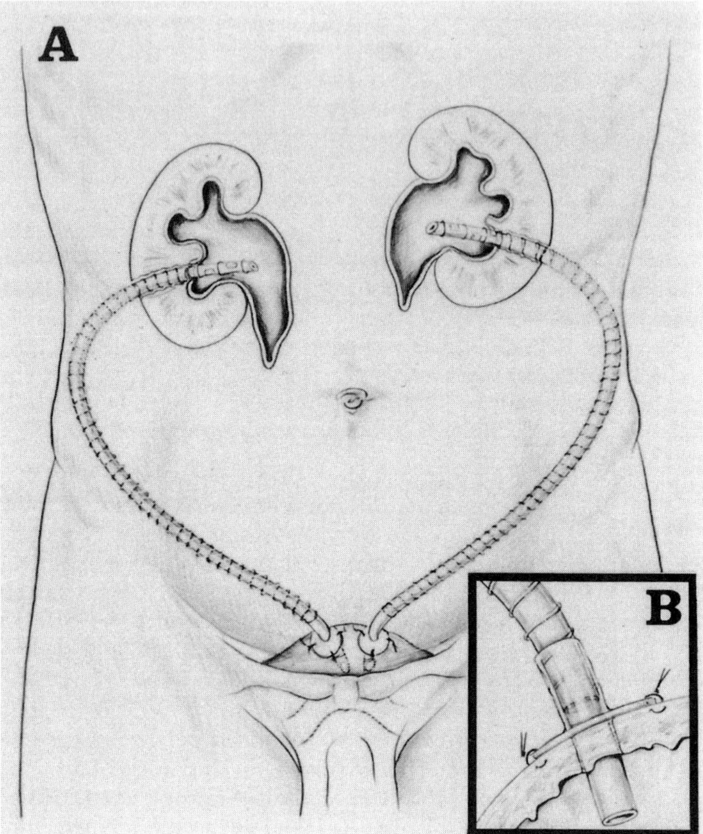

FIGURE 1.—**A,** subcutaneous pyelovesical bypass. **B,** detail of vesical extremity. (Courtesy of Desgrandchamps F, Cussenot O, Meria P, et al: Subcutaneous urinary diversions for palliative treatment of pelvic malignancies. *J Urol* 154:367–370, 1995.)

patients who have a functional bladder. For those who have a nonfunctional bladder, anterior cutaneous nephrostomy produces a single, easily dressed anterior stoma. Because of the risk of long-term graft incrustation, these 2 procedures are currently recommended only for patients who have limited life expectancy.

▶ The authors present a series of patients who had terminal pelvic neoplasms that obstructed the ureters and whose clinical condition did not allow urinary drainage with internal double-J stents. Their success rate with a very low incidence of complications is impressive. As they point out, it is very useful and, indeed, part of our duty to improve the quality of life of patients who have terminal disease. The authors have previously described the pyelovesical bypass procedure,[1] but the anterior cutaneous nephrostomy is new. The latter procedure is perhaps less certain to be a significant contribution for 2 reasons. First, follow-up of these patients is short, so that more

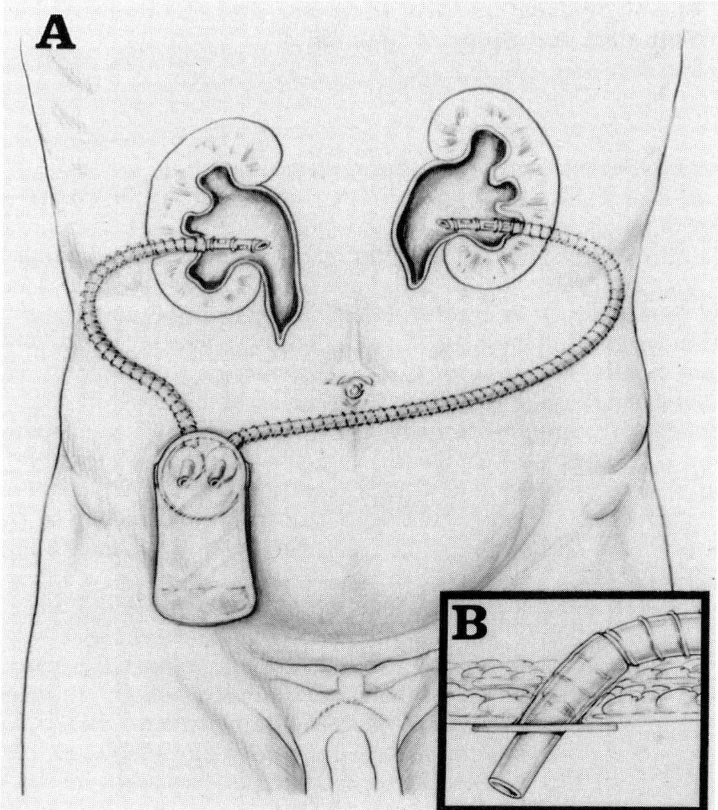

FIGURE 2.—**A,** anterior cutaneous nephrostomy. **B,** detail of cutaneous extremity. (Courtesy of Desgrandchamps F, Cussenot O, Meria P, et al: Subcutaneous urinary diversions for palliative treatment of pelvic malignancies. *J Urol* 154:367–370, 1995.)

complications may occur. Second, the patients require a bag. It has been our experience that most patients with a well-placed percutaneous nephrostomy do not have serious problems. The key to both procedures appears to be the large-bore indwelling catheters with 2 coaxial tubes: a coiled, expanded polytetrafluoroethylene tube with an outer diameter of 9.5 mm that contains a glued silicone tube with an inner diameter of 6 mm (18F). These tubes are different from and larger than those previously used in similar diversions.

S.S. Howards, M.D.

Reference

1.   Desgrandchamps F, Cussenot O, Bassi S, et al: Percutaneous extra-anatomic nephrovesical diversion: Preliminary report. *J Endourol* 7:323, 1993.

Risk of Bowel Dysfunction With Diarrhea After Continent Urinary Diversion With Ileal and Ileocecal Segments

Roth S, Semjonow A, Waldner M, Hertle L (Univ of Münster, Germany)
J Urol 154:1696–1699, 1995   16–2

Objective.—The use of gastrointestinal tract sections to create bladder substitutes poses risks of complications resulting from the choice of surgical technique, sustained absorption phenomena, or reduction of the intestinal absorption area. The section of intestine resected could be related to the rate of occurrence of malabsorption. The terminal ileum and ileocecal valve play important roles in resorption, regulation of bowel evacuation, and compensation for small bowel loss. Patients who had undergone continent diversion with ileal or ileocecal segments were surveyed to determine the risk of subsequent bowel dysfunction.

Methods.—One hundred patients who had undergone continent urinary diversion with ileal and ileocecal segments from 1990 to 1994 were included. Sixty-five patients had ileal resection, and 35 had ileocecal resection; mean follow-up was 16 and 18 months, respectively. The patients were interviewed about the occurrence of diarrhea since hospital discharge.

Results.—Chronic diarrhea lasting more than 6 months was reported by 11% of patients who had ileal resection and 23% of those who had ileocecal resection. Two patients in each group reported spontaneous resolution of this problem. Most patients responded well to treatment with cholestyramine, loperamide, or psyllium. Drug treatment produced no response, however, in 2 patients who had diarrhea after ileocecal resection. These patients had the longest ileum resections, 45–50, cm related to the construction of a nipple valve.

Conclusions.—In patients who are undergoing continent urinary diversion, ileocecal resection appears to have twice the risk of postoperative diarrhea compared with ileal resection. When chronic diarrhea occurs, most patients will respond to symptomatic drug treatment. Diarrhea should be regarded as an acceptable risk that should not affect the decision to perform continent diversion. The patient should understand, however, that there is a possibility of chronic diarrhea after surgery.

▶ The risk of chronic diarrhea is of great concern to all of us who do continent urinary diversions and bladder augmentations. It is well known that removal of the ileocecal valve increases the risk. Removal of a significant length of ileum alters the absorption of fat and bile salts, which can result in diarrhea. One has to be especially concerned if the patient has a history of persistent diarrhea, radiation therapy, or neurologic disease. These authors provide us with useful and disturbing information. The incidence of chronic diarrhea in their patients is higher than most of us acknowledge in our practice and higher than that reported in the medical literature. There have been reports of no diarrhea after creation of a Koch pouch[1] vs. the 11% in this series. Fortunately, most afflicted patients respond to medical treatment with cholestyramine and other drugs. However, even a single patient who is unresponsive would create a very unpleasant situation.

S.S. Howards, M.D.

Reference

1. Åkerlund S, Delin K, Kock NG, et al: Renal function and upper urinary tract configuration following urinary diversion to a continent ileal reservoir (Kock pouch): A prospective 5 to 11-year followup after reservoir construction. *J Urol* 142:964, 1989.

Long-term Metabolic Effects of Urinary Diversion on Skeletal Bone: Histomorphometric and Mineralogic Analysis

Davidsson T, Lindergård B, Obrant K, Månsson W (Univ Hosp, Lund, Sweden; Univ Hosp, Malmö, Sweden)
Urology 46:328–333, 1995   16–3

Background.—Segments of intestine can be used for reconstructive surgery of the urinary tract. Patients who have undergone such surgery, however, are vulnerable to metabolic and acid-base abnormalities, i.e., hyperchloremic metabolic acidosis, as a result of solute resorption across the intestinal mucosa. Metabolic bone disease can occur in patients who have chronic metabolic acidosis of various causes. The possible long-term effects of intestinal urinary diversion on bone metabolism were assessed.

Methods.—Thirty-nine patients who had well-functioning urinary diversions were included. The status of all patients was followed at least 5 years. Twenty patients had conduit urinary diversion, and 19 had cecal continent reservoir; all had normal or near-normal renal function. The patients underwent densitometry to assess bone mineral content. Bone biopsy specimens were obtained and analyzed with histomorphometric technique.

Results.—The 2 patient groups did not differ significantly in bone mineral content from each other or from a reference group. There were no signs of defective bone mineralization or increased bone resorption on histomorphometric analysis. The patients with cecal continent urinary reservoir had a greater than normal trabecular bone volume, whereas the conduit group did not. Both groups had a significantly subnormal appositional rate, with no difference between groups.

Conclusions.—The electrolyte and acid-base changes that occur in patients who have intestinal urinary diversion and normal renal function do not appear to affect long-term bone mineralization. Patients with conduit or continent urinary diversion do appear to have a lower than normal appositional rate. Those with continent urinary diversion also have increased trabecular bone volume, which perhaps reflects a decrease of bone turnover.

▶ This paper is most reassuring. McDougal and Koch have raised considerable concern regarding the chronic effects of urinary diversion on bone metabolism.[1, 2] The authors of this paper present data that were not previously available on analysis of actual bone biopsy specimens of patients with urinary diversion. Fortunately, they found absolutely no effect on bone mineralization. A possible explanation for the difference between this investigation and some of the other studies is that these patients are adults, not growing children. It is also relevant that these patients had good renal function.

S.S. Howards, M.D.

References

1. McDougal WS: Metabolic complications of urinary intestinal diversion. *J Urol* 147:1199–1208, 1992.
2. Koch MO, McDougal WS, Hall MC, et al: Long-term metabolic effects of urinary diversion: A comparison of myelomeningocele patients managed by clean intermittent catheterization and urinary diversion. *J Urol* 147:1343–1347, 1992.

Experience in 100 Patients With an Ileal Low Pressure Bladder Substitute Combined With an Afferent Tubular Isoperistaltic Segment
Studer UE, Danuser H, Merz VW, Springer JP, Zingg EJ (Univ of Berne, Switzerland)
J Urol 154:49–56, 1995   16–4

Background.—Since April 1985, an ileal low pressure bladder substitute has been used after radical cystectomy in men treated at the University of Berne. The functional outcomes of this approach in the first 100 patients were reported.

Patients and Findings.—The patients underwent lower urinary tract reconstruction after cystectomy between April 1985 and April 1993. Median age at surgery was 64 years (range, 40–81 years). All had undifferentiated, invasive urothelial cancer. Treatment consisted of an ileal low-pressure reservoir using the Goodwin cup-patch principle combined with an afferent ileal tubular segment. Early complications occurred in 11% of the patients. Two men died of septicemia after surgery. Fourteen patients needed surgery for late complications after a median follow-up of 27 months. These complications included intestinal obstruction, urethral stricture or tumor recurrence, hernia, and ureteral stenosis. Thirty-two patients eventually died of metastatic bladder cancer, and 7 died of other causes. After 3–12 months, the functional capacity of the bladder substitute was increased to the desired 450–500 mL, paralleled by improving urinary continence. Ninety-two percent of patients were continent by day at 1 year, and 80% were continent at night by 2 years. Four left ureteral strictures were seen on upper tract surveillance with excretory urography, renal ultrasound, and serum creatinine estimation. However, there was no significant upper tract deterioration or ureteral recurrence. On video urodynamics, significant reflux was seen only when the reservoir was overfilled. During voiding, the intra-abdominal pressure increase with straining acted on the reservoir and ureters equally. Therefore no isolated intravesical pressure increase occurred, and there was no reservoir reflux.

Conclusions.—An ileal low-pressure reservoir with an afferent isoperistaltic ileal segment, combined with an open end-to-side ureteroileal anastomosis, permits radical surgery for cancer with resection of the ureters where they cross the iliac vessels. The risk of ureteral stenosis is minimized. The unidirectional peristalsis of the ureters and afferent tubular ileal segment apparently provide sufficient protection of the upper urinary tract. This surgical technique is straightforward. Later conversion to an ileal conduit can be done if necessary. With careful patient selection, rehabilitation, and meticulous follow-up, the functional outcomes of the bladder substitute are similar to other reservoir techniques.

▶ Dr. Studer and associates are certainly among the leaders in the field of continent urinary diversion. They had previously reported that anastomosing the ureters end-to-side into the proximal end of an afferent isoperistaltic ileal limb protects the upper tracts better than does creating a nipple. This paper presents excellent results of a large series of continent ileal bladders. A very modest number of serious complications occurred, and an impressive day-time continence rate at 1 year was achieved. These authors perform the ileal urethral anastomosis by making a large (8–10 mm) hole in the lower wall of the reservoir. They believe that this technique is the reason that they had only 2% urethral anastomotic strictures and that 98% of their patients can void spontaneously. These are indeed impressive results.

S.S. Howards, M.D.

Ureterosigmoidostomy: Is It a Viable Procedure in the Age of Continent Urinary Diversion and Bladder Substitution?
Bissada NK, Morcos RR, Morgan WM, Hanash KA (Ein Shams Univ, Cairo; King Faisal Specialist Hosp, Riyadh, Saudi Arabia)
J Urol 153:1429–1431, 1995   16–5

Introduction.—Ureterosigmoidostomy is an unpopular procedure at many centers. In properly selected patients, it can be a useful form of urinary diversion. The results of standard ureterosigmoidostomy, in which an antireflux technique was used, were reported.

Methods.—Sixty-three patients were included. During follow-up visits at 1, 3, 6, and 12 months, patients underwent tests to determine renal profile and serum level of electrolytes. Urine and feces specimens were analyzed for blood, and upper tract studies were occasionally done. Records were reviewed for demographic data, diagnosis, indications for urinary diversion, perioperative details, continence, metabolic abnormalities, stone disease, and evidence of early and late complications.

Results.—Forty-nine patients had cancer, and 14 had other conditions. All patients underwent standard bowel preparation before surgery. Two patients died after surgery; 1 died of a myocardial infarction, and 1 of respiratory and septic complications. Median follow-up was 41 months. Twenty-four of 47 remaining patients with cancer died during follow-up. In 92% of patients, renal function remained stable. Radiography detected renal deterioration in 23% of patients. Severely impaired function or nonfunction was observed in 7% of renal units. Patients did not take fluids for 2 hours before bedtime. All patients remained dry during the day. Thirty patients were able to stay dry at night without needing to awaken to empty the rectum. To stay dry, 31 patients needed to awaken to empty the rectum 2 or more times at night. No patients had blood in the urine or feces. Hyperchloremic acidosis and/or hypokalemia developed in 4 patients who were not compliant with medications.

Conclusion.—Ureterosigmoidostomy is a good and convenient alternative for select patients who have bladder cancer and cannot undergo other forms of continent urinary diversion or bladder substitution. This approach is not a good alternative for patients who have benign disease and are expected to live for several decades. Patients must have good anal sphincter control, and this method should not be considered for patients who have neurogenic bladder. It should be considered cautiously in patients who have irradiated bowel, diverticulitis, colon polyps, and grossly dilated ureters and renal impairment.

▶ We have always believed that, in highly selected patients, ureterosigmoidostomy is a reasonable procedure. Indeed from time to time, articles such as this appear in the urologic literature that support the selected use of the procedure. The authors performed a large number of ureterosigmoidostomies in a rather brief period. Their results were satisfactory, although it must be mentioned that the follow-up has been short and more renal complications are bound to occur.

S.S. Howards, M.D.

17 Interstitial Cystitis

Absence of Neuropathic Pelvic Pain and Favorable Psychological Profile in the Surgical Selection of Patients With Disabling Interstitial Cystitis
Lotenfoe RR, Christie J, Parsons A, Burkett P, Helal M, Lockhart JL (Univ of South Florida, Tampa)
J Urol 154:2039–2042, 1995   17–1

Background.—Patients who have persistent pain from interstitial cystitis are now treated with simple cystectomy, urethrectomy, and continent supravesical diversion. Patients who have a bladder capacity less than 400 mL while under anesthesia have done better than have those who have a larger capacity. Poor outcomes also are related to persistent pelvic pain after surgery. Comprehensive psychological assessment could determine whether underlying psychopathology negatively affects the medical situation. Long-standing pain might sensitize nociceptive neurons in the dorsal horn and result in ongoing pain. The value of psychological assessment and pain localization studies was determined in patients who had disabling interstitial cystitis and underwent cystectomy, urethrectomy (or cystoprostatectomy), and construction of a continent colonic urinary reservoir in the form of the Florida pouch.

Patients and Methods.—Twenty women and 2 men, aged 31–75 years, underwent surgery after being symptomatic for 2–14 years. The average duration of symptoms was 7 years. Multiple treatments had been tried in all patients. All patients had cystoscopy and underwent bladder biopsies and urodynamic evaluation. The 5 most recent patients were also evaluated by a clinical psychologist and underwent pain localization study by a differential epidural technique that attempts to distinguish between psychogenic and sympathetic or somatic pain.

Results.—The overall surgical cure rate was 73%. Patients younger than 40 years of age did less well than did those who were older. All but 3 of 17 patients who had an anesthetized bladder capacity less than 400 mL, compared with only 1 of 5 who had a larger capacity, were cured. All 5 patients who were symptomatic for less than 4 years were cured. Two of the 7 patients evaluated psychologically were found to have psychogenic pain and were referred to a chronic pain team. The other 5 patients had pain of somatic origin and were considered to be good surgical candidates.

All 5 specially screened patients who underwent surgery were free of symptoms after surgery, compared with 64% of patients who were evaluated only clinically.

Conclusion.—Patients who have interstitial cystitis and have a favorable psychological profile and pain of somatic origin can be expected to do well after cystectomy and continent urinary diversion.

▶ The authors did a large number of radical surgical procedures for interstitial cystitis. We see many patients who have interstitial cystitis at our institution and do significantly fewer total cystectomies. The success rate of their approach with only clinical evaluation was 64%. It is very surprising that the Editors of the *Journal of Urology* did not insist that the authors provide the reader with the duration of follow-up. We have no idea how many of the cures were enduring. When the authors used their "differential epidural technique" to screen 7 patients and then operated on the 5 who "passed" the screen, all 5 were "cured." As the authors acknowledge, this study does not include enough patients to draw firm conclusions. Nevertheless, if this technique proves to be predictive of success after long follow-up in a significant number of patients, it could be a valuable addition to the urologic armamentarium.

S.S. Howards, M.D.

18 Cystic Disease

Apoptosis and Loss of Renal Tissue in Polycystic Kidney Diseases
Woo D (Univ of California, Los Angeles)
N Engl J Med 333:18–25, 1995   18–1

Background.—Polycystic kidney disease is inherited as either an autosomal dominant or autosomal recessive disorder. Affected patients have hundreds or thousands of renal cysts and grossly enlarged kidneys. Although the gene that causes most cases of autosomal dominant polycystic kidney disease has been identified, the primary pathogenic process underlying the loss of normal renal tissue that causes renal dysfunction and failure is not understood. Whether apoptosis, a process of programmed cell death that occurs during embryonic development and the renewal of mature tissues, is a cause of the loss of normal renal tubules in these patients was investigated.

Methods.—Genomic DNA was obtained from the tissues and cultured cells of 16 polycystic kidneys (with and without end-stage renal disease), 12 normal kidneys, and kidneys with other diseases (5 with IgA nephropathy, 3 with nephrosclerosis, 2 with focal glomerulosclerosis, 1 with diabetic nephropathy, 6 with acute tubular necrosis, 6 with acute renal transplant rejection, and 4 with chronic renal transplant rejection). Apoptotic DNA fragmentation was assayed by gel electrophoresis and by in situ end-labeling, with use of the DNA-specific bisbenzimide dye Hoechst 33258 to detect apoptotic nuclei.

Results.—Apoptotic DNA fragmentation was identified in tissues and cultured cells from all patients who had autosomal recessive or dominant polycystic kidney disease. It was not identified, however, in normal kidneys or in the tubules of kidneys with noncystic renal disease. In the kidneys with polycystic disease, apoptotic nuclei were found in the noncystic tubular epithelial cells, in glomerular cells, and in cells lining renal cysts. Apoptotic nuclei were found in the glomeruli of 1 patient who had IgA nephropathy and in 1 patient who had acute transplant rejection, which may be associated with recovery, rather than injury.

Conclusions.—Apoptosis, along with cyst enlargement and interstitial fibrosis, is characteristic of polycystic kidney disease. Because the mature kidney cannot generate new nephrons, apoptosis results in the progressive loss of normal renal tissue.

▶ This study provides further evidence that apoptosis must be added to cyst enlargement and interstitial fibrosis as part of the pathogenesis of polycystic kidney disease. The role of each of these phenomena in the deterioration of the polycystic kidney, however, remains unclear. It is also intriguing that in *cpk* mice with polycystic kidney, apoptosis is found not only in the kidney but also in extrarenal tissue, thereby confirming that polycystic kidney disease is more than a disease of the kidneys.

S.S. Howards, M.D.

19 Bladder Cancer

Hematuria Home Screening: Repeat Testing Results
Messing EM, Young TB, Hunt VB, Newton MA, Bram LL, Vaillancourt A, Hisgen WJ, Greenberg EB, Kuglitsch ME, Wegenke JD (Univ of Wisconsin, Madison; Univ of Colorado, Denver; Blue Cross Blue Shield, Durham, NC)
J Urol 154:57–61, 1995   19–1

Background.—Screening for hematuria by asymptomatic men aged 50 years and older through repeated self-testing of the urine for hemoglobin with a chemical reagent strip can reveal early-stage bladder cancer and other serious urologic disease. The screening interval necessary for repeat testing to detect bladder cancer before it invades the muscle was determined.

Methods and Findings.—The participants were 856 men who had had 14 negative results on daily home tests for hematuria with the chemical reagent strip 9 months earlier. These men again tested their urine at home once a day for 14 consecutive days. Fifty of these men, or 5.8%, had at least 1 positive result during that 14-day testing period. Thirty-eight were further evaluated. Fifteen, or 39.5%, had significant urologic abnormalities. Eight had malignancies. Seven men had bladder cancer with no tumor invasion of the muscularis propria. Thus the overall incidence of bladder cancer in these 856 patients was 0.82%.

Conclusions.—Bladder cancer appears to have a brief preclinical duration. Thus, for screening to be maximally effective in reducing mortality from this malignancy, testing must be repeated every year, at least, so that bladder cancer can be detected before it invades the muscle.

▶ This is one in a series of well-done studies that evaluate the usefulness of home hematuria screening for the detection of bladder cancer.[1,2] The previous investigations have documented that hematuria screening is specific and sensitive. The tests picked up transitional cell carcinomas in 1.2% of the men screened. The purpose of this study was to determine an appropriate interval for rescreening. The data support the authors' contention that 9 months is a reasonable interval. The cost of this program was $102 per individual and $8,570 per cancer detected. This group has clearly documented the usefulness of their approach. Nevertheless, because of logistics and cost considerations, it is unlikely that hematuria home screening will be widely accepted.

S.S. Howards, M.D.

References

1. Messing EM, Young TB, Hunt VB, et al: Home screening for hematuria: Results of a multi-clinic study. *J Urol* 148:289–292, 1992.
2. Messing EM, Young TB, Hunt VB, et al: Urinary tract cancers found by home screening with hematuria dipsticks in healthy men over 50 years of age. *Cancer* 64:2361–2367, 1989.

Results of a Multicenter Trial Using the BTA Test to Monitor for and Diagnose Recurrent Bladder Cancer

Sarosdy MF, DeVere White RW, Soloway MS, Sheinfeld J, Hudson MA, Schellhammer PF, Jarowenko MV, Adams G, Blumenstein BA (Univ of Texas Health Science Ctr, San Antonio; Univ of California-Davis; Univ of Miami, Fla; et al)

J Urol 154:379–384, 1995

19–2

Background.—Although other methods have been evaluated, cystoscopy in combination with urinary cytology remains the most sensitive method of diagnosing recurrence of bladder cancer. In a prospective multicenter study, the Bard BTA (bladder tumor antigen) assay was compared with urinary cytology studies to determine its usefulness for detecting bladder cancer. The specificity of BTA was also evaluated in a separate group of healthy subjects and patients with urologic disease.

Methods.—Urine samples provided by patients with bladder cancer were evaluated for the BTA assay cytology and urinalysis. Positive urinary cytologic findings were defined as urine diagnostic or suggestive of transitional cell carcinoma. Tumor cells were graded for anaplasia and staged. The BTA test was performed on 564 healthy subjects and patients without bladder cancer to determine the specificity of the test. Data were evaluated using the McNemar test.

Results.—The highest disease stage was Ta in 56.6% and T1 in 20.9% of patients. At least one positive cystoscopy result occurred in 151 patients; urinary cytology was positive in 25 cases and the BTA test result was positive in 61. The sensitivity of the antigen test was 40.4% and of urinary cytology was 16.6%. Of the 151 patients, 80% had findings that were confirmed histologically. In this study, for stage Ta and grade 1 tumors, both measures had low to no sensitivity. The antigen test showed increased sensitivity for patients with grade 2 and grade 3 disease; even better sensitivity was shown for patients with stage T2 or greater disease (Table 6). Although there were insufficient data to report valid conclusions, it appears that a combination of tests improved sensitivity. The overall specificity was 95.9% in healthy subjects and ranged from 94.3% to 86.4% for patients with other urologic diseases. The positive predictive value of a positive cystoscopy study was 52%.

Discussion.—The BTA test is superior to urinary cytology for monitoring patients for recurrence of bladder cancer. The test is rapid and easy to use and does not require technical personnel to perform it.

TABLE 6.—Sensitivity by Combined Stage and Grade Groupings, First Positive Visits

Stage/Grade	Visit Count	Test Name	Sensitivity (%)	95% Confidence Interval
All	116	Bladder tumor antigen	41	31.5–50.0
		Voided urinary cytology	16	10.2–24.4
		Both	47	37.2–56.1
Ta/1 (low risk)	29	Bladder tumor antigen	17	5.8–35.8
		Voided urinary cytology	0	0.0–11.9
		Both	17	5.8–35.8
Ta/2 (low risk)	32	Bladder tumor antigen	41	23.7–59.4
		Voided urinary cytology	6	0.8–20.8
		Both	44	26.4–62.3
Ta/3, T1/2 and 3 (high risk)	32	Bladder tumor antigen	47	29.1–65.3
		Voided urinary cytology	19	7.2–36.4
		Both	56	37.7–73.6
T2 or more	14	Bladder tumor antigen	64	35.2–87.2
		Voided urinary cytology	43	17.7–71.1
		Both	71	41.9–91.6
Tis/3	9	Bladder tumor antigen	56	21.2–86.3
		Voided urinary cytology	56	21.2–86.3
		Both	78	40.0–97.2

(Courtesy of Sarosdy MF, DeVere White RW, Soloway MS, et al: Results of a multicenter trial using the BTA test to monitor for and diagnose recurrent bladder cancer. *J Urol* 154:379–384, 1995.)

▶ The last decade has seen any number of new diagnostic testing strategies evaluated for their ability to detect bladder cancer. The report by Sarosdy et al. on the use of the BTA test is the latest in a series that includes conventional cytology, flow cytometry, and quantitative fluorescence image analysis, alone or in combination with antibodies to tumor-associated antigens. Critical to the clinical use of these tests are 2 questions. First, what information are we asking them to provide? Second, what levels of sensitivity and specificity are required for these tests to obviate the need for additional studies, or to serve as the basis for therapeutic decisions?

For example, are we simply trying to determine the presence or absence of tumor? If so, does a positive or negative BTA test result obviate the need for the "benchmark study" cytoscopy? Are we attempting to identify the presence of "occult" carcinoma in situ (CIS)? In this regard, do the BTA results obviate the need for cytology? In actuality, cystoscopy, with its high sensitivity for low-grade disease, combined with cytology for the detection of occult high-grade disease/CIS, proves complementary with respect to the information provided. The increased sensitivity of the BTA test for low-grade disease is of little value in the face of a detection sensitivity of only 40% relative to cystoscopy. This, together with the inability of the BTA test to distinguish high-grade from low-grade disease, prompts me to question how this test will alter diagnostic or therapeutic decision making.

W.A. See, M.D.

The Relationship Among Multiple Recurrences, Progression and Prognosis of Patients With Stages TA and T1 Transitional Cell Cancer of the Bladder Followed For at Least 20 Years

Holmäng S, Hedelin H, Anderström C, Johansson SL (Sahlgrenska Univ Hosp, Göteborg, Sweden; Kärnsjukhuset, Skövde, Sweden; Univ of Nebraska Med Ctr, Omaha)
J Urol 153:1823–1827, 1995   19–3

Introduction.—A 1993 retrospective study was performed on 176 patients treated between 1963 and 1972 for stage Ta and T1 transitional cell bladder cancer. Histopathologic material was retained from an earlier review of the cases in 1977, as well as material obtained after 1977 for the 1993 study. Material submitted at both times was reviewed by the same pathologist, then graded and staged accordingly. Although 163 patients had died by 1993, most had cystoscopy 1 year before death. The relationship between histopathologic results and clinical course was analyzed.

Results.—Thirty-nine of the patients died as a result of their bladder cancer, whereas 123 died of other causes. The surviving 14 patients, 5 of whom had cystectomies, showed no evidence of cancer on most recent follow-up. Broken down by stage, 11% of the 77 patients with Ta tumor died of their cancer, whereas 30% of the 99 patients with T1 cancer died of their cancer. Recurrences persisting on 10 or more cystoscopies occurred in 16 patients, of whom 10 eventually died of bladder cancer. Patients receiving thiotepa instillations showed no improvement in their recurrences. Fourteen of 24 patients with recurrences after 4 years of surgery went on to have muscle invasion or metastases, whereas most patients with initial recurrences eventually became tumor-free within 4 years. Of the 59 patients remaining free of recurrences for 5 years or longer, only 1 had a grade 1 recurrence after 6 years and 1 had carcinoma in situ after 12 years. Only 3 patients of the total had renal pelvic or ureteral tumors on follow-up, 2 of whom had hematuria and 1 asymptomatic patient whose tumor was picked up on screening excretory urography.

Discussion.—Not surprisingly, persistent recurrences on 10 or more cystoscopies are predictive of continuing recurrences until death or complete cystectomy. Late recurrence, occurring more than 4 years after initial treatment, is another indicator of poor prognosis. Repeated cystodiathermy may be sufficient to treat small grade 1 recurrences, but large or multiple recurrences should be treated more aggressively. Thiotepa instillations showed no utility in patients with recurrences. Follow-up cystoscopy would appear to be of limited value beyond 5–10 years after the last recurrence of a solitary, low-grade lesion, and screening urography does not appear to be cost-effective at any point in the follow-up period.

▶ The retrospective study by Holmäng et al. provides interesting insight into the natural history of superficial bladder cancers in the "preintravesical therapy" era. Although the use of multiple primary treatment modalities further complicates extrapolation of their findings to current practice, their relational observations on the duration of tumor recurrences (> 4 years) and tumor biology have relevance to today's patient with bladder tumor. The minimal benefit derived from follow-up cystoscopy in patients tumor-free for 5 or more years, and the low yield from follow-up IV pyelography, may have particular relevance in this era of cost-containment.

W.A. See, M.D.

Partial Allelotype of Carcinoma in Situ of the Human Bladder

Rosin MP, Carins P, Epstein JI, Schoenberg MP, Sidransky D (Johns Hopkins Univ, Baltimore, Md; Simon Fraser Univ, Burnaby, BC, Canada)
Cancer Res 55:5213–5216, 1995   19–4

Background.—There is little published information on the molecular changes underlying cancer of the urinary bladder. It is suggested that tumors develop through progressive stages from noninvasive lesions to invasive lesions, and metastatic tumors. Multiple genetic changes in oncogenes and tumor suppressor genes underlie this progression. The genetic changes in bladder carcinoma in situ were investigated.

Methods.—Thirty-one specimens of bladder carcinoma in situ were microdissected and analyzed for loss of heterozygosity on 13 chromosomal arms using 29 microsatellite markers. These markers were located in regions that have had frequent loss of heterozygosity in primary transitional cell carcinoma of the bladder.

Results.—In 77% of lesions, loss of heterozygosity of chromosome 9 was frequent; 19 of 31 lesions showed deletion on the 9p arm, and 17 of 28 lesions showed deletion on the 9q arm. Fine mapping at 9p21 showed very frequent loss of heterozygosity surrounding the $p16^{INK4A}$ locus, like superficial papillary tumors. Loss of 14q was frequent in these lesions, but was very rare in papillary lesions. Frequent loss of heterozygosity was also observed on 8p, 17p, 13q, 11p, and 4q. Less frequent loss was noted on 11q, 4p, 3p, 18q, and 5q.

Conclusions.—These lesions had many of the genetic changes shown by highly invasive tumors. Carcinoma in situ lesions are significantly different from superficial papillary lesions. Further research is needed to determine which deletions are central to the development of carcinoma in situ lesions.

▶ This paper sheds some light into the genetic changes associated with carcinoma in situ of the bladder. Previously Dalbagni et al.[1] and Spruck et al.[2] have postulated that loss of heterozygosity of 9^q was not a common event in carcinoma in situ (cis), a finding that is not supported by this paper. The authors show that chromosomal 9 abnormalities are common in both superficial papillary transitional cell carcinoma and cis. Furthermore, they identified loss of a gene on chromosome 14^q as being a prerequisite for the development of cis.

J. Sheinfeld, M.D.

References

1. Dalbagni G, Presti J, Reuter V, et al: Genetic alterations in bladder cancer. *Lancet* 342:469–471, 1993.
2. Spruck CH III, Ohneseit PF, Gonzalez-Zulueta M, et al: Two molecular pathways to transitional cell carcinoma of the bladder. *Cancer Res* 54:784–788, 1994.

Molecular Detection of Primary Bladder Cancer by Microsatellite Analysis

Mao L, Schoenberg MP, Scicchitano M, Erozan YS, Merlo A, Schwab D, Sidransky D (Johns Hopkins Univ, Baltimore, Md; Johns Hopkins Hosp, Baltimore, Md)
Science 271:659–662, 1996
19–5

Introduction.—Urine cytology for the diagnosis of bladder cancer can miss up to 50% of tumors. Cystoscopy is not good as a general screening tool for the detection of bladder cancer because it is expensive and invasive. It is possible that microsatellite markers could be useful as clonal markers in the detection of human cancer because simple DNA repeat alterations can be readily detected in clinical samples using the polymerase chain reaction (PCR). Urine samples from 25 patients with bladder lesions suggestive of cancer underwent microsatellite analysis.

Methods.—All patients had symptoms suggestive of bladder cancer and had suggestive lesions at cystoscopy. Urine samples from 25 patients and 5 controls without neoplasm were distributed in blinded fashion for microsatellite analysis and routine urine cytology. Urine and lymphocyte DNA were amplified by PCR. Polymorphic alleles were compared at 10 preselected microsatellite loci that were identified in a previous investigation.

Results.—The urine DNA of 10 patients contained a microsatellite alteration in close agreement with a frequency based on calculations that were determined previously. Eighteen urine DNA samples demonstrated a loss of heterozygosity (LOH), particularly with marker D9S747 from chromosome 9p21. This is consistent with frequent findings of a loss of chromosome 9 in bladder cancer. Analysis of additional dinucleotide markers on chromosome 9p21 (D9S171, D9S162, and IFNA) for LOH confirmed the presence of deletions in urine samples demonstrating the loss of chromosome 9 with marker D9S747. When the code was broken, it was determined that 20 of 25 patients had histologically confirmed bladder cancer. Microsatellite analysis with the 13 markers indicated genetic alterations in 19 of 20 cancer patients. None of the 5 control patients had any microsatellite changes. The same microsatellite alterations and LOH patterns observed in the urine were also seen in the primary tumor. The urine samples showed LOH or microsatellite alterations not present in the biopsy specimens of 2 patients. In both instances, the LOH in at least one locus and loss of the identical allele was shared between the urine sediment and biopsy sample. It is possible that the urine sample contained a more advanced tumor cell clone derived from the same progenitor cell, but was not sampled by the small tumor biopsy. Using light microscopy, neoplastic cells were identified by cytology in 9 of 18 patients for whom molecular analysis was positive and 1 patient for whom molecular analysis was negative.

Conclusion.—Microsatellite analysis could be a powerful tool in the detection of primary bladder cancer. The markers used in this investigation detected 95% of bladder cancers. This approach can be expanded and improved as new markers are identified.

▶ The authors compared the sensitivity of urine cytology and the sensitivity of microsatellite DNA markers in detecting the presence of bladder cancer. The number of samples analyzed is small. Despite the fact that the majority of tumors were of high grade, the sensitivity of urine cytology was low, a problem that needs to be addressed. X immunocytology has a sensitivity of 85% and does not require a blood sample.[1] A comparison of the sensitivity of the microsatellite markers with that of the X immunocytology would have been interesting. Additional and diverse control patients would also be important.

J. Sheinfeld, M.D.

Reference

1. Sheinfeld J, Reuter VE, Melamed MR, et al: Enhanced bladder cancer detection with the Lewis X antigen as a marker of neoplastic transformation. *J Urol* 143:285, 1990.

Autocrine Growth of Transitional Cell Carcinoma of the Bladder Induced by Granulocyte-Colony Stimulating Factor
Tachibana M, Miyakawa A, Tazaki H, Nakamura K, Kubo A, Hata J-I, Nishi T, Amano Y (Keio Univ, Tokyo; Kyowa Hakko Kogyo Co, Ltd, Tokyo)
Cancer Res 55:3438–3443, 1995

19–6

Background.—In patients with cancer, the granulocyte-colony stimulating factor (G-CSF) produced by nonhematopoietic malignant cells can reportedly induce a leukemoid reaction in the host. This phenomenon, which occurs via intense stimulation of leukocyte production, has been linked to aggressive tumor cell growth and a poor clinical outcome. Direct evidence of G-CSF-induced autocrine growth of bladder cancer cells was found.

Methods.—Cancer cells for study were obtained from a 76-year-old man with metastatic transitional cell bladder carcinoma who underwent radical cystectomy. The patient had a peripheral blood leukocyte count of $94,900/mm^3$ and a serum G-CSF level of 103 pg/mL. The cells were cultured and studied by reverse-transcription polymerase chain reaction for the expression of G-CSF and G-CSF receptor mRNA expression.

Results.—A significant amount of G-CSF—5,560 pg/mL—was measured in the culture medium in which the cancer cells were grown. The cultured cells themselves showed significant levels of G-CSF and G-CSF receptor mRNA expression. Furthermore, in binding studies with radiolabeled recombinant G-CSF, high-affinity G-CSF binding receptors were identified on the cultured cells. The addition of exogenous G-CSF stimulated the growth of cultured cancer cells, and the addition of anti-G-CSF antibody inhibited this stimulation.

Conclusions.—Bladder cancer cells can produce G-CSF, which promotes autocrine growth. The expression of G-CSF and G-CSF receptor by cancer cells may play a key role in the malignant progression of nonhematopoietic cancers. The findings underscore the need for caution when G-CSF is considered for clinical use in patients with bladder cancer.

▶ The authors identified the presence of G-CSF production in bladder cancer cells with the expression of a functional receptor. This is a very important paper; however, the findings were based on cells derived from a single patient with metastatic disease. It would be premature to make recommendations on the clinical use of G-CSF in patients with bladder cancer.

J. Sheinfeld, M.D.

Apparent Failure of Current Intravesical Chemotherapy Prophylaxis to Influence the Long-term Course of Superficial Transitional Cell Carcinoma of the Bladder
Lamm DL, Riggs DR, Traynelis CL, Nseyo UO (West Virginia Univ, Morgantown)
J Urol 153:1444–1450, 1995   19–7

Introduction.—Controlled investigations of intravesical chemotherapy in the treatment of superficial bladder cancer are highly variable in entrance criteria, length of follow-up, and methods of reporting results. The only outcome measure that is uniformly reported is the percentage of patients with recurrent tumor. A review of all 22 prospective randomized controlled comparisons of intravesical therapy and surgery was conducted using the percentage of patients with tumor recurrence to provide an objective estimate of the benefit of treatment.

Methods.—A total of 3,899 patients were enrolled in the 22 chemotherapy trials. Of the 22 trials, 13 demonstrated a statistically significant decrease in tumor recurrence as a result of intravesical chemotherapy.

Short-term Reduction in Recurrence.—A total of 1,130 patients were enrolled in 9 controlled thiotepa investigations. Five of 9 investigations achieved statistical significance. There was a 12% reduction in tumor recurrence for patients treated with thiotepa, compared to surgery alone. The greatest reduction in tumor recurrence was observed in the 2 trials that used a single early postoperative thiotepa instillation. There were 1,389 patients enrolled in 5 doxorubicin controlled trials. Three of the trials that reached statistical significance indicated that the greatest benefit of doxorubicin was observed with a single early postoperative treatment. There was a 15% advantage of treatment over surgery alone (38% vs. 53%). A similar comparison of mitomycin C showed a 9% benefit in treated patients, compared to those who had surgery alone. Single instillations of ethoglucid showed a 31% advantage and epirubicin showed a 12% advantage over treatment with surgery alone.

Long-term Protection from Recurrent Tumor.—The 5-year recurrence rates for patients treated with thiotepa, doxorubicin, and mitomycin C were just as high, if not higher, than rates for patients receiving surgery alone. The overall modest decrease of 14% in tumor recurrence rate reported in patients treated with intravesical chemotherapy offered no evidence of beneficial influence on the risk of tumor progression. No survival advantages have been reported for patients treated with intravesical chemotherapy, compared to patients treated with surgery alone.

Bacille Calmette-Guerin (BCG) Immunotherapy.—Complete response rates were more encouraging in patients treated with BCG immunotherapy. An average complete response rate exceeding 70% was reported in patients thus treated. Patient survival rates have been improved in patients treated with BCG immunotherapy. One trial with results on 3-year follow-up showed that the mortality rate was 37% in the control group, compared to 12% in the BCG group.

Conclusion.—This review indicates that current intravesical chemotherapy protocols lower the short-term, 2-year incidence of tumor recurrence by 14%. Early postoperative single instillations seem to be the most effective approach. Surgery alone may be the best treatment for patients with low-grade, stage Ta tumor. Long-term incidence of tumor recurrence, tumor progression, and mortality do not seem to be decreased using intravesical chemotherapy prophylaxis. Concern has been raised about a possible carcinogenicity of intravesical cytotoxic chemotherapy.

▶ This important review of 22 prospective studies of intravesical chemotherapy sends a very important message: intravesical chemotherapy appears to impact on only short-term tumor recurrence rates and does not show any beneficial impact on long-term tumor progression. By way of distinction, the benefits of intravesical BCG therapy appear to persist for 5–10 years. Long-term follow-up of all patients receiving intravesical therapy for superficial bladder tumor is necessary to place these agents in their proper prospective.

G.L. Andriole, M.D.

Adjuvant Treatment With a Vitamin A Analogue (Etretinate) After Trans-urethral Resection of Superficial Bladder Tumors: Final Analysis of a Prospective, Randomized Multicenter Trial in Switzerland
Studer UE, Jenzer S, Biedermann C, Chollet D, Kraft R, von Toggenburg H, Vonbank F (Universities of Berne, Basel, Geneva, et al)
Eur Urol 28:284–290, 1995   19–8

Objective.—A prospective multicenter trial was conducted to determine whether adjuvant treatment with oral etretinate would reduce the recurrence rate of superficial bladder tumors after transurethral resection. Etretinate, an aromatic retinoid, has been found to lower the incidence of carcinogen-induced bladder cancer in rats.

Patients and Methods.—Ninety patients with superficial bladder tumors stage T_a and T_1 grades 1–3 entered the study and were randomly assigned to treatment with etretinate (25 mg twice daily) or to placebo. Eligible patients had undergone resection of all visible bladder tumors. The planned duration of treatment was 2 years. Patients had cystoscopy performed every 3 months and tumor recurrences during therapy were resected.

Results.—Seventy-nine patients were available for analysis, 42 in the placebo group and 37 in the etretinate group. The 2 groups had comparable histologic findings and were similar in age and other characteristics, but a significantly higher number of patients in the placebo group withdrew during the first year of the study because of treatment failure. Mean time to first recurrence of tumor was similar in the placebo (13.5 months) and etretinate (13.6 months) groups. Subsequent tumor recurrence, however, occurred at a mean of 12.7 months in patients given placebo and 20.3 months in those treated with etretinate. Thus the number of transurethral resections was significantly reduced in the active treatment vs. the placebo group. The most common side effect of etretinate, dryness of mucous membranes, was judged tolerable by most patients.

Conclusion.—The number of withdrawals from the placebo group during the first year changed the risk profile of this group to one with a reduced risk of recurrence. Although the 2 groups were almost identical in time to first recurrence, the time to a further recurrence was significantly extended in patients treated with etretinate. Thus the early reappearance of papillary tumors should not be taken as a sign of treatment failure. These tumors should be resected and retinoid therapy continued for at least 2 years. Because etretinate's teratogenic effect is well known, women of reproductive age cannot take the drug. Liver enzymes should be regularly checked because of the possibility of liver toxicity.

▶ This nicely designed, prospective, placebo-controlled, randomized study provides some evidence that oral use of a synthetic retinoid (etretinate) may delay the time to tumor recurrence among selected patients with superficial bladder cancer. Although the differences between the placebo and treated arm are not overwhelming, this study does provide a solid foundation upon which to design subsequent larger studies that may clarify the overall ability of etretinate to reduce superficial bladder tumor recurrences.

G.L. Andriole, M.D.

A Controlled Study of Intravesical Epirubicin With or Without Alpha2b-Interferon as Prophylaxis for Recurrent Superficial Transitional Cell Carcinoma of the Bladder
Raitanen M-P, Lukkarinen O, on behalf of Finnish Multicentre Study Group (Seinäjoki Central Hosp, Finland; Oulu Univ, Finland)
Br J Urol 76:697–701, 1995   19–9

Introduction.—The timing and length of treatment with intravesical chemotherapy and immunotherapy have not been established for patients with superficial transitional cell carcinoma (TCC). A randomized, controlled multicenter trial was conducted to determine the efficacy of intravesical epirubicin with or without alpha 2b-interferon (alpha2b-IFN) as a prophylactic treatment for recurrent superficial TCC of the bladder.

Methods.—Sixty-one men and 20 women, with a mean age of 71 years, were treated at 5 different urology departments in Finland. Tumors were stage Ta and T1 and were well or moderately differentiated grades 1 and 2. All patients had recurrent disease. Patients were randomized into 3 groups: group 1—treated by transurethral resection alone; group 2—treated with 50 mg of epirubicin instilled IV in 50 mL sterile buffer solution, and group 3—treated with 50 mg of epirubicin and 10 MU alpha2b-IFN. The drugs were instilled via catheter into the bladder and retained for 2 hours. For combined treatments, epirubicin was installed first, then followed immediately by IFN. Installations began 1 week after transurethral resection and were performed once weekly for the first month, then monthly for 1 year. Patients were followed every 3 months for the next 2 years. Recurrence rates were calculated.

Results.—Comparing recurrence rates, patients treated with both epirubicin and IFN had the most favorable outcome. Three of 19, 14 of 32, and 19 of 30 patients in group 1, 2, and 3, respectively, were free of recurrence at the end of the first year. Between-group differences were significant. Differences in tumor rates were significant between group 1 and group 3. These differences were notable, but not significant between groups 2 and 3. There were no significant between-group differences during the second year in recurrence rates. Tumor rates were lower in group 3 than in group 1 in the second year. Overall, 7 patients had a progression in stage and 13 had a progression in grade in the second year. Side effects were usually mild and transient, with no significant between-group differences in severity or duration. Six patients died during follow-up: 2 in group 1, 1 in group 2, and 3 in group 3.

Conclusion.—Treatment with epirubicin, with or without alpha2b-IFN, decreased the number of patients with superficial TCC having recurrences and lengthened the disease-free interval. Perhaps because there were too few patients, there were no significant differences in these parameters in group 2 and 3 patients. The chemotherapy approach was particularly helpful in patients with a history of prior recurrences.

▶ This well-designed trial compared the results of treatment with intravesical epirubicin alone or the combination of epirubicin and interferon on short-term tumor recurrence rates. It suggests that the maximal treatment effect may be achieved by the combination of chemotherapy and immunotherapy. However, because of the small number of patients in this study, the differences were not statistically significant. Moreover, the costs of this therapy would have to be considered before its use could be routinely recommended. Finally, comparison with the gold-standard intravesical Bacille Calmette-Guerín therapy would be the true acid test of this form of chemoimmunotherapy.

G.L. Andriole, M.D.

Long-term Follow-up of Patients With Superficial Transitional Cell Carcinoma of the Urinary Bladder Treated by Intravesical Mitomycin C

Pavlotsky A, Eidelman A, Barak F, Walach N, Horn Y (Assaf Harofeh Med Ctr, Zerifin, Israel; Univ of California, San Francisco)
J Surg Oncol 60:191–195, 1995   19–10

Introduction.—The use of mitomycin C (MMC) in the treatment of patients with superficial transitional cell carcinoma (TCC) has produced higher remission rates, compared to other drug regimens. A comparison between response rates or determined end points is complicated because the dosage and frequency of MCC instillation regimens differ greatly. Results of a 5-year follow-up in 86 patients treated with a 36-week course of intravesical MMC were evaluated.

Methods.—All patients had undergone transurethral resection for histologically proved TCC of the urinary bladder. Tumors were of various grades and were either stage 0 TaN0M0 or stage A T1N0M0. During the 36-week induction period, patients received 15 MMC instillations and 3 cystoscopic procedures. A transurethral resection and the initial intravesical chemotherapy procedure were repeated if periodic cystoscopy revealed a recurrent tumor. Patients in remission at the end of the 36-week induction period were started on maintenance therapy of monthly fractionations for 9 months and cystoscopy every 3 months, then were treated at 2-month intervals for 12 more months with cystoscopy every 6 months. The intravesical chemotherapy procedure was repeated from the beginning if cystoscopy revealed recurrence. The protocol was completed in 30 months for patients with no recurrence since the initial induction regimen.

Results.—Patients received a total of 3,196 intravesical chemotherapy instillations and underwent 767 cystoscopies. No tumor was present in 660 (86%) cystoscopy evaluations. There were 107 (14%) cystoscopies that were positive for tumor. Of 86 patients, 58 (67%) followed protocol as originally prescribed. Treatment was discontinued in 15 (17%) patients because of disease progression and in 13 (15%) because of patient refusal to continue with instillations after undergoing more than 2 courses. Treatment was not discontinued because of toxicity in any patients. There was no clinical evidence of toxicity related to MCC administration. At the 2-year follow-up, 64 patients remained eligible for long-term evaluation. Of these, 54 (84.4%) were in complete remission. At 3 year follow-up, 38 of 45 (84.4%) remaining patients were in remission. At 5 year follow-up, 21 of 26 patients (80.8%) remained on the prescribed protocol with no evidence of tumor. Twenty-seven patients with no response to previous treatment with other drugs responded to MMC.

Conclusion.—Therapeutic results and complete response rates were superior in patients with superficial TCC treated with long-term intravesical chemotherapy with MMC. These findings compared favorably with previous trials. Long-term results in this patient cohort indicate that complete response can be estimated on the basis of cystoscopic and clinical grounds without the need for random bladder biopsies.

▶ The results of this study are encouraging, but one must consider that the authors treated a relatively favorable subgroup of patients with superficial disease and at 5 years of follow-up, only about one third of the initial group of patients were available for evaluation. Moreover, this fairly intensive regimen of intravesical chemotherapy would be quite expensive if administered in the United States and is sufficiently cumbersome that only 67% of the patients followed the protocol of instillations as originally planned. Because of these limitations, it is difficult to come to any definitive conclusions regarding the long-term ability of mitomycin to control superficial bladder cancer.

G.L. Andriole, M.D.

Preventive Effect of a *Lactobacillus casei* Preparation on the Recurrence of Superficial Bladder Cancer in a Double-Blind Trial
Aso Y, Akaza H, Kotake T, Tsukamoto T, Imai K, Naito S, and the BLP Study Group (Univ of Tokyo, Japan; Univ of Tsukuba, Japan; The Center for Adult Diseases, Osaka, Japan; et al)
Eur Urol 27:104–109, 1995   19–11

Background.—BLP, a preparation containing about 1×10^{10} of viable *Lactobacillus casei* organisms per gram, has long been used in Japan for the treatment of intestinal dysfunction. Recent research has demonstrated antitumor activity against murine bladder tumors when BLP is given orally. The value of BLP in preventing the recurrence of superficial bladder cancer was investigated in a double-blind, placebo-controlled study.

Methods.—One hundred thirty-eight patients with superficial transitional cell carcinoma of the bladder after transurethral resection were enrolled in the study. Patients were grouped according to whether they had

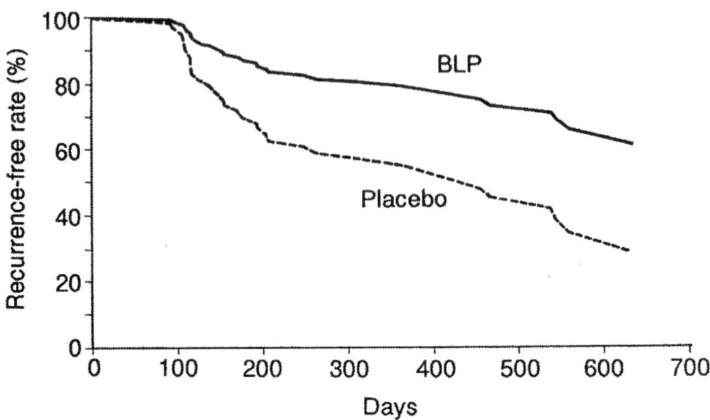

FIGURE 3.—Corrected cumulative recurrence-free rates for the placebo-treated and BLP-treated patients in subgroups A and B, as determined by Cox multivariate analysis. (Courtesy of Aso Y, Akaza H, Kotake T, et al: Preventive effect of a *Lactobacillus casei* preparation on the recurrence of superficial bladder cancer in a double-blind trial. *Eur Urol* 27:104–109, 1995. S. Karger AG, Basel, publisher.)

multiple primary tumors, recurrent single tumors, or recurrent multiple tumors. Patients in each group were assigned randomly to receive BLP or placebo.

Findings.—The prophylactic effect of BLP was better than placebo in the first 2 subgroups. In the third subgroup, the results of BLP and placebo were not significantly different. A Cox multivariate analysis indicated that BLP outcomes were significantly better than placebo outcomes. Three patients given BLP and 3 given placebo had slight, tolerable adverse reactions (Fig 3).

Conclusions.—The oral administration of BLP appears to be safe and effective in preventing recurrences of superficial bladder cancer. Additional research is needed to clarify this agent's mechanism of action.

▶ *Prospective, randomized,* and *double-blind* are adjectives that precede the titles of many well-designed clinical trials. However, trial design constitutes but one of the serial steps required to definitively address a clinical question. Equally, if not more important, is the method of statistical analysis of the trial results. Analysis based upon intent to treat, absence of data editing, and adherence to the original statistical design are critical elements for the valid and meaningful interpretation of clinical data. This trial, having found no difference in outcome among the overall group, and having insufficient numbers of patients for meaningful analysis based upon prerandomization stratification, combined stratification groups predicated upon the authors' impressions of similarity. When a secondary analysis failed to demonstrate a statistically significant effect of treatment on outcome, a tertiary analysis was employed to correct for intergroup differences in recurrence risk factors. These acknowledged manipulations of the data preclude any statement regarding the efficacy of oral BLP as recurrence prophylaxis in patients with superficial bladder cancer.

W.A. See, M.D.

Intravesical Adjuvant Chemotherapy for Superficial Transitional Cell Bladder Carcinoma: Results of 2 European Organization for Research and Treatment of Cancer Randomized Trials With Mitomycin C and Doxorubicin Comparing Early Versus Delayed Instillations and Short-Term Versus Long-Term Treatment
Bouffioux C, Kurth KH, Bono A, Oosterlinck W, Kruger CB, De Pauw M, Sylvester R, and the Members of the European Organization for Research and Treatment of Cancer Genitourinary Group (Univ Hosp, Leige, Belgium; Univ Hosp, Ghent, Belgium; European Organization for Research and Treatment of Cancer Data Ctr, Brussels, Belgium; et al)
J Urol 153:934–941, 1995   19–12

Introduction.—The European Organization for Research and Treatment of Cancer has completed parallel, prospective, randomized studies utilizing intravesical mitomycin C and doxorubicin, respectively, as adjuvant treatment after transurethral resection of superficial transitional cell carcinoma of the bladder. The goal was to compare treatment given on the day of resection with that delayed for 7–15 days, and also to compare treatment durations of 6 and 12 months.

Patients.—A total of 965 patients having totally resectable (stage Ta or T1) papillary transitional cell cancer were admitted to the 23 trials. Patients who had received non-study drugs intravesically at least 3 months previously were accepted.

Treatment.—Patients were randomly assigned to receive instillations of 30 mg of mitomycin C or 50 mg of doxorubicin starting either on the day of resection or 7–15 days later. The drug was retained in the bladder for at least an hour. Instillations were repeated at weekly intervals for 4 weeks and then every month for 5 months. Patients then were again randomly assigned to receive 6 further monthly instillations or no maintenance treatment.

Results.—There was no major local toxicity in either study, and no life-threatening systemic toxicity occurred. After an average follow-up of nearly 3 years, 43% of patients given early treatment and 49% of those whose treatment was delayed had at least 1 recurrence. Half the patients not given maintenance treatment and 43% of those so treated had recurrences. Patients who received delayed treatment for 6 months only tended not to do as well as those in the other groups. There were no significant treatment-related differences in duration of survival. Multivariate analysis confirmed a higher recurrence rate in patients given delayed, shorter-term treatment. Treatment could not be related to the development of distant disease or the appearance of a second primary neoplasm.

Conclusions.—Adjunctive intravesical treatment starting on the day of resection appears to be advantageous for patients with bladder cancer. Maintenance treatment for a second 6 months is seemingly beneficial only when initial treatment is delayed.

▶ The precise cause, or causes, of the idiosyncratically high rate of superficial bladder tumor recurrence remains enigmatic. As a consequence, many of the decisions regarding the use of intravesical chemotherapy for recurrence prophylaxis have been empirically, rather than scientifically, based. This report by the European Organization for Research and Treatment of Cancer clarifies 2 important issues regarding the timing and duration of the administration of intravesical chemotherapy. Their observations, together with reports on the clonality of bladder cancer,[1] provide growing evidence that intraepithelial tumor dissemination, occurring as a consequence of concomitant tumor morselization and urothelial trauma,[2] contributes to recurrence rates. Whether the small observed benefit from immediate drug instillation correlates with the relative contribution of implantation to overall recurrence, or with the efficacy of this strategy to prevent implantation, awaits further study.

Although perioperative administration of intravesical chemotherapy offers optimal benefit, it is critical to remember that Bacillus of Calmette-Guérin should never be administered in the "posttraumatic" setting. To do so significantly increases the risk of serious, potentially life threatening morbidity.[3]

W.A. See, M.D.

References

1. Sidransky D, Frost P, von Eschenbach A, et al: Clonal origin of bladder cancer. *N Engl J Med* 326:737–749, 1992.
2. See WA, Chapman PH, Williams RD: Kinetics of transitional tumor cell line 4909 adherence to injured urothelial surfaces in (F-344) rats. *Cancer Res* 50:2499–2504, 1990.
3. Lamm DL, van der Meijden APM, Morales A, et al: Incidence and treatment of complications of BCG intravesical therapy in superficial bladder cancer. *J Urol* 147:596–600, 1992.

Vascular and Other Serious Infections With *Mycobacterium bovis* After Bacillus of Calmette-Guérin Therapy for Bladder Cancer
Hellinger WC, Oldenburg WA, Alvarez S (Mayo Clinic, Jacksonville, Fla)
South Med J 88:1212–1216, 1995   19–13

Introduction.—Although intravesical application of bacillus of Calmette-Guérin (BCG)—a live attenuated strain of *Mycobacterium bovis*—can be an effective therapy for bladder cancer, serious complications occur in some cases. One patient had a mycotic abdominal aortic aneurysm and another had *M. bovis* bacteremia after BCG therapy.

Case Report 1.—Man, 71, had 2 courses of weekly intravesical BCG therapy for recurrent superficial bladder cancer. The therapy was stopped when he experienced 3 days of malaise after several monthly instillations of BCG, administered when the second weekly BCG course was completed. A year later, a pseudoaneurysm of the right lower extremity required bypass revision. Recurrent pseudoaneurysms of the bypass graft led to removal of all prosthetic material. Although bacterial cultures of the aneurysm were without growth, the patient experienced fever, failure of the wound to heal, and secondary wound infections. Laboratory data and CT examination of the abdomen and pelvis suggested mycotic abdominal aneurysm as a cause of fever and malaise and mycobacterial cultures of the excised aneurysm grew *M. bovis*. The patient remains well 1 year after treatment with appropriate antibacterial antibiotics.

Case Report 2.—Man, 71, with multiple medical problems, had fulguration for transitional cell carcinoma of the bladder, followed by BCG therapy. Within 8–12 hours, a fever developed, which lasted several days and recurred at 7- to 14-day intervals. When he was hospitalized again with fever about 9 months later, a mycobacterial culture of blood yielded growth of *M. bovis*. The patient's fever resolved after 2 weeks of treatment with isoniazid and ethambutol, therapy that continued for 1 year.

Discussion.—Treatment with BCG has been considered the therapy of choice for bladder carcinoma in situ and is used in some other forms of the disease as well. Both local and systemic reactions to BCG have been reported, and these reactions have been major in some cases. Infection with *M. bovis* at sites distant from the bladder can occur months or even years after BCG therapy, particularly in immunosuppressed patients. Questions that remain to be answered are when and how to refrain from further BCG therapy and the optimal use of antimycobacterial chemotherapy and corticosteroid therapy.

▶ It is well known that infectious complications can occur after treatment of bladder cancer with BCG. Lamm and associates reviewed 2,500 patients treated with BCG.[1] They found that minor local reactions such as cystitis and hematuria were almost universal. Transient low-grade fever and malaise occurred in about 25% of patients. More severe reactions including fever (> 38.5%), granulomatous prostatitis, epididymo-orchitis, hepatitis, and sepsis were experienced by a total of approximately 5% of patients. A disturbing feature of the above-reported cases is the late appearance of these reactions months after cessation of therapy.

S.S. Howards, M.D.

Reference

1. Lamm DL: Complications of bacillus Calmette-Guérin immunotherapy. *Urol Clin North Am* 19:565–572, 1992.

Does Neoadjuvant Cisplatin-Based Chemotherapy Improve the Survival of Patients With Locally Advanced Bladder Cancer: A Meta-Analysis of Individual Patient Data From Randomized Clinical Trials

Ghersi D, Stewart LA, Parmar MKB, Coppin C, Martinez Pineiro J, Raghavan D, Wallace MA (British Med Research Council Cancer Trials Office)
Br J Urol 75:206–213, 1995
19–14

Background.—Many clinicians use neoadjuvant chemotherapy in the routine treatment of locally advanced bladder cancer. Although results of phase II studies are encouraging, there is yet no conclusive evidence that chemotherapy improves survival. To investigate further, a meta-analysis or quantitative overview was undertaken to assess more reliably whether neoadjuvant chemotherapy improves survival in locally advanced bladder cancer.

Materials.—Individual data from 497 patients (301 deaths) included in 4 randomized trials comparing local definitive treatment alone with neoadjuvant or concurrent single-agent cisplastin followed by local definitive treatment were analyzed. In another similar randomized trial of cisplastin and doxorubicin, summary data were available for 325 patients (127 deaths).

Results.—Meta-analysis of individual patient data provided an overall hazard ratio of 1.02 in favor of local therapy alone, giving an estimated 1% detriment in 2-year survival from the use of chemotherapy, from 50% to 49%. However, the confidence intervals indicated that these overall results were consistent with a possible absolute improvement in absolute survival of 7%, or with a detriment of 8% in the 2-year survival rate. When this analysis was supplemented with the summary data from 1 trial, the hazard ratio was 0.91 in favor of chemotherapy for an estimated absolute improvement in 2-year survival of 3%. However, the confidence interval suggested that these results were consistent with an improvement at 2 years of 9%, or conversely, a possible reduction of survival of 3%. The only prognostic factor that suggested a differential treatment effect (interaction) across groups was age, with chemotherapy appearing to be more effective in patients younger than 60 years.

Conclusions.—Despite combining the results of all known randomized trials, there is still insufficient information to reliably address the question of whether neoadjuvant chemotherapy improves survival in locally advanced bladder cancer. Hence, neoadjuvant cisplastin-based chemotherapy cannot currently be recommended for routine use in patients with locally advanced bladder cancer and any further clinical trial should include a "no chemotherapy" control arm.

▶ No studies have documented salutary effect of neoadjuvant or adjuvant chemotherapy from locally advanced bladder cancer. To date, results of trials are conflicting, and debates continue on whether to use any chemotherapy at all—as well as on the timing of administration. The proponents of neoadjuvant therapy state that chemotherapy is better tolerated when administered before a major operation, finding of p0 at the time of surgery indicates a good prognosis, and micrometastatic disease is eradicated early. Supporters of adjuvant therapy claim that a more tailored approach can be used in patients who are at higher risk of progression.

This manuscript focuses on meta-analysis to aid in the determination of the value of neoadjuvant chemotherapy. Unfortunately, most of the trials do not have sufficient power to detect small (i.e., less than 15%) differences in survival. One can conclude from the majority of these smaller studies that there is no major improvement in survival rate (i.e., greater than a 30% improvement). Meta-analysis, when properly performed, can provide meaningful information. However, it requires very precise statistical procedures as well as the inclusion of all potentially eligible trials. Meta-analysis has been used in studies of advanced prostate cancer to determine the value of combined androgen blockade, but the results of such analyses have been subject to significant criticism. The take-home message from this trial is that there is no major improvement in overall survival rate from neoadjuvant therapy. Regardless, toxicity seems to be minimal. The Southwest Oncology Group has currently completed a trial that should answer this question in a more definitive manner.

E.D. Crawford, M.D.

Local Control of Muscle-Invasive Bladder Cancer: Preoperative Radiotherapy and Cystectomy Versus Cystectomy Alone
Cole CJ, Pollack A, Zagars GK, Dinney CP, Swanson DA, von Eschenbach AC
(Univ of Texas MD Anderson Cancer Ctr, Houston)
Int J Radiat Oncol Biol Phys 32:331–340, 1995   19–15

Purpose.—Preoperative radiotherapy for patients with muscle-invasive bladder cancer has largely been abandoned in the United States because of improved results with radical cystectomy alone. Local control of muscle-invasive bladder cancer with 2 modalities, preoperative radiotherapy and radical cystectomy (PREOP) and radical cystectomy (CYST) alone, was evaluated retrospectively.

Methods.—The PREOP group consisted of 338 patients with stages T2–T4 transitional cell carcinoma of the bladder treated between 1960 and 1983. A mean total dose of 49.3 ± 0.2 Gy was administered at 2 Gy per fraction 4–6 weeks before cystectomy. There were 232 patients in the CYST group, treated between 1985 and 1990; radical cystectomy alone has been the primary treatment modality for this cancer in the study institution since 1985. Analysis was restricted to the 301 patients who completed PREOP and the 220 who completed CYST planned treatments.

Results.—Preoperative radiotherapy had a significant impact on local control for patients with stage T3b disease. Actuarial 5-year local control in the 92 patients in the PREOP group with stage T3b disease was 91%, compared to 72% for the 42 similar patients in the CYST group. At 5 years, the PREOP patients also had fewer distant metastases, more freedom from disease, and greater overall survival. There were no differences between the groups for stages T2 or T3a, and there were not enough patients in stage T4 in the PREOP group for a meaningful comparison. Pretreatment hemoglobin, blood urea nitrogen, and treatment type were independently predictive of local control.

Conclusions.—Any biases in the study would likely favor the CYST group because they were treated with more modern surgical techniques, and 80% of them received multiagent chemotherapy. Therefore, the differences favoring PREOP over CYST may be underestimated, and preoperative radiotherapy should be considered as an adjunct to chemotherapy and surgery for patients with clinical stage T3b disease.

▶ Preoperative radiation in combination with radical cystectomy for the management of invasive bladder cancer has been relegated to historical interest only. In an attempt to improve upon the results of cystectomy, preoperative radiation in various doses was introduced in the late 1960s. However, the results came under intense scrutiny, and randomized trials of preoperative radiation and cystectomy with cystectomy alone suggested similar survival rates. The Southwest Oncology Group conducted a large randomized trial to address its value.[1] There appeared to be no survival advantage to adding preoperative radiation. However, this study was criticized because few patients had T3 disease, and survival (not local control) was used as an end point.

This current retrospective review documents a significant impact on local control for stage T3b disease. Retrospective reviews are fraught with difficulties and generally carry little statistical significance. In addition, subset analysis (T3b), as utilized in this manuscript, further weakens its validity. Nevertheless, there may be some value to preoperative radiation therapy in a subset of patients. Clinical staging is inaccurate and hinders a correct designation of who may benefit. I doubt that this report is going to change current management practices of invasive bladder cancer. There is more contemporary interest in both neoadjuvant and adjuvant chemotherapy as methods to improve overall survival.

E.D. Crawford, M.D.

Reference

1. Crawford ED, Das S, Smith JA, Jr: Preoperative radiation therapy in the treatment of bladder cancer. *Urol Clin North Am* 14:781–787, 1987.

Early Complications and Survival Following Short-Term Palliative Radiotherapy in Invasive Bladder Carcinoma
Holmäng S, Borghede G (Sahlgrenska Univ, Göteborg, Sweden)
J Urol 155:100–102, 1996   19–16

Introduction.—Elderly patients with muscle invasive bladder cancer who are unfit for cystectomy may be given a short course of moderate dose external beam radiotherapy. The short-term outcome of such treatment was examined in a series of 96 patients.

Patients and Methods.—A review of files for the period between 1981 and 1992 yielded 69 men and 27 women treated with a short course of pelvic radiotherapy. All but 13 patients were age 75 or older and all but 3 had histopathologic evidence of detrusor muscle invasion. Clinical stage was T2MO in 13 cases, T3MO in 36, T4MO in 26, and T2–4M+ in 21. Thirty-eight patients had documented ureteral obstruction. Two fractionated irradiation regimens were used in the patient group. Fifteen received 5 Gy 4 times to a maximum of 20 Gy and 81 were treated with 7 Gy 3 times to a total of 21 Gy. Both treatments were given every 2 days. Follow-up was complete until 1994 or death.

Results.—Side effects of treatment were documented in 45 patients, 22 of whom were hospitalized for a median of 10 days. Seven of the 12 deaths that occurred within 5 weeks of treatment were the result of unexpectedly rapid progressing disease. None of the 17 patients who had severe local symptoms before radiotherapy appeared to experience significant symptomatic improvement after treatment. Two patients were hospitalized with late complications, 1 with proctitis and another with rectal stenosis.

Conclusion.—These elderly patients who were treated with short-term moderate dose radiotherapy for invasive bladder carcinoma had a median survival of 6 months. This survival rate is similar to that obtained when no treatment is given. Only those with clinical stage T2MO disease had a longer survival (median 27 months). Because of the acute side effects of treatment, its lack of palliative value, and its potential to hasten death, short-term radiotherapy appears to be of little benefit to such patients.

▶ This retrospective study shows that elderly patients who are not surgical candidates do not benefit from palliative radiotherapy for invasive bladder carcinoma. It is encouraging that 12 of the 14 patients who had hematuria before the institution of radiation therapy had relief of this problem, but all of these patients died within 4 months so it is difficult to be certain that this would have been an enduring effect. It seems that palliation for elderly nonsurgical candidates with invasive bladder cancer may be best achieved by repetitive use of local therapies such as transurethral resection, laser fulguration, and other symptomatic measures.

G.L. Andriole, M.D.

Tumor-associated Antigens as Prognostic Factors for Recurrence in 382 Patients With Primary Transitional Cell Carcinoma of the Bladder

Allard P, Fradet Y, Têtu B, Bernard P, and the Quebec Urology Research Group (Laval Univ, Quebec, Canada)
Clin Cancer Res 1:1195–1202, 1995   19–17

Background.—Although transurethral resection (TUR) is effective in removing superficial transitional bladder carcinomas, about half the patients have recurrences within 2 years of the initial resection. Intensive follow-up cystoscopies are needed to prevent recurrences from invading the muscle layer of the bladder wall. Although several prognostic factors have been identified for tumor recurrence, they do not predict recurrence in individuals accurately enough to modulate the follow-up policy based on risk of recurrence. The prognostic value of the expression of 19A211, M344, T138, and T43 antigens was assessed in patients for whom initial TUR was done to remove primary superficial bladder tumors.

Methods.—All patients with primary superficial bladder tumors treated by endoscopic resection in 15 hospitals were enrolled from 1990 to 1992. Immunostaining for 19A211 and M344 was done on paraffin-embedded material and for T43 and T138, on frozen tissue. Follow-up consisted of the standard schedule of cystoscopies. A total of 2,254 follow-up cystoscopies were performed on 368 of the 382 patients initially enrolled.

Findings.—Tumor recurrence was found in 55.7% of the patients. Ninety percent of the primary tumors demonstrated positivity to 19A211. The expression of this antigen was associated with a reduction in first recurrence hazard and recurrence rate. Fifteen percent of the tumors showed T138 positivity. The expression of this antigen was related to an increase in first recurrence hazard and recurrence rate. Seventy-one percent of the tumors were positive for M344, whose expression was correlated with increased tumor rate. The expression of T43 was uncorrelated with recurrence end points.

Conclusions.—The expression of 19A211, M344, and T138 antigens was associated with tumor recurrence in a large cohort with primary superficial bladder cancer. The prognostic value of these antigens was independent of primary tumor features.

▶ In attempts to interpret the significance of immunohistologically expressed antigens in bladder cancer, it is important to consider what these molecules represent. The assumption is that they are antigens specific for bladder tumors and may indicate future behavior. These substances are the expression of a tumor's phenotype. Whether they reflect the propensity for tumor cells to be more motile or even potentially more infiltrative is unclear. Correspondingly, whether their detection will ultimately be useful in determining the risk for recurrence and in choosing how to treat patients will require further investigation.

The application of this technique with some degree of uniformity can be problematic, especially if archival tissue cannot be used. The standardization of staining techniques and the rigorous control of objective assessments of tissue samples are mandatory for effective applicability.

The observation of these molecules on histologically "normal" epithelium taken from areas in the bladder that were endoscopically normal is highly important conceptually. It suggests that stem cells, which give rise to transitional cell cancers, may colonize other areas of the bladder, accounting for recurrent disease. This would suggest that intravesical treatments are more frequently necessary in preventing the at least 50% likelihood that cancers may recur.

In this regard, several reports have described limited efficacy of intravesical treatments in preventing recurrence in the long term and virtually no efficacy in preventing tumor progression. Predictive factors such as high grade, infiltration of the lamina propria, association with carcinoma in situ, multiplicity of disease, and persistence or rapidity of recurrence may themselves be indicators for the development of tumor progression. Within this context, it will be of importance to document the greater predictive value of molecules such as those examined in the present study to determine whether they provide a diagnostic advantage in assessing the likelihood of recurrence and progression, and also whether their expression is sufficient cause to prompt adjustments in our therapeutic approach.

M.J. Droller, M.D.

Tumor Angiogenesis Correlates With Lymph Node Metastases in Invasive Bladder Cancer

Jaeger TM, Weidner N, Chew K, Moore DH, Kerschmann RL, Waldman FM, Carroll PR (Univ of California, San Francisco; Univ of Heidelberg, Germany)
J Urol 154:69–71, 1995   19–18

Background.—Tumor tissue neovascularization, or tumor angiogenesis, is believed to play a crucial role in tumor growth, proliferation, and eventually metastasis. Microvessel density or count is correlated with clinical outcome in carcinoma of the skin, breast, lung, and prostate. The possible association between tumor angiogenesis and nodal metastasis was determined.

Methods.—Microvessel counts were made in 41 bladder cancers of stages T2 to 4,NX,MO. Immunostaining of endothelial cells for factor VIII-related antigen was done to identify microvessels, which were scored in certain regions showing active neovascularization. The scoring was done by counting a 200× field or by using a 10 × 10 square ocular grid.

Findings.—The microvessel count was related to the presence of occult lymph node metastases. Twenty-seven patients with no lymph node metastases had a mean microvessel count of 56.2 microvessels per 200× field, or 28.6 microvessels per grid. A mean of 138.1 microvessels per 200× field, or 74.7 microvessels per grid, were documented in the 14 patients with histologically proved lymph node metastases. Area and grid counting were well correlated. Tumor T stage, grade, and the presence of vascular or lymphatic invasion were unassociated with the presence of lymph node metastases.

Conclusions.—Determining the number of microvessels counted per 200× field or grid areas within the most neovascular regions of the invasive bladder carcinomas may provide strong prognostic indication of metastatic disease in pelvic lymph nodes. Further research is needed to determine whether the microvessel counts of tumor material obtained in the initial transurethral resection predict the risk of lymph node metastases. The ability of microvessel count to predict distant relapse in the absence of lymph node metastases also needs to be investigated.

▶ The apparent predictive association between the presence of metastases and microvessel count (angiogenesis) in various cancers is predicated on the assumption that those factors that promote angiogenesis are related to those that promote the development of metastatic disease. In this report, several observations suggested possible variance from this assumption. First, there was no correlation between tumor microemboli in bladder wall vessels and lymphatics and the occurrence of lymph node metastases. Second, would angiogenesis not be correlated more with hematogenous metastases rather than spread to lymph nodes?

One might also consider questions involving methodology. Can one distinguish the process of angiogenesis creating numerous small vessels that are then counted as such in cross-section vs. the development of just a few vessels with a spiral configuration, which may loop in and out of the plane of section? Because areas were selected on the basis of their most populous vascular appearance, might a selection bias have been introduced into a study such as this? Also, could prior transurethral resection have created an inflammatory response that itself induced angiogenesis? Transurethral resection specimens were not evaluated to see if the proposed correlation was validated in "virgin" tissue.

Several reports have questioned proposed correlations between angiogenesis (as determined by microvessel score) and the aggressiveness of a cancer. Although the correlation proposed in this study is of interest, more work needs to be done to validate the correlation, to refine it so that it may be applicable in the individual patient, and to understand the association implied between new vessel formation and the occurrence of metastatic disease.

M.J. Droller, M.D.

Bladder Cancer Among French Farmers: Does Exposure to Pesticides in Vineyards Play a Part?

Viel J-F, Challier B (Dept of Public Health, Biostatistics and Epidemiology Unit, Faculty of Medicine, Besançon, France)
Occup Environ Med 52:587–592, 1995

19–19

Background.—As many as a million individuals in France, many of them farm workers, are potentially exposed to pesticides. Deaths from bladder cancer are most prevalent in the south of France, where vineyards are predominantly located. Aromatic amines, which are used in manufacturing pesticides, have been related to bladder cancer in dyestuff workers. Past studies of bladder cancer in farm workers have yielded mixed results.

Objective.—An attempt was made to relate bladder cancer to pesticide exposure in French vineyard workers, males ranging from 35 to 74 years of age. The 837,413 farmers and farm laborers included in the study were followed for 3 years. Exposure was estimated at the geographic level using the pesticide exposure index (PEI).

Findings.—Mortality from bladder cancer overall was comparable to the national norm; the standardized mortality ratio was 0.96. These deaths were significantly associated with the PEI on both univariate and multivariate analysis. The risk ratio was 1.17 in univariate analysis and 1.14 in multivariate analysis.

Conclusion.—These observations lend some support to the claim that exposure to pesticides in vineyards may increase the risk of dying of bladder cancer.

▶ Epidemiologic studies are difficult to do, mainly because of problems in acquiring reliable data. In this study of an association between bladder cancer and working in vineyards, only bladder cancer mortality was assessed because there are no registries for the general incidence or prevalence of bladder cancer. In this type of study, however, there would appear to be the need to identify marker molecules of carcinogens to which these workers were exposed, so that the degree of exposure (duration, intensity) could be correlated with incidence of disease and the risk be more precisely determined. Considerations of lagtime between exposure and disease expression are also important. A wide range of ages was studied. Whether those in the younger portion of the spectrum would have had as much risk (in association with intensity) or whether sufficient time had passed to allow cancer to develop, is unclear. Host factors might also play a role. Those who have the enzymatic capability to metabolize carcinogens in innocuous forms would undoubtedly have an advantage.

One would presume that carcinogens contained in pesticides would expose workers in this industry to a higher risk for the development of bladder cancer. One cannot presume, however, that it would necessarily lead to the development of an aggressive form of bladder cancer unless confounding variables such as host factors, type of exposure, and type of cancer produced could be well documented.

M.J. Droller, M.D.

Combination Chemotherapy With Intra-arterial Cisplatin and Doxorubicin Plus Intravenous Methotrexate and Vincristine for Locally Advanced Bladder Cancer

Naito S, Kuroiwa T, Ueda T, Hasuo K, Masuda K, Kumazawa J, and Kyushu Univ Urological and Radiological Oncology Group (Kyushu Univ, Fukuoka, Japan)

J Urol 154:1704–1709, 1995   19–20

Background.—Systemic chemotherapy yields response rates of 50% to 70% in patients with advanced bladder cancer. This has led to the proposal that neoadjuvant chemotherapy could be used to sterilize micrometastases, improve cure rate, or preserve the bladder. Although some early benefit of neoadjuvant chemotherapy has been reported, there is the potential for serious toxicity. A phase 2 study of neoadjuvant combination chemotherapy for locally advanced bladder cancer was conducted.

Methods.—The study included 36 patients with locally advanced bladder cancer, i.e., stage T2–T4N0M0. None had received any systemic or intra-arterial chemotherapy. All received the new neoadjuvant combination chemotherapy regimen, which included a relatively low dose of intra-arterial cisplatin and doxorubicin given with angiotensin II, plus IV methotrexate and vincristine. The patients received at least 2 courses of chemotherapy at an interval of 4 weeks.

Results.—There were 12 clinical complete responses and 17 partial responses. All but 1 of the patients with a complete response had bladder preservation, and all 11 of these patients were disease-free at a median follow-up of 33 months. The possibility of clinical complete response was significantly influenced by the size and grade of the primary tumor. Nine of the 17 patients with a clinical partial response underwent bladder-sparing surgery, and 6 of 9 had no evidence of disease at a median follow-up of 26 months. Just 2 of 7 patients with no clinical response had no evidence of disease at a median follow-up of 12 months. Pathologic response rate was 42% and pathologic complete response rate 17%. The neoadjuvant chemotherapy regimen carried no significant toxicity.

Conclusions.—A relatively low-dose combination chemotherapy regimen appears to be a safe and effective treatment for patients with locally advanced bladder cancer. When a clinical complete response is achieved, bladder preservation may be possible. The toxicity associated with this neoadjuvant chemotherapy regimen is acceptable.

▶ This paper describes a bladder preservation strategy using chemotherapy. Two of the drugs, cisplatin and doxorubicin, were given intra-arterially, bilaterally, into the pelvis and the other 2 drugs, methotrexate and vincristine, were given intravenously. The authors report an 80% response rate (partial or complete), and 11 patients obtained an apparent durable complete response in the bladder.

The results reported are slightly better, although probably not statistically different from other neoadjuvant strategies using either systemic chemotherapy by itself or systemic chemotherapy combined with local radiation.[1] The discriminating factor of this article is the use of intra-arterial chemotherapy. This method of drug delivery has been used for bladder cancer for well over 10 years, with a particular interest in Japan. In the United States, interest has waned greatly. One of the problems is that there are so many variables connected with the chemotherapy that cannot be controlled that making a comparison to IV delivery is extremely difficult.[2] The only true way to tell whether intra-arterial delivery of some of the agents is better than IV delivery would be with a prospective randomized trial. Several hundred patients would probably be necessary to detect a meaningful difference. This is unlikely to happen. Variables, such as placement of the intra-arterial catheter, degree of atherosclerosis affecting flow in the involved vessels, addition of vasoconstricting agents such as angiotensin, intrinsic vascularity of the tumor, inherent chemo-sensitivity of the tumor, and patient selection, are all key variables. In a personal experience, some patients appeared to do remarkably well with intra-arterial cisplatin, but the additional expense and potential neurotoxicity seemed to outweigh the uncertain benefit afforded.

The best results reported for bladder preservation strategy have been with the use of intra-arterial cisplatin and concurrent radiation therapy by Eapen and associates.[3] A complete clinical response rate of 90% was identified in 97 patients.

Is there something dramatic about the potential increased dose delivery of cisplatin that can be accomplished intra-arterially? I am not convinced that anyone knows for sure at this time. Data such as that presented in the abstracted article are intriguing, but not conclusive. In the United States, with increased difficulty in performing clinical research such as this, I believe it is unlikely that anyone will undertake a trial of intra-arterial treatments.

J.E. Montie, M.D.

References

1. Tester W. Caplan R. Heaney J, et al: Neoadjuvant combined modality program with selective organ preservation for invasive bladder cancer: Results of radiation therapy oncology group phase II trial 8802. *J Clin Oncol* 14:119–126, 1996.
2. Given RW, Parsons JT, McCarley D, et al: Bladder-sparing multi modality treatment of muscle-invasive bladder cancer: A five year follow-up. *Urology* 46:449–505, 1995.
3. Eapen LS, Crook D, Huan J, et al: Intraarterial cisplatin (IAC) and concurrent pelvic radiation (PR) in the management of transitional bladder cancer: An organ preservation strategy. *Proc Annu Meet Am Soc Clin Oncol* 14:A625, 1995.

Pelvic Lymphadenectomy (Staging) in Patients With Bladder Cancer Laparoscopic Versus Open Approach
Poulsen J, Krarup T (Aalborg County Hosp, Denmark)
Scand J Urol Nephrol 172:19–21, 1995   19–21

Background.—The extent of disease is a chief determinant of outcome after radical surgery for urinary bladder carcinoma. Cure is less probable if regional lymph node metastases are present. Evaluation of the metastatic status of carcinoma of the bladder or prostate has usually been performed by diagnostic sampling of pelvic lymph nodes. Morbidity from open and laparoscopic lymph node dissection was compared.

Methods.—Pelvic lymph node dissection was performed in 40 patients with bladder carcinoma. Of the 40 patients, 21 had an open procedure and 19 had a laparoscopic procedure. Postoperative analgesia, complications, and length of hospital stay were compared.

Results.—The number of harvested lymph nodes and percentage of patients with positive lymph nodes were similar for both groups. Among patients who underwent an open procedure, complications included 2 lymphoceles, 1 wound infection, and 1 ureteral lesion. The median hospital stay was 8 days. Among patients who had a laparoscopic procedure, 1 patient was changed to an open procedure because of perioperative bleeding. Other complications included 1 omental snip prolapse through a portincision, and 1 scrotal hematoma. The median hospital stay was 1 day. Patients who had a laparoscopic procedure required significantly less postoperative analgesia.

Discussion.—In these patients, there was significantly lower morbidity after laparoscopic lymph node dissection. Laparoscopic lymphadenectomy is safe and well tolerated by most patients, who experience relatively little pain and a rapid recovery.

▶ There is little argument in 1996 that a laparoscopic pelvic lymphadenectomy can be done safely, has comparable yield in terms of nodes to an open procedure, and causes less discomfort to the patient with quicker return to usual activities. It also takes longer and usually costs more. This study is difficult to evaluate in one respect because the later cystectomy was not done at comparable times after the lymphadenectomy in the 2 arms; the relative degree of pelvic fibrosis at later laparotomy would be interesting to compare.

I don't think initial laparoscopic lymphadenectomy is attractive for patients with bladder cancer unless the patient is selected to be at very high risk for metastasis, such as clinical T3b or worse tumor. Our management philosophy is such that if lymph node metastases are noted on an imaging study, initial chemotherapy is used. The main determinant for survival in this patient population is how well they respond to the chemotherapy. If they don't respond to the chemotherapy, no degree of surgery is going to work. On the other hand, in patients without gross adenopathy, the cystectomy is usually continued even if positive nodes are found because some patients with low volume nodal disease are cured with surgery alone. In addition, adjuvant chemotherapy may provide a benefit.

J.E. Montie, M.D.

Laparoscopic Nephroureterectomy for Upper Tract Transitional Cell Cancer: The Washington University Experience
McDougall EM, Clayman RV, Elashry O (Washington Univ, St Louis)
J Urol 154:975–980, 1995
19–22

Introduction.—For patients with benign disease requiring removal of the kidney, laparoscopic nephrectomy is a recognized form of therapy; however, the use of the technique in patients with upper tract transitional

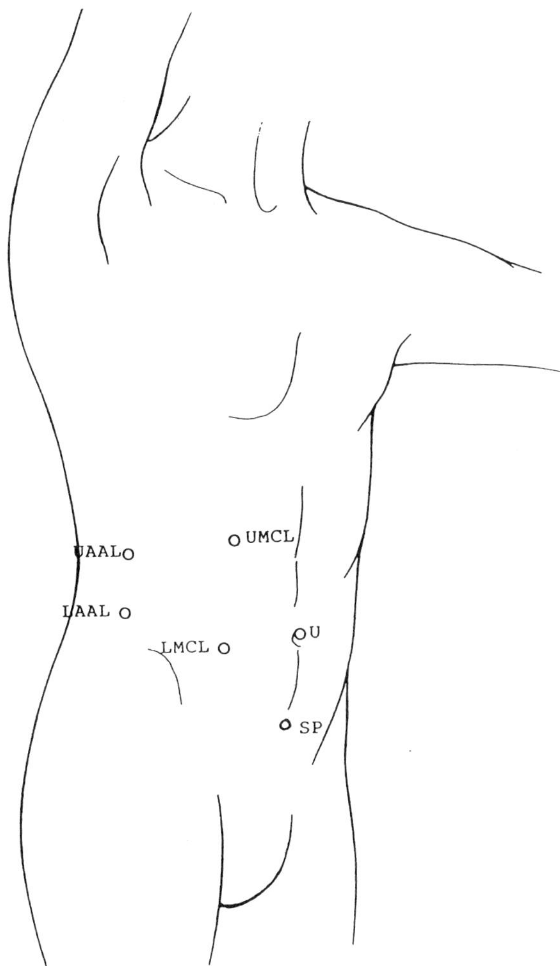

FIGURE.—Port placement for laparoscopic nephroureterectomy. *Abbreviations: U*, 12-mm umbilical port; *UMCL*, 12-mm upper midclavicular line port; *LMCL*, 5-mm lower midclavicular line port; *SP*, 12-mm suprapubic port; *UAAL*, 5-mm upper anterior axillary line port; *LAAL*, 5-mm lower anterior axillary line port. (Courtesy of McDougall EM, Clayman RV, Elashry O: Laparoscopic nephroureterectomy for upper tract transitional cell cancer: The Washington University experience. *J Urol* 154:975–980, 1995.)

cell cancer has been controversial. Ten patients who had laparoscopic nephroureterectomy for upper tract transitional cell carcinoma were compared with patients undergoing open nephroureterectomy for the same disease.

Methods.—Ten patients who had laparoscopic nephroureterectomy for upper tract transitional cell carcinoma were reviewed to determine operative time, surgical specimen weight, pathologic stage, postoperative analgesia, when normal oral intake resumed, postoperative recovery, and follow-up. They were compared with 8 patients who had open surgical nephroureterectomy. Laparoscopic nephroureterectomy involves the placement of a 12-mm trocar at the umbilicus, a 12-mm port below the costal margin, a 5 mm-port placed 2–3 cm below the level of the umbilicus, and a 12-mm trocar above the symphysis pubis (Figure).

Results.—Open nephroureterectomy took half as much time as laparoscopic nephroureterectomy. However, compared to the open surgical group, the patients who had the laparoscopic procedure resumed oral intake sooner, had a shorter hospital stay, and required less postoperative analgesia. The laparoscopic group completely recovered 5 times more rapidly than the open surgical group (6 weeks compared to 7.4 months). The open surgical group needed more than twice as much time to return to normal activities as the laparoscopic group, 2.7 weeks compared to 6 weeks.

Conclusion.—For patients with upper tract transitional cell carcinoma, laparoscopic nephroureterectomy is a feasible treatment option and is equal to open nephroureterectomy. The operative time is longer and there is need for significant laparoscopic experience on the part of the surgeon.

▶ Laparoscopic nephrectomy is feasible, and there is little reason to doubt that good results can be obtained in appropriately selected patients. The described technique assures removal of the entire ureter, including the intramural ureter. It is also clear that the procedure is a formidable one, even in the hands of some of the most experienced urologic laparoscopic surgeons in the world. I suspect a laparoscopic nephroureterectomy is an appropriate procedure for only a few surgeons possessing the breadth of expertise required. I also believe laparoscopic surgery is here to stay and will gradually increase in volume in concert with advances in technical support equipment. I am not as convinced as the authors are that more than a handful of urologists will command the needed credentials to do this surgery in the near future. Although theoretically the number and type of cases that could be performed laparoscopically is more than is currently done now, the reality is that relatively few cases in most centers are approached this way and it will be only a slow transition into more widespread use.

J.E. Montie, M.D.

20 Prostate and Benign Prostatic Hyperplasia

Benign Prostatic Hyperplasia Specific Health Status Measures in Clinical Research: How Much Change in the American Urological Association Symptom Index and the Benign Prostatic Hyperplasia Impact Index is Perceptible to Patients?
Barry MJ, Williford WO, Chang Y, Machi M, Jones KM, Walker-Corkery E, Lepor H (Massachusetts Gen Hosp, Boston; Veterans Affairs Med Ctr, Perry Point, Md; Med College of Wisconsin, Milwaukee; et al)
J Urol 154:1770–1774, 1995   20–1

Background.—Two self-administered questionnaires have been proposed by the American Urological Association (AUA) Measurement Committee to determine the health status significance of benign prostatic hyperplasia (BPH). The AUA symptom index measures symptom frequency, and the BPH impact index measures the health impact of symptoms. It is important to determine what changes in scores are perceptible to patients. Score changes on these indexes were correlated with patient global ratings of improvement in a large, randomized, double-blind trial of 4 BPH treatment strategies—placebo, finasteride, terazosin, and the combination of finasteride and terazosin.

Methods and Findings.—A total of 1,218 men were included in the study. Absolute score changes from baseline were compared with global ratings of improvement at 13 weeks. Men rating themselves as being slightly improved had a mean reduction of 3.1 points on the AUA symptom index. The mean decrease on the BPH impact index was 0.4 points. Baseline scores greatly affected this association.

Conclusions.—Individual researchers can use the data in this paper to select the index thresholds they wish to detect in their own studies. When comparing the outcomes of 2 or more treatments, the authors recommend presenting confidence intervals around differences in point estimates of the outcome measures so that readers will have more information than *P* values alone. Providing absolute differences in scores is also preferred when reporting changes in these indexes over time.

Percentage differences in scores are apparently not more closely related to patient global improvement ratings.

▶ The take-home message of this work is that the American Urological Association (AUA) symptom index and the benign prostatic hyperplasia impact index correlate well with patients' global assessment of their lower urinary tract symptoms thus making these 2 indices valuable tools in clinical trials. In this era of multiple emerging and competing options of management of lower urinary tract symptoms, the availability of these indices is, indeed, fortunate. They provide uniform and universal scales of outcomes that investigators can use in comparative clinical trials. I take exception to an important facet of this study. As mentioned in another editorial in this Year Book, patients in the cooperative Veterans Administration Trial 359 may not have had true prostatic enlargement resulting from benign prostatic hyperplasia. The ranges of prostate volumes of men in that VA study were not significantly different from prostate volumes of normal men of comparable age in an Omstead County Epidemiological Study.[1] Patients do not know whether their prostate glands are enlarged, nor do they know if they have true benign prostatic hyperplasia or some other urinary condition. They do know they have urinary tract symptoms, making this issue one of somatics from the patient's point of view. Nonetheless, as scientists we should not continue to consistently assign all lower urinary tract symptoms in aging men to the specific disease benign prostatic hyperplasia without proof that they in fact have prostate gland enlargement.

H.L. Holtgrewe, M.D.

Reference

1. Chute CG, Panser LA, Girman CJ, et al: The prevalence of prostatism: A population based survey of urinary symptoms. *J Urol* 150:85–89, 1993.

Health Status and Quality of Life of British Men With Lower Urinary Tract Symptoms: Results From the SF-36
Hunter DJW, McKee M, Black NA, Sanderson CFB (London School of Hygiene & Tropical Medicine)
Urology 45:962–971, 1995   20–2

Background.—Approximately 25% of all men of at least middle age have moderate or greater urinary symptoms of benign prostatic hyperplasia, yet the effect of these symptoms on health status and well-being have not been well characterized. The general health status and quality of life of men with urinary symptoms was assessed using the SF-36. The SF-36 is a validated, self-administered questionnaire used to measure general health status and quality of life. It has not been used to examine these issues in community-living men with lower urinary tract symptoms.

Methods.—Eight randomly chosen general practices in the North West Thames region provided lists of men aged 55 years and older. A database of 2,000 patients was created and the patients were surveyed for urinary tract symptoms. The response rate was 78%. Respondents were categorized by symptom severity and then resurveyed via the SF-36.

Findings.—The response rate to the SF-36 was 84%. Half of all men with moderate or greater urinary tract symptoms reported some interference in activities of daily living. Increasing symptom severity was associated with decreased physical activity, social functioning, vitality, mental health, and perception of general health status. There was a stronger association between being bothered by symptoms and scores on the SF-36, than there was with symptoms. Men who were bothered by their lower urinary tract symptoms had worse health status in all aspects except physical activity than the general population.

Conclusions.—General health status and quality of life were investigated in a group of British men of at least 55 years with lower urinary tract symptoms. There was a decrease in general health status and quality of life with increased urinary symptom severity and with the extent that these symptoms bothered the patient. There was a great deal of individual variation in how men respond to their symptoms.

▶ This study gives solid scientific confirmation to what those of us who have managed older men with lower urinary tract symptoms have come to recognize—that severity of symptoms correlates with a negative impact on quality of life and perception of general health status. In an era when few men are seen with major complications of urinary tract obstruction making surgery mandatory, relief of symptoms and improvement of impaired quality of life have become central to the treatment of their lower urinary tract symptoms. But of the 2, relief of symptoms or improvement in impaired quality of life, clearly the latter is more critical to patients and should be the determining force in their selection of therapy as they balance (with the assistance of their urologist) the probability of quality-of-life improvement against the possible harms and risks of the various strategies of management available in 1996.

H.L. Holtgrewe, M.D.

Transurethral Resection of the Prostate Versus Open Prostatectomy: Long-term Mortality Comparison
Crowley AR, Horowitz M, Chan E, Macchia RJ (Brooklyn Va Med Ctr and Scientific/Academic Computing Ctr, Brooklyn, NY; State Univ of New York at Brooklyn)
J Urol 153:695–697, 1995   20–3

Introduction.—Transurethral prostatic resection is a common procedure in the United States, but its safety has been questioned in recent years. To determine the long-term impact of transurethral vs. open prostatectomy on mortality rates, the medical records of 1,315 patients who underwent prostatectomy for benign disease from 1978 through 1987 were reviewed.

Patients and Methods.—The patients were treated at a single institution, with 1,125 having the transurethral procedure and 190 having open prostatectomy. Charts were complete and follow-up was adequate for 421 in the transurethral group and 106 in the open prostatectomy group. Long-term mortality was compared in the 2 groups overall and in a healthiest subgroup. Data collected included age, preoperative medical illnesses, urinary retention, type of anesthesia, health status, and cause of death.

Results.—The 2 operative groups, were similar in mean age, American Society of Anesthesiologists category distribution, and significant preoperative risk factors. Men in the open surgery group were almost twice as likely to require a catheter for urinary retention preoperatively and had a somewhat higher incidence of hypertension. With an average follow-up of 70.7 months, 77% of patients in the transurethral group were still alive; 78% of those who underwent open prostatectomy were still alive at an average follow-up of 71.4 months. Thus overall mortality was almost identical for the 2 groups. In the transurethral group, men without preoperative medical illness had a significantly better long-term survival than those with preoperative conditions, a finding not present in the open

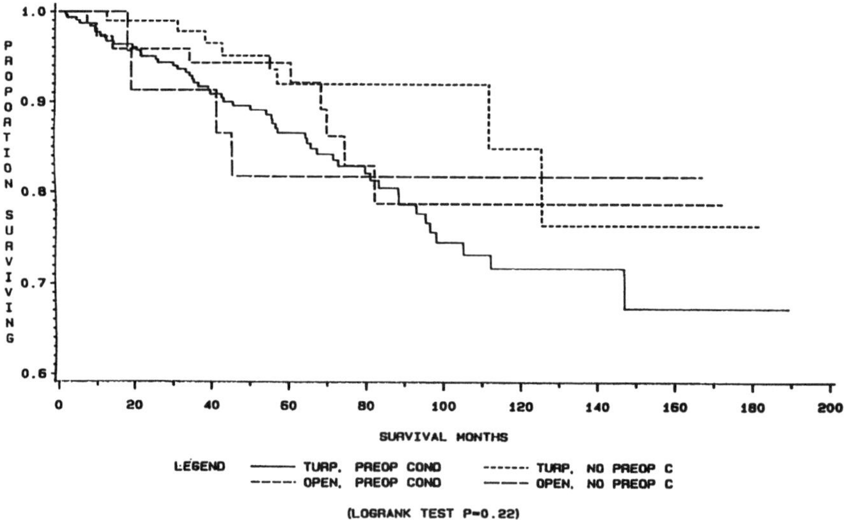

FIGURE 2.—Kaplan-Meier survival analysis (cardiac deaths censored). Numbers of censored patients without preoperative condition at 0, 20, 60, 80, and 120 months were 95, 92, 55, 27, and 12, respectively, for patients undergoing transurethral prostatectomy (TURP), and 24, 21, 14, 10, and 6, respectively, for those undergoing open surgery. Numbers of censored patients with preoperative condition were 304, 286, 166, 107, and 44, respectively, in transurethral resection group, and 74, 67, 45, 22, and 7, respectively, in open surgery group. (Courtesy of Crowley AR, Horowitz M, Chan E, et al: Transurethral resection of the prostate versus open prostatectomy: Long-term mortality comparison. *J Urol* 153:695–697, 1995.)

prostatectomy group. The healthiest subset of patients showed no significant survival difference, whatever procedure was used (Fig 2).

Conclusion.—Preoperative condition was a better predictor of long-term survival than type of procedure (transurethral vs. open surgery) in patients undergoing prostatectomy, and the significance of this factor was greater in the transurethral prostatectomy group. Studies showing increased long-term mortality after transurethral prostatectomy may have included more patients with significant cardiovascular disease in the transurethral groups than in the open procedure groups.

▶ The Roos et al.[1] article, which appeared in the *New England Journal of Medicine* in 1989, created much anxiety among patients and their urologists when discussing surgical options for benign prostatic hyperplasia. It seemed a self-fulfilling prophecy that patients who underwent transurethral resection of the prostate (TURP) would have more significant postoperative mortality than patients who underwent open prostatectomy. This is because patients who were too sick or frail to undergo open procedures would have a TUR. This article should put this issue to rest. After correction for co-morbidities, there is no difference in long-term mortality with these 2 time-honored methods of surgical treatment of bladder outlet obstruction.

S. Kaplan, M.D.

Reference

1. Roos NP, Wennberg JE, Malenka DJ, et al: Mortality and reoperation after open and transurethral resection of the prostate for benign prostatic hyperplasia. *New Engl J Med* 320:1120, 1989.

Does Catheter Traction Reduce Post-Transurethral Resection of the Prostate Blood Loss?
Walker EM, Bera S, Faiz M (Milton Keynes General NHS Trust, Milton Keynes, UK)
Br J Urol 75:614–617, 1995   20–4

Objective.—Traction on an indwelling catheter has been advocated to control postoperative bleeding after transurethral resection of the prostate (TURP), but its effects have yet to be evaluated. A prospective randomized trial was conducted to determine whether traction on a catheter after TURP reduces postoperative bleeding.

Study Design.—From 1992 to 1993, 115 consecutive patients undergoing TURP were assigned to receive either traction or no traction on the catheter. At the end of resection, a three-way 22 Ch Simplastic catheter was inserted and filled to approximately twice the volume of the resected prostate. For patients selected for traction, a 1.36 g of traction was applied to the catheter for 30 minutes using a pulley and weight system. Blood loss was measured during and for 2 hours after surgery.

Outcome.—In the group who did not receive traction, blood loss was greatest in the first 30 minutes after resection with a mean of 36.9 mL. Traction during this period significantly reduced blood loss to a mean of 14.8 mL. When traction was removed, blood loss was not significantly altered and there was no additional rebound bleeding. Operative blood loss correlated significantly with the duration of resection and weight of the prostate resected.

Conclusion.—Postoperative catheter traction is a useful technique to control post-TURP bleeding and is a valuable adjunct to careful operative hemostasis.

▶ Most of us have observed for a long time that traction can sometimes decrease bleeding immediately after TURP. This study confirms the observation. Of course, TUR is becoming less and less popular, and the newer techniques cause less bleedng. I suspect that the issue of traction after partial prostatectomy will become moot.

J.B. deKernion, M.D.

Transurethral Resection Versus Incision of the Prostate: A Randomized, Prospective Study
Riehmann M, Knes JM, Heisey D, Madsen PO, Bruskewitz RC (Univ of Wisconsin Hosp and Clinics, Madison; William S Middleton Mem Veterans Hosp, Madison, Wisc)
Urology 45:768–775, 1995   20–5

Introduction.—During the last 2 decades, transurethral incision of the prostate (TUIP) has become an increasingly popular alternative to transurethral resection (TURP) for patients with symptomatic benign prostatic hyperplasia (BPH). Although randomized studies of TUIP vs. TURP have been reported, follow-up times have been short. The longer-term results of 1 such study were assessed.

Methods.—The randomized, prospective trial included 120 patients with symptoms of bladder outlet obstruction caused by small benign prostates—estimated resectable weight was less than 20 g in every case. The patients were randomly assigned to undergo either TUIP or TURP. Before and at intervals after surgery, the patients were assessed in terms of urinary symptoms, sexual function, and uroflowmetric findings. Overall surgical outcome was evaluated in 112 patients at a mean follow-up of 34 months.

Results.—Both the TUIP and TURP groups showed improvements in mean urinary peak flow rates throughout the study period. The TURP group tended to have higher peak flow rates, although the difference was not statistically significant. Both groups at all follow-up intervals showed significant declines in irritative, obstructive, and total symptom scores. At no point were these scores significantly different between groups.

TABLE 1.—Comparison of TURP and TUIP

	Operating Time (min)	Blood Loss* (mL)	Catheter Time (days)	Postoperative Stay (days)
TURP				
Mean	55	190	2.5	4.3
Range	5–135	25–700	1–12	2–14
TUIP				
Mean	23	54	1.4	3.0
Range	7–95	5–300	1–3	1–8
P value	<0.0001	<0.0001	<0.0001	<0.0001

* Estimated blood loss.

Abbreviations: TURP, transurethral resection of the prostate; *TUIP*, transurethral incision of the prostate.

(Reprinted by permission of the publisher from "Transurethral resection versus incision of the prostate: A randomized, prospective study," by Riehmann M, Knes JM, Heisey D, et al: *UROLOGY* 45, pp. 768–775, Copyright 1995 by Elsevier Science, Inc.)

Both groups reported significant and similar subjective improvement at follow-up. Of the patients who were sexually active before and after surgery, 35% of the TUIP group and 68% of the TURP group had postoperative retrograde ejaculation. Further treatment for benign BPH-related infravesical obstruction was needed by 23% of the TUIP group and 16% of the TURP group, a nonsignificant difference. Operating time, blood loss, catheter time, and postoperative stay were all significantly less with TUIP (Table 1).

Conclusions.—For patients with BPH causing bladder outlet obstruction and small prostates, TUIP and TURP appear to be equally effective. The increased use of TUIP, an underutilized procedure, has great potential to reduce health care costs.

▶ Transurethral incision of the prostate (TUIP) has been termed "the most underutilized procedure" in urology. The results reported herein suggest that improvements in both subjective and objective parameters are equal for TUIP and TURP in carefully selected patients. Nevertheless, a number of caveats should be noted. Transurethral incision of the prostate should be done only in small prostates (in this series < 20 g) with short prostate urethras (in this series < 3 cm). The incidence of retrograde ejaculation is significantly less for TUIP than for TURP (in this series 35% vs. 68%). In our own experience, when utilizing a single incision at the 5 o'clock position, the incidence of retrograde ejaculation is less than 10%. Finally, the number of retreatments for both groups was unusually high. For the TUIP group, 8 patients required a TUR of the bladder neck. This reflects the potential hazards of performing TURP in small prostates. In the TUIP group, 23% of patients required a subsequent treatment of bladder outlet obstruction: 12 had a TURP, 1 had a second TUIP and required medication. Although the upfront cost of a TUIP is less than that of a TURP, this significant retreatment rate may make TUIP a less attractive option for patients and their insurance carriers.

S. Kaplan, M.D.

A Prospective Randomized Comparison of Transurethral Resection to Visual Laser Ablation of the Prostate for the Treatment of Benign Prostatic Hyperplasia

Cowles RS III, Kabalin JN, Childs S, Lepor H, Dixon C, Stein B, Zabbo A (Atlanta Ctr for Urology, Ga; Palo Alto Veterans Affairs Med Ctr, Calif; Stanford Univ, Calif; et al)
Urology 46:155–160, 1995   20–6

Introduction.—Bladder outlet obstruction caused by benign prostatic hyperplasia (BPH) is conventionally managed by transurethral resection of the prostate (TURP), a major operation that entails significant morbidity. An alternative approach is visual laser ablation of the prostate (VLAP) using a neodymium:yttrium-aluminum-garnet laser.

Objective and Methods.—The effectiveness and safety of the 2 procedures were examined in 115 men older than 50 years with symptomatic BPH who were accessed at 6 sites in the United States. Fifty-nine of them were randomly assigned to undergo TURP, wheres 56 patients in the VLAP group received an average of 10,200 J of energy in 5.5 intraprostatic laser applications. Most patients received a sequence of 4 applications midway between the verumontanum and bladder neck.

Results.—Transurethral resection of the prostate took considerably longer than VLAP (45 vs. 23 minutes). In both groups spinal anesthesia was used in a majority of cases, but general anesthesia was used more often in the VLAP group. Symptoms were eliminated more consistently by TURP 1 year postoperatively, but average symptom scores at last follow-up decreased in both groups (Table III). Peak urine flow increased in both groups, but the postvoid residual urine volume decreased less in the

TABLE III.—Principal Clinical Outcomes at 12 Months

Variable	VLAP (n = 55)	SD	TURP (n = 57)	SD	P Value
AUA-6 symptom score	−9.0 (−27 to 8)	8.9	−13.3 (−29 to 7)	7.5	< 0.04
Peak urine flow (cc/s)	5.3 (−5.9 to 26.6)	6.9	7.0 (−16.8 to 27.8)	9.5	0.27
Postvoid residual urine volume (cc)	−55.4 (−425 to 220)	124.3	138.8 (−728 to 130)	162.3	< 0.01
Quality of life: Patients improved	43 (78.2%)		53 (93.0%)		0.03

Abbreviations: VLAP, visual laser ablation of the prostate: *TURP,* transurethral resection of the prostate: *AUA,* American Urological Association.
(Reprinted by permission of the publisher from Cowles RS III, Kabalin JN, Childs S, et al: A prospective randomized comparison of transurethral resection to visual laser ablation of the prostate for the treatment of benign prostatic hyperplasia. *Urology* 46:155–160. Copyright 1995 by Elsevier Science, Inc.)

VLAP group. After 1 year, 93% of patients having TURP and 78% of those in the VLAP group reported an improved quality of life. Forty per cent of patients undergoing TURP had a greater than 2.2 g/dL decrease in hemoglobin, compared to a single patient who underwent VLAP. Serious treatment-related complications occurred in 11% of patients undergoing VLAP and 36% of patients undergoing TURP.

Conclusions.—Laser ablation is an effective means of relieving bladder outlet obstruction secondary to BPH. The low-energy technique removes less tissue than TURP, but the procedure causes less morbidity and is clinically effective.

▶ This article by some of the giants of laser prostatectomy documents the efficacy of VLAP (a low-energy coagulation necrosis technique) with conventional TURP. It demonstrates that the complication rate with VLAP is significantly less than with TURP (11% vs. 36%, $P < 0.01$). It also shows it is inferior to TURP in reduction of symptom scores and postvoid residual urine decreases, and in avoidance of urinary retention. I am surprised that maximum flow rates in the TURP group did not improve more. The VLAP was safer and quicker. It is of great interest that, although more patients with VLAP had dysuria (14% vs. 10%, $P = 0.58$), more patients who underwent TURP had pain (12% vs. 4%, $P = 0.16$). Neither of these were statistically significant differences. Often laser therapy is criticized for allegedly causing more dysuria and pain than does TURP. Many papers on TURP probably downplay the postoperative symptoms. Quality-of-life improvement was superior in the TURP group (93% vs. 78%, $P = 0.03$). The low-energy levels used in this VLAP study, between 5,760 and 11,520 mean J, are *much* less than subsequent treatment schema and adversely impacted on the results. This study demonstrates that low-energy VLAP, on balance, compares favorably with TURP. Subsequent higher energy level laser techniques (both coagulative and evaporative) are discussed in the paper by Narayan et al.[1] and show even better laser results.

D.L. McCullough, M.D.

Reference

1. Narayan P, Tewari A, Aboseif S, et al: A randomized study comparing visual laser ablation and transurethral evaporation of prostate in the management of benign prostatic hyperplasia. *J Urol* 154:2083–2088, 1995.

A Multicenter, Randomized, Prospective Study of Endoscopic Laser Ablation Versus Transurethral Resection of the Prostate

Anson K, Nawrocki J, Buckley J, Fowler C, Kirby R, Lawrence W, Paterson P, Watson G (Middlesex Hosp, London; Brighton Gen Hosp, Sussex, England; Royal Infirmary, Glasgow, Scotland; et al)

Urology 46:305–310, 1995

Objective.—A prospective, randomized, multicenter study was planned to compare endoscopic laser ablation of the prostate (ELAP) with conventional transurethral resection (TURP) in 151 patients having bladder outflow obstruction secondary to benign prostatic hyperplasia (BPH).

Patients.—Seventy-six patients 52–84 years of age were randomly assigned to ELAP, and 75 to TURP. The average age was 68 years. All patients were more than 50 years of age, had urine flow rates consistent with outflow obstruction, and had an estimated prostatic urethra more than 2.4 cm long. A total of 137 patients were followed for 1 year or longer.

Methods.—Endoscopic laser ablation of the prostate was performed using the Urolase fiber and the Nd-YAG laser after cystourethroscopy had excluded synchronous bladder lesions. Laser energy of 60 W was delivered for 1 minute at the 2-, 5-, 7-, and 10-o'clock positions midway between the verumontanum and bladder neck. An additional round of 4-quadrant treatment was delivered if the prostatic urethral length exceeded 4.0 cm.

Efficacy.—Symptom scores and maximal flow rates indicated that both treatments were significantly effective. Symptoms were relieved more consistently at 1 year in patients having TURP, and maximum flow rates were higher than after the laser procedure. In addition, residual urine volume

TABLE V.—List of Major Complications for All Patients Treated

	TURP (n = 75)	ELAP (n = 76)
Failed treatment	—	5
Dysuria	6	25
Clot retention	5	1*
Secondary hemorrhage	3	—
Epididymo-orchitis	1	2
Deep vein thrombosis	2	1
Pulmonary embolus	1	—
Laparotomies	—	3*
Myocardial infarction	1	—
Cerebrovascular accident	—	1

* One episode of clot urinary retention, which was managed conservatively, occurred 24 days after an ELAP procedure. Three patients required laparotomies at various times after ELAP.

Abbreviations: TURP, transurethral resection of the prostate; *ELAP,* endoscopic laser ablation of the prostate.

was reduced more in the patients undergoing TURP. Retrograde ejaculation was described by 33% of patients in the ELAP group and 63% of those having TURP 1 year after treatment.

Safety.—One death in each group was unrelated to treatment. The hemoglobin decreased less after ELAP than in the TURP patients, 16% of whom required blood transfusion. Urinary tract infection and dysuria, however, were more frequent in the ELAP group (Table V).

Conclusions.—These preliminary findings suggest that TURP is more effective than ELAP in relieving symptoms of bladder outlet obstruction in patients with BPH. The latter procedure is, however, a useful alternative to TURP.

▶ The authors report a relatively large, prospective, randomized study comparing endoscopic laser ablation of the prostate (ELAP) and TURP with 1-year follow-up. The results reported are consistent with what most urologists in the community believe: ELAP works but not as well as TURP. However, a number of phenomena occurred in this study that should be highlighted. (1) The tranfusion rate for the TURP group was 16%. This is significantly higher than that reported for more contemporary series of TURP. (2) The urinary tract infection rate was much higher in the ELAP group. This is a common theme in laser prostatectomy series and probably reflects longer postoperative catheterization time. (3) The improvements in urodynamic parameters in the ELAP group are significantly less than in the TURP group. In fact, the improvement on peak uroflow (Qmax) of 5.5 mL/sec at 1 year is more consistent with reported increases with other "coagulation necrosis" techniques such as thermotherapy, and transurethral needle ablation (TUNA).

S. Kaplan, M.D.

Neodymium: YAG Laser Coagulation Prostatectomy: 3 Years of Experience With 227 Patients
Kabalin JN, Bite G, Doll S (Palo Alto Veterans Affairs Med Ctr, Calif; Stanford Univ, Calif)
J Urol 155:181–185, 1996   20–8

Introduction.—Laser coagulation prostatectomy with neodymium:YAG (Nd:YAG) wavelength appears to be a safe procedure of particular value in the management of high-risk patients. A cohort of 227 men who underwent Nd:YAG for symptomatic bladder outlet obstruction was prospectively followed for the long-term efficacy and durability of the procedure.

Methods.—The patients were treated with the Urolase right-angle firing laser fiber between October 15, 1991 and October 15, 1994. A known histologic diagnosis of prostate cancer was present in 101 patients. Before treatment, excess or resectable benign prostatic hyperplasia tissue was estimated on the basis of cystoscopic appearance and digital palpation. Application of the laser produces coagulation necrosis of treated tissue, followed by dissolution and slough. In the last 156 cases, a 40-W power setting was combined with continuous 90-sec spot application times. Patients were followed for complications, voiding outcomes, and symptom scores.

Results.—With a median follow-up of 26 months, all measured voiding parameters showed significant improvement. At least a 50% improvement in peak urinary flow rate or symptom score was present in 80% to 90% of patients at 1, 2, or 3 years postoperatively. Voiding outcomes in patients with prostate cancer did not differ significantly from those in the group as a whole. Only 4 men reported that their symptoms were worse than before surgery. Overall, 87% felt that their quality of life was improved after the procedure. Complications included reoperation for residual prostate tissue (5.3%), bladder neck contracture (4.4%), prostatitis (2.6%), and urethral stricture (1.8%). When postoperative ejaculatory function was evaluated in 135 sexually active patients, 98 reported preservation of antegrade ejaculation and 37 reported new retrograde ejaculation.

Conclusion.—The voiding outcomes in the series of patients treated with Nd:YAG laser coagulation prostatectomy compared favorably to those reported for standard electrocautery resection of the prostate. Resolution of symptomatic bladder outlet obstruction persisted for at least 3 years, and the laser procedure has the advantage of minimal morbidity.

▶ The Stanford group has been the leading proponent of laser coagulation prostatectomy. In numerous previous reports, the improvements in both symptoms and flow rates have consistently approached that of contemporary transurethral resection series. Unfortunately, results reported from other multicenter series (see Abstract 20–7) have not approached the results reported herein. This reflects a common problem in assessing new technologies. Most initial reports are single investigator, single center, nonrandomized trials. In addition, new technologies undergo evolution with time. For example, in this series, the incidence of retrograde ejaculation was 27%, which is much higher than earlier reports from the same group. This result reflects increased thermal energy applied to the prostate and bladder neck. Ultimately, given the cost of laser technology and the advent of equally efficient, less expensive methods of performing prostatectomy, the role of laser coagulation prostatectomy in the future remains to be determined.

S. Kaplan, M.D.

Transurethral Microwave Thermotherapy versus Transurethral Resection for Symptomatic Benign Prostatic Obstruction: A Prospective Randomized Study With a 2-Year Follow-Up
Dahlstrand C, Waldén M, Geirsson G, Pettersson S (Sahlgrenska Univ Hosp, Göteborg, Sweden)
Br J Urol 76:614–618, 1995   20–9

Introduction.—No matter what the diagnostic technique, there is an age-related increase in benign prostatic hypertrophy (BPH). The common symptoms are classified as obstructive and irritative. There are varying degrees of outflow obstruction and between 30% and 70% of patients undergoing transurethral resection of the prostate (TURP) describe little or no obstruction. In patients with mild obstruction and few symptoms, the "gold standard" TURP procedure has less than favorable results. Thus, the appropriate treatment for patients with BPH is still under question and new treatment methods are still of interest. Recently, the transrectal microwave thermotherapy method has been modified for a transurethral approach. The results of a randomized trial of patients treated with either TURP or thermotherapy were evaluated.

Methods.—To be included in the study, the men had to have a prostate length of 35–50 mm and a Madsen and Iversen score of at least 8. A total of 72 patients with benign prostatic hypertrophy were randomly divided into a TURP (n=35) or a thermotherapy (n=37) group. Diagnostic tests were obtained before and 3, 6, 12, and 24 months postoperatively. Although the TURP procedures were performed by senior surgeons, only 1 surgeon performed the outpatient thermotherapy procedure using materials and software capable of delivering 60 W of microwave energy. Before the thermotherapy treatment, 50 mg of indomethacin and 400 mg of norfloxacin were given. After treatment, norfloxacin was continued twice daily for 5 days, indomethacin was given twice for 1 day and postprocedure catheters were used only if the patient was unable to void before discharge.

Results.—The randomization procedure resulted in 2 statistically similar groups. The 2-year follow-up was complete for all but 10 patients. The average time for the TURP procedure was 48 minutes followed by a 4-day hospital stay. Four patients who underwent thermotherapy were dissatisfied with their results. Two underwent repeat thermotherapy and 2 underwent TURP. Both treatment methods improved the symptom score, residual volume of urine, the rate of free flow of urine, and infravesical obstruction. The latter 2 variables showed greater improvement after TURP. Serious complications, leading to further surgeries, occurred only in patients undergoing TURP.

Conclusion.—Thermotherapy and TURP deliver similar results in patients with benign prostatic hypertrophy and the positive outcomes continue for 2 years. The improvement after thermotherapy, sufficient to improve micturition to levels typical of asymptomatic elderly men, was not as obvious as the improvement with TURP.

▶ This excellent study has evaluated a new outpatient therapy for symptomatic benign prostatic hyperplasia and compared it to a known surgical standard. The authors highlight the reduced morbidity of the new treatment as well as its durability for a 2-year follow-up period. The objective improvements in pressure flow parameters after transurethral microwave thermotherapy (TUMT) were not as dramatic as in those treated by TURP where tissue was directly removed. I would agree in principle with the contention that TURP may overcorrect the bladder outlet obstruction at the potential cost of higher morbidity, whereas the lesser morbid treatment of TUMT may allow voiding parameters to return into a range comparable to an age-matched asymptomatic population. Clearly, further multicenter studies on larger numbers of patients followed for a longer period of time are appropriate to validate this important observation.

A. Patel, M.S., F.R.C.S. (Urol.)

Microwave Hyperthermia in Benign Prostatic Hypertrophy: A Controlled Clinical Trial
Venn SN, Montgomery BSI, Sheppard SA, Hughes SW, Beard RC, Bultitiude MI, Lloyd-Davies RW, Tiptaft RC (St Thomas' Hospital, London; Worthing Hosp, Worthing, England)
Br J Urol 76:73–76, 1995   20–10

Introduction.—Microwave hyperthermia has been used for a decade in treating bladder outflow obstruction (BOO) caused by benign prostatic hypertrophy (BPH), but few studies have examined the value of hyperthermia relative to sham treatment. A controlled clinical trial enrolling 96 patients with BPH sought to determine the effects of microwave hyperthermia on subjective and objective measures of BOO.

Patients and Methods.—Before study entry and at 3 and 6 months after treatment, patients underwent a full subjective and objective assessment of their condition. Examinations conducted before enrollment in the trial included urine culture and cytology, ultrasonography of the urinary tract, and urodynamic studies. Excluded were patients with previous surgery on the lower urinary tract and those with evidence of prostate or bladder cancer. Forty-eight patients were randomly assigned to microwave hyperthermia and 48 to a sham treatment.

Results.—Ninety-three patients were evaluated at 3 months and 62 at 6 months. Symptom scores showed an overall improvement of 40%, with no significant difference between treated and control groups (Table 4). The only significant difference observed was in the American Urological Association bothersome score at 3 months. For both treatment and control groups, the median pressure of the detrusor at maximum urinary flow and the median change in urinary flow rate (Table 5) showed no significant

TABLE 4.—Median Percentage Change in the Symptom Scores for the Treated and Control Groups After Treatment

| | 3 months | | 6 months | |
	Treated	Control	Treated	Control
Number	47	46	42	20
Madsen score (range)	42 (100–14)	38 (100–20)	44 (100–33)	35 (100–67)
AUA (range)	17 (88–83)	30 (95–60)	21 (100–116)	35 (68–83)
AUA b (range)	12 (100–67)	60 (100–100)	17 (100–180)	55 (100–50)

Abbreviations: AUA, American Urological Association score: *AUA b:* bothersome score.
(Courtesy of Venn SN, Montgomery BSI, Sheppard SA, et al: Microwave hyperthermia in benign prostatic hypertrophy: A controlled clinical trial. *Br J Urol* 76:73–76, 1995.)

TABLE 5.—Changes in Urinary Flow Rate and Residual Urine Volumes After Treatment With or Without Microwave Hyperthermia

	Treated			Control		
	Better	Same	Worse	Better	Same	Worse
Urinary flow rate change > 5 mL	3	43	1	1	45	0
Residual urine volume change	5	31	6	5	33	7

(Courtesy of Venn SN, Montgomery BSI, Sheppard SA, et al: Microwave hyperthermia in benign prostatic hypertrophy: A controlled clinical trial. *Br J Urol* 76:73–76, 1995.)

changes from baseline to the follow-up periods. Multivariate analysis using subjective improvement as the outcome variable and 10 subjective and objective factors as predictors yielded no predictor of improved outcome.

Conclusion.—In this study of the potential benefits of microwave hyperthermia, both treatment and control groups experienced significant subjective improvement. No predictor indicated which patients were likely to improve, however, and objective assessment of BOO found hyperthermia to have no advantages over sham treatment. The placebo effect appears to be important in BOO caused by BPH.

▶ The authors describe a randomized clinical trial comparing sham treatment with microwave hyperthermia of the prostate using a helical antenna and a new microwave frequency (434 MHz). The large subjective placebo effect they have observed can certainly be influenced by the natural history of clinical BPH and the selection of patients with moderate-to-severe symptoms who are most likely to benefit from intervention. It is unfortunate that only half of the control group were available for follow-up at 6 months. The lack of objective change in the "treated" group is probably related to an inadequate thermal dose from this particular device. Optical interstitial thermometry mapping studies in the critical evaluation of any new tissue heating therapy for BPH are certainly to be recommended. This study reemphasizes the need for careful evaluation of new physical treatment modalities for symptomatic BPH by sham studies and the authors are to be commended in this respect. The quality of such sham studies can be improved further only by prospective blinded design of both treatment and outcome evaluation and by determining the efficiency of the blinding procedure 6–12 months after the treatment has been completed.

A. Patel, M.S., F.R.C.S. (Urol.)

The Prediction of Clinical Outcome From Transurethral Microwave Thermotherapy by Pressure-Flow Analysis: A European Multicenter Study

Tubaro A, Carter SSC, de la Rosette J, Höfner K, Trucchi A, Ogden C, Miano L, Valenti M, Jonas U, Debruyne F (L'Aquila Univ, Rome; "La Sapienza" Univ, Rome; Charing Cross Hosp, London; et al)

J Urol 153:1526–1530, 1995   20–11

Introduction.—For benign prostatic obstruction, transurethral microwave thermotherapy is a minimally invasive treatment. Contradictory data exist on outcomes, and treatment is difficult to forecast for patients. To evaluate any predictive parameters that might identify patients who would respond best to microwave thermotherapy, a retrospective analysis was conducted on 100 patients who had transurethral microwave thermotherapy for benign prostatic obstruction.

Methods.—Patients with benign prostatic obstruction received microwave thermotherapy and were divided into 2 groups: those who had a constrictive obstruction and those who had a compressive obstruction. Treatment was 60 minutes with a maximum power output of 60 W and a total possible power deposition of 197 kJ. The C10 catheter had the microwave applicator located 10 mm below the Foley balloon. Clinical outcomes were compared at 6 months. Data were analyzed for changes in uroflowmetry, symptom score evaluation, and residual urine.

Results.—At entry, patients had a maximum flow rate of 15 mL/sec or less, residual urine volume of 300 mL or less, and a Madsen-Iversen score of 8 or more. In both groups, the change in Madsen-Iversen score was the same. In the constrictive group, maximum flow rate increased from 8.71 ± 2.62 to 14.73 ± 4.04 mL/sec and residual urine decreased from 96.00 ± 72.85 to 40.34 ± 56.33 mL. In the compressive group, maximum flow rate increased from 8.54 ± 2.26 to 10.41 ± 4.52 mL and residual urine decreased from 109.86 ± 67.09 to 84.65 ± 81.45 mL. In 68% of the constrictive, and in 15% of the compressive group, there was success, with an increase of 50% or more in maximum flow and a good Madsen-Iversen score.

Conclusion.—Patients being considered for thermotherapy should be selected by pressure-flow criteria to improve the overall clinical results. An analysis of the type of obstruction could be performed at a urodynamic laboratory when pressure-flow tracings are evaluated.

▶ This retrospective analysis suggests that responders to transurethral microwave thermotherapy (TUMT) may be selected on the basis of pretreatment urodynamic characterization of voiding dysfunction with pressure-flow cystometry. The authors suggest that those with constrictive obstruction are most likely to benefit from this new treatment. I believe that it is hard to justify routine (and expensive) invasive studies of this nature in daily clinical practice, until the positive predictive value of such testing has been validated by prospective multicenter studies using standardized urodynamic protocols and techniques in patients with symptomatic benign prostatic hyperplasia. Furthermore, in today's restrictive fiscal health care climate, such tests can only be prohibitive to the overall cost/benefits of this new outpatient treatment unless the outcomes are at least as good and as durable as those achieved by treatments that do not require initial pressure-flow studies.

A. Patel, M.S., F.R.C.S. (Urol.)

A Comparative Study of Transurethral Resection of the Prostate Using a Modified Electro-Vaporizing Loop and Transurethral Laser Vaporization of the Prostate

Kaplan SA, Te AE (Columbia Univ, New York)
J Urol 154:1785–1790, 1995   20–12

Purpose.—A number of alternatives to transurethral resection of the prostate for patients with benign prostatic hyperplasia (BPH) have been proposed, with the goals of reducing morbidity, hospital stay, and cost. The results of laser therapy for BPH have been variable; most reported techniques have used noncontact coagulation with low-power or higher-energy contact vaporization of the prostate. A modified transurethral resection technique using the VaporTrode vaporizing electrode was compared with transurethral laser vaporization of the prostate using the Ultraline fiber.

Methods.—The study included 58 patients with moderate-to-severe symptoms of prostatism. Twenty-nine consecutive patients underwent transurethral electrovaporization of the prostate beginning in 1994. They were compared with 29 consecutive, noncurrent patients who had transurethral laser evaporation of the prostate. Safety and efficacy were evaluated at baseline, 1 week, and 1 and 3 months. The 2 treatment groups were compared for operative time, postoperative catheterization time, American Urologic Association (AUA) symptom score, peak urine flow, and postvoid residual urine.

Results.—In the patients undergoing electrovaporization, AUA symptom score declined from 15.3 at baseline to 5.3 at 1 month and 4.9 at 2 months. Their mean peak urine flow increased from 8.2 to 14.9 mL/sec at 1 month and 15.6 mL/sec at 3 months. For the patients treated with laser vaporization, AUA symptom score decreased from 14.7 to 10.1 at 1 month and 7.6 at 3 months, while peak urine flow increased from 9.7 to 13.7 at 1 month and to 14.9 mL/sec at 3 months. These differences were not significant. However, mean catheterization time was 14.7 hours in the electrovaporization group compared to 79.6 hours in the laser group. Just 3 patients in the electrovaporization group had postoperative irritative symptoms, compared to 19 patients in the laser group. None of the patients in the electrovaporization group required repeat catheterization because of urinary retention, compared to 6 in the laser group.

Conclusions.—Initial experience suggests that electrovaporization of the prostate has some important advantages over laser vaporization. Although the 2 procedures are equally effective, electrovaporization appears to have a lower rate of postoperative morbidity. The long-term efficacy and safety of electrovaporization as a treatment for symptomatic BPH are being evaluated in a multicenter clinical trial.

▶ This retrospective study has compared a new electrosurgical prostate treatment with an established form of high-energy laser vaporization of the prostate. In the short term, advantages in favor of electrovaporization resulted from reduced catheterization time and a lower incidence of postoperative irritative symptoms. The explanation for these findings is not entirely clear and, in my view, may relate to differences in energy utilization and depth of tissue coagulative necrosis, which ultimately influences healing time.[1] At 3 months, however, subjective and objective outcomes were equivalent. Prospective double-blinded randomized comparisons with the community gold standard of transurethral resection of the prostate and longer follow-up are essential to validate the initial promise of this new electrosurgical treatment.

A. Patel, M.S., F.R.C.S. (Urol.)

Reference

1. Marks LS, Dorey F, Treiger B, Patel A: Electrovaporization vs laser prostatectomy: Comparison of anatomic and clinical outcomes. *J Urol* 155 (Suppl 24): 316A, 1996.

A Randomized Study Comparing Visual Laser Ablation and Transurethral Evaporation of Prostate in the Management of Benign Prostatic Hyperplasia
Narayan P, Tewari A, Aboseif S, Evans C (Univ of Florida, Gainesville; Univ of California, San Francisco)
J Urol 154:2083–2088, 1995   20–13

Background.—The Nd:YAG laser is increasingly used in place of transurethral electroresection as a treatment for symptomatic benign prostatic hyperplasia (BPH). Two methods are currently used. The coagulative method applies laser energy in a noncontact mode, and the treated tissue eventually necroses and sloughs. The operating time is relatively short, but one third of patients have prolonged urinary retention and many will require retreatment. The evaporative technique utilizes a high-power density laser output in contact with tissue.

Objective.—The 2 methods of transurethral laser treatment were contrasted in 64 consecutive patients with symptomatic BPH. Thirty-two patients were randomly assigned to evaporative treatment, and 32 to a modified coagulative technique. Six and 3 patients, respectively, had urinary retention at the time of treatment. Baseline American Urological Association (AUA) symptom scores were comparable in the 2 treatment groups.

Results.—The AUA scores decreased significantly in both groups of patients. Average scores were more than 50% lower at 1 month, and at 1 year were approximately 75% below baseline. Peak flow rates improved significantly in both groups, but significantly greater improvement occurred with evaporative treatment in the first year of follow-up. Total applied energy was significantly greater in this group. Sixteen percent of patients assigned to coagulative treatment but none of those treated by evaporation required reoperation. Prolonged irritative symptoms were similarly frequent in the 2 groups.

Conclusion.—Transurethral evaporative laser treatment fails less often than does the coagulative method, and provides superior clinical results for at least the first year.

▶ The authors provide good evidence that vaporization techniques provide significantly better long-term flow rates and a reoperative rate of 0% vs. a reoperative rate of 16% in the coagulation group. I have long favored vaporization techniques and have used them exclusively the last 2 years and agree that prolonged catheterization is rarely necessary in such patients. Creation of an "instant lumen" as accomplished with a standard transurethral resection of the prostate (TURP) is a worthy goal and one that evaporative laser techniques achieve. It appears that the additional time and effort required by the evaporative technique are worth the effort in virtually eliminating reoperations.

D.L. McCullough, M.D.

Randomized Double-Blind Study Comparing the Efficacy of Terazosin Versus Placebo in Women With Prostatism-Like Symptoms

Lepor H, Theune C (New York Univ; Med College of Wisconsin, Milwaukee)
J Urol 154:116–118, 1995   20–14

Background.—Terazosin is a long-acting selective α1-blocker that appears to be safe and effective in the treatment of benign prostatic hyperplasia (BPH). This agent has been found to significantly increase peak urinary flow rate and reduce symptom scores in men with BPH. Its efficacy against prostatism-like symptoms in women was investigated.

Methods.—Twenty-nine women aged 47–79 years were enrolled in the randomized, double-blind study. Fourteen received terazosin, and 15, placebo. Enrollment criteria included an American Urologic Association (AUA) symptom index exceeding 8, postvoid residual volume of less than 300 mL, and no history of stress urinary incontinence or recurrent urinary tract infection.

Findings.—In the placebo group, the AUA symptom score was 12.7 at baseline and 10.7 at the most recent follow-up. The corresponding scores in the active treatment group were 16.4 and 13.6. The between-group differences in AUA score change were not significant statistically or clinically.

Conclusions.—This pilot study suggests that α1-blockers are ineffective for alleviating prostatism-like symptoms in unselected female patients. The pathophysiology for this symptomatology is gender-specific. Selective α-blockers have been found to be useful in about 50% of men. Male nonresponders and women with prostatism-like symptoms may have a similar disease process.

▶ This is a well-done, prospective, randomized study. It is curious that, in spite of randomization, the treatment group had statistically significantly higher baseline scores. They also had higher symptom scores and lower flow rates, but these changes were not significant. It was logical to expect that α-blockers might help women with voiding difficulties and increased AUA symptom scores. Unfortunately, this was not the case.

S.S. Howards, M.D.

Five-Year Follow-Up of Patients With Benign Prostatic Hyperplasia Treated With Finasteride
Geller J (Univ of California, San Diego)
Eur Urol 27:267–273, 1995
20–15

Introduction.—Finasteride, a 5α-reductase inhibitor, prevents formation of dihydrotestosterone, the major mitogen regulating prostatic cell growth. Treatment with finasteride for 1–3 years has been shown to reduce prostate volume significantly, increase maximal flow rates, and reduce symptoms in patients with benign prostatic hyperplasia (BPH). The longer-term effects of finasteride treatment were investigated in 18 patients who underwent reevaluation after 5 years of treatment.
Methods.—Eighteen patients with BPH who had participated in 2 double-blind clinical trials of finasteride were offered open extension treatment and completed at least 60 months of treatment. These patients and 18 other patients who discontinued treatment at 6–54 months were evaluated for prostate volume, maximum urinary flow rate, and symptom score (including assessments of nocturia, frequency greater than every 2 hours, strength of stream, urinary urgency, urinary intermittency, and incomplete bladder emptying). Clinical improvement was indicated by a decrease of at least 2 units in the symptom score and/or an increase in the maximum urinary flow rate of 3 mL/sec.
Results.—The 18 patients who completed 5 years of treatment demonstrated an average 24% decrease in prostate volume, which mainly occurred during the first 12 months of treatment. There was only a modest decrease in the maximum urinary flow rate between 1 and 5 years of treatment. The significance of the change could not be assessed because there were no reliable baseline measurements of maximum urinary flow rate. There was a highly significant decline in symptom scores, with the majority of the decrease occurring within the first 12 months, but followed by further significant decreases. Of the 18 patients completing 5 years of

therapy, 12 had clinical improvement, 6 had stable BPH, and none had progressive disease. Among the 18 patients who discontinued treatment earlier, 83% demonstrated clinical improvement or stability. Sexual dysfunction was the only side effect, which occurred in 11 patients and could be attributed to finasteride treatment in 3.

Conclusions.—Treatment with finasteride for 5 years arrested the process of BPH in all of the patients, resulting in reduced prostate volume and symptomatic improvement or stability. Further study is needed to confirm these findings in a larger cohort and to identify reliable criteria that will identify patients in whom BPH is likely to progress.

Proscar: Five-Year Experience

Moore E, Bracken B, Bremner W, Geller J, Imperato-McGinley J, McConnell J, Roy J, Tenover L, Vaughan D, Pappas F, Cook T, Gormley G, Stoner E (Merck Research Labs, Rahway, NJ)
Eur Urol 28:304–309, 1995   20–16

Background.—Recent studies have demonstrated that finasteride (Proscar) lowers levels of dihydrotestosterone (DHT), reduces prostate size, and improves urinary flow and symptoms in patients with benign prostatic hyperplasia (BPH). The longest follow-up data to date on patients treated with finasteride for 5 years in the open extension phase of previously reported trials were analyzed.

Patients and Methods.—Eighty-five patients who had participated in double-blind trials of finasteride therapy continued into the fifth year of the open-label study. Seventy of these men had safety data available for analysis and 54 had complete efficacy data. The mean age of the patients at the start of the double-blind studies was 67 years. Efficacy and safety were evaluated every 4 months and prostate size was measured with MRI every 6 months from year 1 through year 3 and annually thereafter. Also assessed were serum testosterone and DHT concentrations, serum prostate-specific antigen (PSA), urinary flow rate, and BPH symptoms.

TABLE 1.—Summary of Efficacy Variables

	Baseline	Year 1 (n = 54)	Year 5 (n = 54)
Median prostate volume, cm^3	79.9	53.5	48.5
Median DHT, ng/dl	47.0	9.9	9.5
Median PSA, ng/dl	2.1	1.4	1.0
Maximum urinary flow*, cm^3/s	10.8	12.9	12.3
Total mean symptom score†	—‡	7.3	6.3

* Urinary flow machine changed from month 7 to 18.
† Range = 0 (absence of symptoms) to 35 (worst response to all symptoms).
‡ The baseline symptom score questionnaire was different in the 2 studies.
Abbreviations: DHT, dihydrotestosterone; *PSA,* prostate-specific antigen.
(Courtesy of Moore E, Bracken B, Bremner W, et al: Proscar: Five-year experience. *Eur Urol* 28:304–309, 1995. S. Karger AG, Basel, publisher.)

Results.—After 5 years of continuous finasteride treatment, prostate volume showed a mean reduction of 30% from baseline. The median percent change from baseline in PSA was 53.7%; median DHT fell from 47.0 ng/dL at baseline to 9.5 ng/dL at year 5, a median decrease of 76.6%. Improvements were also sustained in maximum urinary flow and mean symptom scores (Table 1). No serious drug-related events were reported in years 3–5. The most common reasons for discontinuing finasteride treatment were lack of clinical improvement, decreased libido and impotence, and cardiovascular adverse events.

Conclusion.—With 5 years of follow-up, finasteride is confirmed to be an effective and well-tolerated treatment for BPH. Adverse sexual experiences were reported by approximately 10% of patients, but the incidence of such side effects did not increase with increasing duration of treatment. The benefits of finasteride are sustained during long-term treatment and represent a reversal of the natural progression of BPH.

Can Finasteride Reverse the Progress of Benign Prostatic Hyperplasia? A Two-Year Placebo-Controlled Study
Andersen JT, Ekman P, Wolf H, Beisland HO, Johansson JE, Kontturi M, Lehtonen T, Tveter K, and the Scandinavian BPH Study Group (Univ of Copenhagen, Denmark)
Urology 46:631–637, 1995   20–17

Introduction.—Clinical studies with 6–12 months of follow-up have shown finasteride, a potent inhibitor of 5α-reductase, to reduce prostate volume and relieve the obstructive and irritative symptoms of benign prostatic hyperplasia (BPH). In a multicenter study patients were followed for 2 years to determine the drug's safety, efficacy, and ability to reverse the progress of BPH.

Patients and Methods.—The double-blind, placebo-controlled trial involved 707 patients enrolled at 59 centers. All patients were in general good health and had moderate symptoms of BPH; the mean age of the group was 65.5 years. After a 1-month, single-blind placebo run-in period, patients were randomly assigned to finasteride (5 mg once daily) or placebo for 24 months. Patients completed a symptom questionnaire at baseline and at scheduled follow-up visits. Urinary flow rates were obtained at these visits for all patients and prostate volume measured in a subset of 416 patients. Postvoiding residual urine volume and serum prostate-specific antigen were measured in all patients at screening and at 12 and 24 months.

Results.—Placebo-treated patients experienced a small improvement in total symptom score in the first 12 months but returned to baseline scores at 24 months. In contrast, patients in the finasteride group continued to show improvement throughout the treatment period. The difference between the groups was significant at 12 and 24 months. Prostate volume decreased a mean of 19% in the finasteride group and increased a mean of

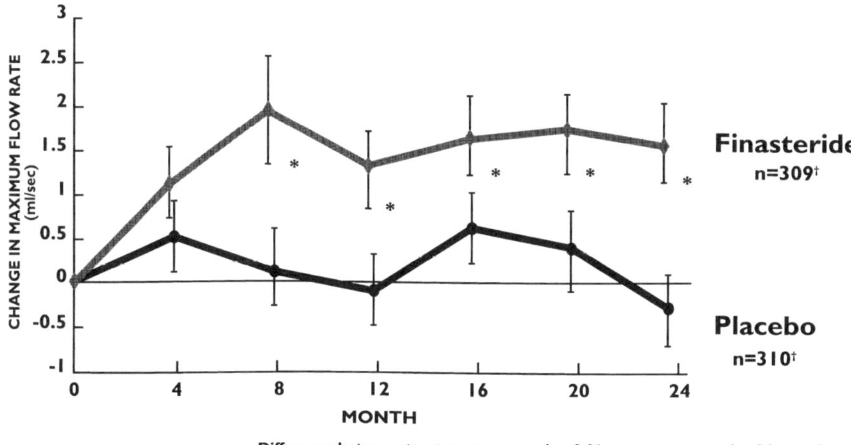

FIGURE 3.—Changes in maximum urinary flow rate (mL/sec) from baseline. Means ± 95% confidence interval. All patients treated analysis. (Reprinted by permission of the publisher from "Can finasteride reverse the progress of benign prostatic hyperplasia? A two-year placebo-controlled study," by Andersen JT, Ekman P, Wolf H, et al: *UROLOGY* 46:631–637, Copyright 1995 by Elsevier Science, Inc.)

12% in the placebo group. Maximum urinary flow rate increased significantly in the finasteride group compared to the placebo group (Fig 3). The median percent change from baseline in PSA was +6% with placebo and −52% with finasteride, a significant difference. The 2 groups were similar in proportion of patients who discontinued treatment and who had adverse side effects.

Conclusion.—Finasteride was effective and generally well tolerated when used to treat BPH. Patients given placebo reported initial improvement but no long-term benefits, whereas finasteride-treated patients maintained reductions in prostate volume and increases in maximum urinary flow rate over the 2-year study period. Treatment with finasteride can thus reverse the natural progression of BPH.

▶ These 3 articles (Abstracts 20–15, 20–16, 20–17), regarding the effect of finasteride on the prostate, all conclude that the effect is durable over several years. All 3 articles report a decrease in the volume of a prostate. In the 5-year studies by Geller and Moore et al., a 30% reduction was noted and in the 2-year study by Andersen et al., which involved a much larger series of patients, a reduction of 19% was noted.

There had been some concern that finasteride inhibiting the transformation of testosterone to dihydrotestosterone might increase testosterone to the point that regrowth of the gland would occur over time. As noted by Moore and Geller, testosterone increased by approximately 10% in the double-blind study but remained essentially within normal limits over their 5-year study. However, the size of the prostate does not correlate well with the degree of bladder outlet obstruction or the patient's symptoms.

All 3 series report an increase in urinary flow rate. This increase was maintained for several years. However, the increase in flow rate was only modest. Moore et al. reported 1.5 cc/sec improvement (from a baseline of 10.8) to 12.3. Over time, this apparently increased by 2.3 cc/sec. Andersen et al. also noted a modest improvement in flow rate from 10.2 cc/sec at baseline by 1.5 cc at the end of the 2-year period of study. All of these were considered to be statistically significant, although I would wonder whether a patient would really notice such a modest improvement in flow rate. Note that the flow rate at the end of the study would still be considered by others to be indicative of bladder outlet obstruction.

All 3 studies indicate that patient symptoms improved. However, it should be noted that the symptom score questionnaire was changed for the open study, as noted by Geller and Moore et al., from the one used in the initial dosing study reported in 1992.[1] In that study the baseline symptoms score was 18 (out of a possible 35 points) and there was again a modest but considered statistically significant reduction in symptoms.

Therefore, because of the change in the symptom score, it is a little difficult to compare the symptom improvement reported by Geller and Moore et al., but, nevertheless, the reduction in symptoms was persistent throughout the 5-year study. In the Andersen et al. study, the total symptom score was a possible 54 points and the obstructive symptom score range was 0 to 30. The baseline for the total symptom score in this group was 13.4 and there was an a-2 reduction at 24 months. The symptoms score was 8.8 but there was a reduction of 1.5 at 2 years. Therefore, all 3 studies report mildly to moderately symptomatic patients with a modest reduction in symptoms.

Geller reported a sexual dysfunction rate of 10% and an additional 11% drop-out rate because of drug ineffectiveness. Andersen et al. reported a drop-out rate of 18% because of adverse effects and inadequate response. Sexual dysfunction was 19% in the finasteride group as opposed to 10% in the placebo group. Moore et al. reported a lower drop-out rate from ineffective response to drug but did note a 10% incidence of sexual dysfunction. However, in all 3 studies, the sexual dysfunction occurred early in the study. As noted by Moore, over a 5-year period, there was only a small increase in the incidence of sexual dysfunction.

It would appear, therefore, that finasteride in mildly to moderately symptomatic patients will modestly improve patient symptoms and flow rate or at least the patient's disease will remain stable over a several year period and will not progress. It is my feeling that patients who are severely symptomatic should undergo a transurethral resection of the prostate or a similar invasive procedure.

However, Lepor,[2] reported at the Annual Meeting of the American Urological Association (AUA), May 4–9, 1996, on behalf of the VA Cooperative Study, in which finasteride and terazosin monotherapy were compared with the combination of terazosin and finasteride, as compared with placebo in men with clinical BPH, that there was little difference between the improvement of the AUA Symptom Score or peak flow rate, when comparing finasteride to placebo. However, in all fairness to the authors noted here, this was only a 52-week study, and we will also have to wait to read the published paper before coming to a definite conclusion.

The question could be raised—should patients with mild-to-moderate symptoms be given finasteride as a prophylaxis against progression of obstructing prostatic hyperplasia? What is unknown is how many patients with mild-to-moderate symptoms will need to have intervention because of progression of their symptoms or complication of BPH (i.e., acute urinary retention). Geller mentions in his article that there have been small studies reporting approximately 30% of patients requiring intervention over a 5-year period. What is needed is a long-term prospective study of untreated patients to determine the natural history of the disease.

The use of finasteride for a long time does have some side effects (i.e., sexual dysfunction). However, it is extremely difficult to get objective data on patients being treated with medications or those undergoing transurethral resection of the prostate in regard to sexual dysfunction. The other limiting factor in a prophylactic program would be the cost-effectiveness. If finasteride cost only a few pennies, such a prophylactic program might be considered. However, it does not cost just a few pennies, and if the vast majority of patients with mild-to-moderate symptoms do not progress to a point requiring intervention, then such a program could be extremely costly with only modest effectiveness.

W.K. Mebust, M.D.

References

1. The Finasteride Study Group: Finasteride (MK-906) in the treatment of benign prostatic hyperplasia. *The Prostate* 22:291–299, 1993.
2. Lepor H, for the VA Cooperative Studies BPH Study Group, New York, NY (presented by Dr. Lepor): A department of Veterans Affairs (VA) cooperative randomized placebo controlled clinical trial of the safety and efficacy of terazosin and finasteride monotherapy and terazosin/finasteride combination therapy in men with clinical BPH. Presented at the Annual Meeting of the American Urological Association, Orlando, Fla, May 4–9, 1996. (Abstract 1105.)

The Effects of Finasteride on Hematuria Associated With Benign Prostatic Hyperplasia: A Preliminary Report
Puchner PJ, Miller MI (Columbia Univ, New York)
J Urol 154:1779–1782, 1995   20–18

Background.—Finasteride has been proved effective in relieving the obstructive voiding symptoms associated with benign prostatic hyperplasia (BPH) and in reducing prostate size. However, there have been no studies of finasteride's effect on hematuria, a bothersome symptom associated with BPH.

Methods.—Eighteen patients treated with finasteride, 5 mg daily, for gross hematuria associated with BPH were studied retrospectively. Patients ranged in age from 66 to 86 years. A grading system was developed to assess hematuria.

Findings.—Hematuria was classified as grade 1 in 6 patients, grade 2 in 7 patients, and grade 3 in 5 patients. One patient had severe urgency and frequency just after beginning therapy and stopped taking finasteride. With discontinuation of the drug, his symptoms subsided. No significant adverse effects occurred in the remaining 17 patients. Twelve patients were followed for 4–25 months, and 5 were followed for 3 months or less. Eleven of the 12 patients in the former group improved with finasteride treatment, as evidenced by a better hematuria grade.

Conclusions.—Finasteride is clearly beneficial in the treatment of gross hematuria associated with BPH. The best results were achieved in patients who had undergone prostatectomy and in those with relatively frequent bleeding. Further research is needed to confirm the current findings.

▶ Intermittent gross hematuria to which no other cause can be assigned but benign prostatic hyperplasia is a frustration to both patient and urologist. This is especially true if the patient has no other symptoms that would justify operative intervention. The authors' findings certainly support the policy of instituting finasteride therapy under these circumstances before resorting to prostatectomy. The authors' conjecture regarding the use of finasteride before prostatectomy to reduce intraoperative and postoperative bleeding is intriguing. It would make for an interesting prospective, randomized trial— that is, if sufficient patients undergoing prostatectomy could be found in this era of alternative benign prostatic hyperplasia management.

H.L. Holtgrewe, M.D.

Doxazosin for the Treatment of Benign Prostatic Hyperplasia in Patients With Mild to Moderate Essential Hypertension: A Double-Blind, Placebo-Controlled, Dose-Response Multicenter Study
Gillenwater JY, for the Multicenter Study Group (Univ of Virginia, Charlottesville; Lovelace Scientific Resources Inc, Albuquerque, NM; Univ of Oklahoma, Oklahoma City; et al)
J Urol 154:110–115, 1995   20–19

Background.—Recent research has indicated that doxazosin is safe and effective in patients with benign prostatic hyperplasia (BPH). This agent is a highly selective antagonist of all α1-adrenergic receptor subtypes, including the α1A receptor thought to be the main subtype in the prostate. The efficacy and saftey of doxazosin in men with BPH and mild-to-moderate essential hypertension were investigated.

Methods and Findings.—Two hundred forty-eight hypertensive men aged 45 years or older were included in the 16-week, multicenter, double-blind, placebo-controlled, parallel-group dose-response study. Compared to placebo, doxazosin in doses of 4, 8, and 12 mg produced a significant increase in maximum urinary flow rate. The 8-and 12-mg doses also increased mean flow rate. The improvement in maximum flow rate was significant within 1 week of starting active treatment. Also, doxazosin significantly reduced patient-assessed total, obstructive, and irritative BPH symptoms compared to placebo. At all doxazosin doses, blood pressure was significantly lower than with placebo. Forty-eight percent of patients taking doxazosin and 35% taking placebo reported adverse events, which were primarily mildly to moderately severe.

Conclusions.—Doxazosin is significantly better than placebo in increasing urinary flow and reducing the total, obstructive, and irritative symptoms of BPH. This agent also resulted in a clinically significant reduction in blood pressure in the current series of hypertensive patients. Because of its rapid onset of efficacy and convenient once-daily dosing, this drug should be easier to comply with than other agents. Also, it does not adversely affect lipid profiles or glucose tolerance.

▶ Given the high frequency with which hypertension and lower urinary tract symptoms co-exist in the aging male population, two-for-one therapy with a selective long-acting alpha blocker is both logical and cost-efficacious. However, I must take exception to one facet of this study. The authors evaluated men with hypertension and lower urinary tract symptoms that may, or may not, have been the result of benign prostatic hyperplasia. Although the authors reported performing urodynamic studies on their patients, they do not state whether the combination of high pressure and low flow, substantiating true obstruction, was a criterion for entry into the study. Neither do they make any comment on prostate gland size as determined by either digital rectal examination or sonography. Absent these data how are we to know that patients with only bladder dysfunction of aging and without significant prostate enlargement attributable to benign prostatic hyperplasia were not a part of the studied cohort? I think the time has come to abandon the concept that all older men with lower urinary tract symptoms have BPH. What the authors have documented in this well-conducted study is that men with hypertension and lower urinary tract symptoms can be effectively treated for both with alpha blockers—which, of course, is the issue of greatest importance to our patients.

H.L. Holtgrewe, M.D.

Magnetic Resonance Angiography in Prostatodynia
Terasaki T, Watanabe H, Saitoh M, Uchida M, Okamura S, Shimizu K (Kyoto Prefectural Univ, Japan; Shimadzu Corp, Kyoto, Japan)
Eur Urol 27:280–285, 1995   20–20

Objective.—Three-dimensional magnetic resonance venography (MRV) was used to visualize the prostate and pelvic cavity of patients with prostatodynia and to compare the venous return in those patients with that of normal individuals.

Methods.—Three-dimensional MRV, using a 1.5-tesla SMT-150X machine and a surface-received-only coil, was performed in 8 normal controls, aged 25–30 years, and in 12 patients with prostatodynia aged 19–47 years. Symptoms included suprapubic pain in 5 patients, inguinal pain in 3, perineal pain in 3, testicular pain in 2, loin pain in 2, penile pain in 1, ejaculation pain in 1, and urinary frequency in 4. Although prostate size and shape was normal in all patients, 7 had severe prostate tenderness on digital rectal examination. T2-weighted spin-echo sequences were obtained in the coronal plane in 3-mm slices and processed using a maximum-intensity projection algorithm.

Results.—Normal individuals had fine, symmetrically running deep dorsal vein branches and internal pudendal veins originating from the pudendal plexus located in the posterior area of the pelvis. The anterior and lateral capsular vein diameters of the patients were thicker and were difficult to distinguish from one another. There was a significant dilatation of the pudendal and venous plexuses in 10 of 12 patients suggesting venous congestion. Similar results were seen on repeated three-dimensional MRV in 2 controls and 2 patients after 3–12 months.

Conclusion.—These results suggest that prostatodynia may be caused by intrapelvic venous congestion.

▶ This is an interesting paper, which suggests that prostatodynia is a disease with a definite pathophysiology. There has always been uncertainty as to whether or not prostatodynia is a pathologic state or a psychic disorder. It has been attributed to spasm of the pelvic floor muscles, reflux of urine, and stress. Some authors have noted that, at transrectal ultrasound, there is a sonolucent zone in prostatodynia,[1] but this finding is also often present in normal individuals. If the authors' findings are correct, then prostatodynia is associated with significant alterations in venous blood flow. This of course still leaves the primary cause unknown.

S.S. Howards, M.D.

Reference

1. Peeling WB, Griffiths GJ: Imaging of the prostate by ultrasound. *J Urol* 132:217–224, 1984.

Incidence of Erectile Impotence Secondary to Transurethral Resection of Benign Prostatic Hyperplasia, Assessed by Preoperative and Postoperative Snap Gauge Tests
Tscholl R, Largo M, Poppinghaus E, Recker F, Subotic B (Kantonsspital Aarau, Switzerland)
J Urol 153:1491–1493, 1995   20–21

Introduction.—The most common procedure for men with bladder outlet obstruction from benign prostatic hyperplasia is transurethral prostatectomy. Erectile impotence has been cited as one of the side effects; however, data are contradictory. Before and after transurethral resection, men were tested for potency.

Methods.—A snap-gauge test was given to 98 men claiming to have an adequately rigid erection. The evening before their operation, the men placed a band, locked by 3 snap-release fasteners, snugly around the base of their penises. Those who broke all 3 snap-release fasteners were considered to be potent. The fourth day after their operation, the men again underwent the snap-gauge test. They were retested 3 months later at home. They were considered impotent as a consequence of the operation if they failed the second postoperative test.

Results.—After the fourth day of the transurethral resection, 64 of the 98 men remained potent, whereas 34 were impotent. Three months later, the 34 men were tested and of those, 26 were potent and 8 were impotent. As a consequence of the transurethral resection of the prostate, 8 of 98 men, or 8.3%, became impotent. Six of the 8 impotent men were older than 65 years. Six of the 8 men had a prostatic adenoma that was so small that 10 g or less of benign prostatic hyperplasia tissue could be resected.

Conclusion.—There is a low impotence risk of transurethral resection of the prostate, still considered to be the most efficient procedure to relieve prostatic bladder outlet obstruction. Age was the variable that was most strongly associated with impotence. The inverse effect of the weight of the resected tissue is less understood.

▶ Other recent publications have suggested that the impotence rate following transurethral resection of the prostate (TURP) is between 4% and 10%. By selecting the snap-gauge test with a sensitivity in the 60% to 80% range, it would be difficult to accurately identify the low percentage rate of impotence believed to be secondary to TURP. By administering the test at 3 time periods before and after TURP (and not including all patients in the study at each time point), this tendency to misread the potency rate after TURP is amplified.

R.C. Bruskewitz, M.D.

Urodynamic Results of Laser Treatment in Patients With Benign Prostatic Hyperplasia. Can Outlet Obstruction Be Relieved?

de Wildt MJAM, Slaa ET, Rosier PFWM, Wijkstra H, Debruyne FJM, de la Rosette JJMCH (Univ Hosp Nijmegen, The Netherlands)
J Urol 154:174–180, 1995   20–22

Background.—Laser treatment of the prostate recently became available for patients with benign prostatic hyperplasia (BPH). The advantages of this modality are decreased hospital stay, minimal bleeding, no fluid absorption, rapidity, technical simplicity, and the chance of preserving antegrade ejaculation. Preliminary findings have been encouraging. The ability of laser treatment to relieve bladder outlet obstruction was investigated in a urodynamic study.

Methods.—Since November, 1992, 125 patients were treated with 3 different laser systems. Data on advanced urodynamic studies with pressure-flow analysis done before and 6 months after laser treatment were available in 40 patients.

Findings.—Significant improvement in all obstruction parameters was documented, including detrusor pressure at maximum flow rate, urethral resistance relation, theoretical cross-sectional urethral area, minimal detrusor pressure, and linear passive urethral resistance relation. There was also significant subjective improvement in the international prostate symptom score, and 82% to 92% of the patients were no longer considered to have obstruction after treatment. The outcomes associated with the 3 devices did not differ.

Conclusions.—The results of laser treatment in patients with outflow obstruction are comparable to those obtained with transurethral resection of the prostate. Randomized trials with urodynamic assessments and pressure-flow analyses are needed to assess the ability of this treatment modality to provide long-lasting relief of obstruction for each fiber.

▶ The authors demonstrate that free beam laser ablation of the prostate is effective in statistically improving important urodynamic parameters including detrusor pressure at maximum flow and maximum flow rate. For the ultrasound-guided laser (TULIP), statistically significant improvements were not noted. Also, the patients were tested 6 months after treatment. Presumably these significant urodynamic improvements would not be apparent as rapidly after laser prostatectomy as after transurethral resection of the prostate.

R.C. Bruskewitz, M.D.

Association Between Family History of Benign Prostatic Hyperplasia and Urinary Symptoms: Results of a Population-Based Study

Roberts RO, Rhodes T, Panser LA, Girman CJ, Chute CG, Guess HA, Oesterling JE, Lieber MM, Jacobsen SJ (Mayo Clinic and Found, Rochester, Minn; Merck Researach Labs, Blue Bell, Pa)
Am J Epidemiol 142:965–973, 1995   20–23

Background.—Benign prostatic hyperplasia is a major cause of hospitalization and surgery in men 65 years and older. There is little information published on risk factors for benign prostatic hyperplasia and little attention paid to family history of this condition as a possible factor. The relation between family history of an enlarged prostate and urinary symptoms suggestive of benign prostatic hyperplasia was examined.

Methods.—A group of 2,119 randomly selected men between 40 and 79 years completed a questionnaire that elicited information about urinary symptoms, worry about urinary function, chronic diseases, and demographics. Family history of an enlarged prostate was obtained and peak urinary flow rates were measured.

Results.—Of 2,119 subjects, 440 had a family history of an enlarged prostate. The odds of having moderate-to-severe urinary symptoms were adjusted for age and were higher among subjects with a family history of an enlarged prostate. The odds remained higher after controlling for age and worry about urologic function. This risk was greater for subjects with a relative with an enlarged prostate diagnosed at a younger age. Family history also increased the risk of having an impaired peak urinary flow rate.

Conclusions.—Men who have a family history of an enlarged prostate may be at higher risk of having symptoms that are suggestive of benign prostatic hyperplasia. This risk may be greater in men with relatives with an enlarged prostate diagnosed at a younger age. These findings may help determine early interventions.

▶ Previous studies have shown either a weak association or no association between prostate size and urinary symptoms. The authors show an association between a family history of enlargement and symptoms in the individual male. A closer look at this paper reveals that 81% of the prostate enlargement in family members was manifested by a history of transurethral resection of the prostate (TURP). In the United States, TURP has been performed primarily for symptoms and not for prostate size with most men having smaller weights of tissue resected. An alternate conclusion to this paper would be that the symptoms are more common in men whose male relatives have undergone TURP.

R.C. Bruskewitz, M.D.

21 Prostate Cancer

The Burden of Prostate Cancer From Diagnosis Until Death
Otnes B, Harvei S, Fosså SD (Baerum Hosp, Oslo, Norway; Cancer Registry
of Norway, Oslo; Norwegian Radium Hosp, Oslo, Norway)
Br J Urol 76:587–594, 1995   21–1

Introduction.—About one half of the Norwegian men with prostate
cancer die of their disease. Patients with prostate cancer frequently have
significant and protracted suffering, requiring vast resources for their care.
The need for treatment and care in men treated conservatively for prostate
cancer from diagnosis to death was retrospectively quantified.

Methods.—Using Norway's Cancer Registry and the Register of Deaths
of Statistics, 174 men who resided in 2 cities and died of prostate cancer
between 1987 and 1991 were identified. The locale has a 10% incidence
of prostate cancer and a survival rate similar to that of the rest of the
country. All patients treated with a curative intent were excluded. Metastatic status, stage, histologic data, treatment and care details, and complications were recorded for all patients.

Results.—Ninety-five percent of the patients were symptomatic at the
time of diagnosis and nearly two thirds died of the disease. The crude
survival rate was 44 months. The average hospital stay for all but 2
patients was 1 month. One third needed either residential or home nursing
care. Hospitalizations for complications or continued catheterizations occurred in half the patients. Sixty-six percent underwent surgery, 76% had
androgen ablation, 16% had irradiation, and half received analgesics
including opiates for 37%. If the androgen ablation procedure failed
(29%), prednisone was given.

Conclusions.—The burden on the patient was considerable. Prostate
cancer led to more surgeries and a greater use of analgesics, irradiation,
and prednisone. When compared with other diseases, prostate cancer
resulted in nearly twice the hospital time as well as an increased reliance on
nursing care.

▶ With the popular backlash against aggressive diagnosis and treatment of
prostate cancer, we all benefit from remembering the enormous burden this
tumor can place on individuals and society. In this study, the authors detail
many of the unpleasant medical complications experienced by men dying of
prostate cancer. Not examined is their decrement in health-related quality of

life, nor the monetary costs associated with care, both of which no doubt represented significant personal hardship. In the current environment of watchful waiting for prostate cancer, we must ask ourselves what it is we are watching and waiting for. If it is for signs or symptoms of progression, we must consider that a painless death from competing causes of mortality often does not occur before a tortuous decline to a painful and undignified death from prostate cancer. Both quantity and quality of life must be included in the patient's decision of how aggressively to pursue and fight this disease.

M.S. Litwin, M.D., M.P.H.

Prostate Cancer Mortality in Patients Surviving More Than 10 Years After Diagnosis

Hugosson J, Aus G, Bergdahl C, Bergdahl S (Göteborg Univ, Sweden)
J Urol 154:2115–2117, 1995   21–2

Background.—Prostatic cancer usually is a slow-growing neoplasm and commonly follows a protracted course. A few studies following patients for up to 10 years have indicated a fairly benign course, at least for patients having low-grade, low-stage tumors. Some have questioned the value of curative treatment, but few data are available on the course of disease after 10 years in patients given deferred treatment. A recent lifelong follow-up study revealed unexpectedly high mortality from low-stage, low-grade prostatic cancers.

Objective.—To validate these findings, the causes of death were reviewed in 490 patients in Göteborg, Sweden, who had prostate cancer diagnosed between 1960 and 1979, and who lived longer than 10 years after diagnosis. The mean follow-up was 15 years.

Observations.—Seventy-five patients remained alive at last follow-up. Sixty-two percent of the 415 deaths resulted directly or indirectly from prostatic cancer. The average interval between diagnosis and death was 167 months in patients dying of prostatic cancer and 181 for the others. Although the number of patients living longer than 10 years has more than doubled in the period reviewed, the relative risk of death from prostatic cancer has not changed appreciably. The average age at diagnosis remained constant for patients who died of prostatic cancer.

Implication.—These findings suggest that treatment of localized prostatic cancer (other than stage T1a) should not be deferred in patients who otherwise are expected to live for an appreciable time.

▶ Although prostate cancer is often indolent, this article illustrates that many men with diagnosed prostate cancer die of it. The usual rationale for observational management is that competing causes of mortality are likely to occur more quickly than tumor progression. Yet the patients in this study who died of other causes surprisingly lived 14 months longer than those dying of prostate cancer. Hence, in patients with long life expectancies at diagnosis, the possibility of early death from prostate cancer must be considered despite the usually protracted course of this disease.

M.S. Litwin, M.D., M.P.H.

Digital Rectal Examinations and Prostate Cancer Screening: Attitudes of African American Men
Gelfand DE, Parzuchowski J, Cort M, Powell I (Wayne State Univ, Detroit; Harper Hosp, Detroit)
Oncol Nurs Forum 22:1253–1255, 1995   21–3

Background.—African-American men have an 85% greater chance of prostate cancer being diagnosed and a 114% greater chance of dying from the disease than white men. Despite this, the participation rate of African-American men in prostate cancer screenings remains low. Negative feelings about digital rectal examination (DRE) have been cited as a major barrier to their participation in prostate screening. The relationship between attitudes toward DRE and participation in prostate screenings was studied in African-American men participating in a year-long, community-based survey, the Detroit Education and Early Detection program.

Methods.—The survey was conducted during prostate cancer screenings with a prostate-specific antigen (PSA) blood test held at churches with African-American members in Detroit. Self-administered, structured questionnaires examining attitudes toward DRE, past experiences with DRE, and fear of cancer were completed by 613 African-American men aged 40–70 years (mean, 54.8 years). The men had relatively high income levels and educational backgrounds.

Findings.—Sixty percent of the men indicated a positive attitude toward DRE, 31% had a neutral attitude, and 9% had a negative attitude. Attitudes toward DRE became more positive when men believed that DRE was a normal part of a physical examination and became more negative when fear of cancer increased. Multiple regression analysis showed that older, more educated, and higher-income men were more positive toward DRE than younger, less-educated, and lower-income men. Fear of cancer, education, and accepting DRE as a normal part of a physical examination explained 13% of the variance in attitudes toward DRE.

Implication.—Digital rectal examination does not necessarily deter African-American men from participating in prostate cancer screenings. Fear of cancer may be a more important factor in their failure to take advantage of cancer screening. Plans for prostate cancer screening should include both DRE and PSA, and DRE should be included in annual routine physical examination for all African-American men older than 50 years and, perhaps, for men older than 40 years.

▶ This article from Wayne State University is one of many outstanding recent contributions that furthers our understanding of prostate cancer in African-American men. The findings show that African-American men do not necessarily avoid prostate cancer screening because of negative attitudes about DRE. This work dispels a common misconception that black men are more likely to avoid screening because of a reluctance to undergo DRE. The clinical take-home message is that we should advocate and include DRE in our outreach to the African-American community regarding the early detection of prostate cancer.

J.W. Moul, M.D.

Prostate Cancer Risk in U.S. Blacks and Whites With a Family History of Cancer
Hayes RB, Liff JM, Pottern LM, Greenberg RS, Schoenberg JB, Schwartz AG, Swanson GM, Silverman DT, Brown LM, Hoover RN, Fraumeni JF Jr (Natl Cancer Inst, Bethesda, Md; Emory Univ, Atlanta, Ga; New Jersey State Dept of Health, Trenton; et al)
Int J Cancer 60:361–364, 1995   21–4

Introduction.—The most common cancer among black Americans is prostate cancer, and their mortality from this condition is twice that of whites. Whether genetic factors contribute to the disparity in mortality between these groups was determined.

Methods.—Study participants included 981 case patients and 1,315 controls, aged 40–79 years, who resided in one of the following geographic regions: Fulton or Dekalb County, Georgia; metropolitan Detroit; or in New Jersey. In-person interviews were used to gather demographic information, information about work history, and a family history of cancers. Odds ratios (ORs) were established for each contributing factor using regression analysis, and the ORs were adjusted for marital status, income, education, and socioeconomic status.

Results.—A first-degree relative with prostate cancer is a risk factor (OR = 3.2), and both blacks and whites had increased ORs. This risk was not affected by education, income, or marital or socioeconomic status. Prostate cancer is associated with some cancers such as leukemia, breast cancer, uterine cancer, and colon cancer. The overall risk with a family history of any cancer was similar for both races.

Discussion.—Because no environmental factors were associated with the three-fold increase in risk for prostate cancer among those patients with a history of prostate cancer in a first-degree relative, hereditary factors must be involved. However, this increased risk was present for both blacks and whites, suggesting that genetic susceptibility does not explain the ethnic disparity in risk. Occasionally prostate cancer has been associated with the Li-Fraumeni syndrome, which is caused by a germline mutation in *p53*. Some prostate cancers involve this somatic mutation. Because the familial risks were similar for both blacks and whites, the increased prevalence of prostate cancer among blacks must result from underlying behavioral or environmental factors.

▶ This important paper from the National Cancer Institute reports a large, well-conducted, population-based case-control study to assess the significance of a family history of prostate cancer. Twenty four of 448 (5.4%) black patients with prostate cancer reported a first-degree relative with prostate cancer compared with 43 of 457 (9.4%) whites. The OR (increased risk associated with prostate cancer in a first-degree relative) was 3.4 and 3.1, respectively, for blacks and whites. Because the familial risk was similar by race, the authors concluded that the ethnic disparity in prostate cancer occurrence is likely caused by environmental or behavioral rather than genetic determinants.

This epidemiologic study is generally supported by the sparce molecular genetic studies stratified by race in prostate cancer. Our group has not found significant racial differences in the incidence of *ras*,[1] c-*erb*B-2,[2] cathepsin-D,[3] epidermal growth factor receptor,[3] *p53*,[4] *bcl-2*,[5] *p16*,[6] and *Ki-67* proliferation.[7] Conversely, racial differences in polymorphic CAG repeats in the androgen receptor gene affecting androgen metabolism have been reported.[8] More work is necessary to determine whether racial differences in prostate cancer are truly the result of the environment and/or behavior or the result of more subtle genetic alterations that may potentiate these determinants.

J.W. Moul, M.D.

References

1. Moul JW, Friedrichs PA, Lance RS, et al: Infrequent *ras* oncogene mutations in human prostate cancer. *Prostate* 20:327–338, 1992.
2. Kuhn EJ, Kurnot RA, Sesterhenn IA, et al: Expression of the c-*erb*B-2 oncoprotein in prostate cancer. *J Urol* 150:1427–1433, 1993.
3. Moul JW, MayGarden SJ, Ware JL, et al: Cathepsin-D and epidermal growth factor receptor (EGFR) immunohistochemistry does not predict recurrence of prostate cancer patients undergoing radical prostatectomy. *J Urol* 155:982–985, 1996.
4. Bauer JJ, Sesterhenn IA, Mostofi FK, et al: *p53* nuclear protein expression is an independent prognostic marker in clinically localized prostate cancer patients undergoing radical prostatectomy. *Clin Cancer Res* 1:1295–1300. 1995.
5. Bauer JJ, Sesterhenn IA, Mostofi FK, et al: Elevated levels of apoptosis regulator proteins p53 and bcl-2 are independent prognostic biomarkers in surgically treated clinically localized prostate cancer patients. *J Urol* (in press).
6. Gaddipati JP, McLeod DG, Sesterhenn IA, et al: Mutations of the *p16* gene product are rare in prostate cancer. *Prostate* (in press).
7. Bettencourt M, Bauer JJ, Sesterhenn IA, et al: *Ki-67* expression is a prognostic marker of prostate cancer recurrence after radical prostatectomy. *J Urol* (in press).
8. Coetzee GA, Ross RK: Re: Prostate cancer and the androgen receptor (letter). *J Natl Cancer Inst* 86:872, 1994.

Prostate-Specific Antigen Values at the Time of Prostate Cancer Diagnosis in African-American Men

Moul JW, Sesterhenn IA, Connelly RR, Douglas T, Srivastava S, Mostofi FK, McLeod DG (Walter Reed Army Med Ctr, Washington, DC; Uniformed Services Univ of the Health Sciences, Bethesda, Md; Armed Forces Inst of Pathology, Washington, DC)

JAMA 274:1277–1281, 1995   21–5

Background.—African-American men have a 50% higher incidence of prostate cancer than do white men after adjusting for age, and the highest incidence in the world. Hormonal, genetic, nutritional, and socioeconomic factors all have been considered. Serum levels of prostate-specific antigen (PSA) in military patients with newly diagnosed prostate cancer were determined to assess the importance of access to care and socioeconomic status.

Study Population.—Complete records were available for 541 patients treated for newly diagnosed prostatic adenocarcinoma at Walter Reed Army Medical Center from 1990 through 1994. Data on tumor volume were analyzed in 91 patients having radical prostatectomy in 1993 and 1994.

Observations.—Geometric mean PSA levels were significantly higher in black than in white patients (14.0 ng/mL vs. 8.3 ng/mL). Blacks had higher levels for all categories of age, stage, and tumor grade. Blacks were 2.2-fold more likely than whites to have a PSA exceeding 10 ng/mL.

Radical Prostatectomy Cohort.—Comparable numbers of blacks and whites underwent biopsy on the basis of PSA screening. Black patients had tumor volumes more than twice as large as those of whites, but differences in prostate weight were not significant. There was no racial difference in prostatitis. On linear regression analysis, tumor volume predicted the PSA levels, but race no longer was a significant factor.

Conclusion.—Even given equal access to health care, African-American men with prostate cancer have higher PSA levels at the time of diagnosis than do white patients of similar age who have comparably advanced disease.

▶ This article concludes that in a system of equal access to health care, (1) PSA levels are higher in African-Americans, (2) this difference persists when analyzed by stage, and (3) the reason for this discrepancy may be higher tumor volume in patients of similar age. When combined with other data suggesting that blacks have disease develop at an earlier age, the natural extension of this finding is that increased efforts for early diagnosis may result in improved outcomes for African-American men.[1]

For a variety of reasons, efforts to enroll African-Americans in primary and secondary prevention programs have not been as successful as those to enroll U.S. whites.[2] Among these reasons are a distrust of the research process, a traditional lack of community involvement, economic, disincentives, and barriers to access to care.

Further efforts are necessary to confirm Moul and colleagues' conclusions, especially as more recent case-control studies have suggested that serum PSA values are similar in both whites and African-Americans when adjusted for age.[3] Regardless, these findings provide compelling evidence that health care professionals should direct significant efforts toward developing closer relationships with the African-American community in an attempt to reduce the burden of prostate cancer on this segment of the population.

I.M. Thompson, M.D.

References

1. Optenberg SA, Thompson IM, Friedrichs P, et al: Race, treatment, and long-term survival from prostate cancer in an equal-access medical care delivery system. *JAMA* 274:1599–1605, 1995.
2. Swanson GM, Ward AJ: Recruiting minorities into clinical trials: Toward a participant-friendly system. *J Natl Cancer Inst* 87:1747–1759, 1995.
3. Whittemore AS, Lele C, Friedman GD, et al: Prostate-specific antigen as predictor of prostate cancer in black men and white men. *J Natl Cancer Inst* 87:354–360, 1995.

Race, Treatment, and Long-Term Survival From Prostate Cancer in an Equal-Access Medical Care Delivery System
Optenberg SA, Thompson IM, Friedrichs P, Wojcik B, Stein CR, Kramer B
(Brooke Army Med Ctr, San Antonio, Tex; Natl Cancer Inst, Bethesda, Md)
JAMA 274:1599–1605, 1995   21–6

Background.—In blacks, the death rate from breast or prostate cancer exceeds the death rate in whites even when the rates are controlled for stage, socioeconomic class, and grade. For example, the 5-year survival rate for men with regional prostate cancer is 87% in whites and 69% in blacks. Explanations for such differences include tumor behavior, treatment differences, and access to care. Recent studies indicate that fewer blacks think cancer is preventable and are less likely to participate in screenings (even if free), or seek medical care. Treatment and outcome differences were examined in patients in the Department of Defense (DOD) system, because this population generally has similar access, screening, and treatment protocols.

Methods.—Twenty years of the DOD tumor registry were reviewed for patients with prostate cancer. Independent variables included ethnicity, stage, age, risk factors, and treatment. Survival endpoints were determined. The outcomes of interest included tumor stage and grade, differences between races, risk factors, recurrences, and treatment wait time, as well as the effect of these factors on survival. A total of 1,606 patients were identified; 7.5% were black and the remaining were white.

Results.—Behavioral risk factors and tumor grade or size were not different between the 2 races. However, blacks began active treatment later and had a higher relative risk of cancer at younger ages. They also demonstrated a significantly higher stage and progression to distant disease than whites. The time from diagnosis to the beginning of treatment was not different between the races. Within any stage, there was no difference in the type of treatment. Survival was not affected by race. However, stage, grade, and age affected survival. There was a longer survival for metastatic disease in blacks when the rates were controlled for stage.

Conclusion.—The DOD patients had equal access to the medical care system. There were no stage-specific differences in treatment between the races for patients with prostate cancer. In fact, for high-stage disease, the survival rates for blacks may actually surpass the rates of whites.

▶ Because I am in the U.S. Military health care system myself, know the authors, and have a particular interest in the subject, I am honored to review this paper. The take-home message is that if African-American men are afforded the same access and care, there is no significant difference in stage-adjusted outcome. For the sake of African-Americans with prostate cancer, I hope these results are true and these findings will be duplicated. However, the results are different from those from other recent work.[1, 2] Pienta and associates found that stage-adjusted survival in Detroit was worse for African-American men; however, they could not adjust for treatment received.[1] Our group recently reported on black and white military patients all treated by radical prostatectomy.[2] Even after adjustment for pretreatment serum prostate-specific antigen and acid phosphatase values, and for pathologic stage and grade, blacks still had worse disease-free survival. The disparity of results might be explained by sample bias in the Optenberg et al. study. The Automated Central Tumor Registry (ACTUR) database that they used underrepresents the total number of prostate cancer patients seen during the study (1973–1994) period. They report a cohort of 1,606 patients with 7.5% black, yet at Walter Reed Hospital alone (where I work and part of ACTUR), we have identified *approximately* 2,200 prostate cancer patients, *21%* of whom are black during this interval. Their underreporting, particularly for the blacks, may have skewed the results. For example, if more blacks were lost to follow-up that had disease recurrence and/or cancer death, this could seriously compromise their conclusions. More study needs to be done in this important area.

J.W. Moul, M.D.

References

1. Pienta KT, Demers R, Hoff M, et al: Effect of age and race on the survival of men with prostate cancer in the metropolitan Detroit tri-county area, 1973–1987, *Urology* 45:93–102, 1995.
2. Moul JW, Douglas TH, McCarthy WF, et al: Black race is an adverse prognostic factor for prostate cancer recurrence following radical prostatectomy in an equal-access health care system. *J Urol* 155:1667–1673, 1996.

Vasectomy and Prostate Cancer: Results From a Multiethnic Case–Control Study
John EM, Whittemore AS, Wu AH, Kolonel LN, Hislop TG, Howe GR, West DW, Hankin J, Dreon DM, Teh C-Z, Burch JD, Paffenbarger RS Jr (Stanford Univ, Calif; Northern California Cancer Ctr, Union City; Univ of Southern California, Los Angeles; et al)
J Natl Cancer Inst 87:662–669, 1995   21–7

Purpose.—Several studies have reported that vasectomy is associated with an increased risk of prostate cancer. The epidemiologic evidence is inconsistent, however, and in previous study populations, white men have been overrepresented. To further evaluate this association, a large population of black and white men living in the United States, and Chinese and Japanese men living in the United States or Canada were enlisted for a case-control study. Participants newly diagnosed with prostate cancer were questioned regarding personal history, date of vasectomy (if incurred), and various potential risk factors. Differences in serum concentrations of prostate-specific antigen, androgens, and sex hormone–binding globulin (SHBG) between control subjects who had or had not undergone vasectomy were also analyzed.

Results.—A history of vasectomy was not significantly associated with prostate cancer risk for the multiethnic group as a whole, based on a population of 1,642 patients with prostate cancer and 1,636 control subjects. Nor was any significant association apparent in odds ratios for white, black, or Chinese men. Vasectomy history was associated with a statistically nonsignificant increased risk of prostate cancer for Japanese men; this risk was limited to men that were more educated or had localized cancers. Neither age at the time of vasectomy nor time elapsing since vasectomy proved significant. A higher ratio of dihydrotestosterone to testosterone and a lower serum concentration of SHBG appeared among control subjects who had undergone vasectomy as compared with those who had not.

Discussion.—The contention that vasectomy is associated with an increased risk of prostate cancer was not supported. The strengths of this study design include its population-based approach, inclusion of men from different geographic regions and ethnic backgrounds, exclusion of patients with possible undiagnosed prostate cancer, and case ascertainment that was independent of vasectomy status. The statistically nonsignificant increased risk of prostate cancer with vasectomy found for Japanese men is probably a result of chance. The low serum SHBG values suggest increased tissue availability of testosterone, whereas the higher ratio of dihydrotestosterone to testosterone suggests greater conversion of testosterone to this metabolite. Therefore, large longitudinal studies of the long-term effects of vasectomy on endocrinologic characteristics are indicated.

▶ The possible association between vasectomy and prostate cancer has been the focus of an epidemiologic debate for a number of years. Of concern has been the relative increase in vasectomy use over the past 20–30 years and the possible dramatic impact on prostate cancer incidence. In those studies that have found an association, it has been, at best, weak. A number of major biases may also lead to a higher likelihood of case-finding in men who have had a vasectomy, one of which is that they are more likely to have seen a urologist in the past (at the time of a vasectomy) and therefore may be more likely to have had a rectal examination or a determination of their prostate-specific antigen level.

John and colleagues' study is a major landmark in this subject because the study was purposely multiethnic, with a substantial number of African-Americans, and because it is notable for the endocrine studies. Not only was there no association between vasectomy and prostate cancer, but the authors found that prostate-specific antigen levels were no different between vasectomized and nonvasectomized men. Although the ratio of dihydrotestosterone to testosterone was significantly higher in all ethnic groups, it must be emphasized that there was no significant difference in testosterone and dihydrotestosterone in men who had and had not undergone vasectomy. This and other recent rigidly conducted studies give credence to the conclusion that there is a low likelihood of an association between vasectomy and prostate cancer.

I.M. Thompson, M.D.

Prostate Cancer in Relation to Diet, Physical Activity, and Body Size in Blacks, Whites, and Asians in the United States and Canada
Whittemore AS, Kolonel LN, Wu AH, John EM, Gallagher RP, Howe GR, Burch JD, Hankin J, Dreon DM, West DW, Teh C-Z, Paffenbarger RS Jr (Stanford Univ, Calif; Univ of Hawaii, Manoa, Honolulu; Univ of Southern Calif, Los Angeles; et al)
J Natl Cancer Inst 87:652–661, 1995   21–8

Introduction.—A case-control population-based study of prostate cancer was carried out among blacks, whites, and Asian-Americans living in the United States and Canada to identify the roles of lifestyle pattern and interethnic differences in disease risk. The case patients were 1,655 men aged 84 years or younger with primary carcinoma of the prostate, identified through the cancer registries of Los Angeles, San Francisco, Hawaii, Vancouver, and Toronto. Control subjects were matched one to one with patients by age, ethnicity, and residence. Data were obtained in both groups by a common questionnaire given in the home regarding current diet history, use of vitamin supplements, waist girth, and activity patterns, along with past height, weight, and activity patterns. Of the 1,127 control subjects who had prostate-specific antigen (PSA) levels obtained, only those with normal levels were matched to case patients, with the remaining patients matched to controls with unknown PSA levels.

Results.—Although a positive association was shown between high-fat diets and prostate cancer risk in all ethnic groups, a clear risk gradient with increasing fat intake was only demonstrated in Asian-American men. Saturated fats were more strong in this association than monounsaturated fats. The general association of saturated fats and prostate cancer became even stronger when comparisons were restricted to patients with high-grade lesions and controls with normal PSA levels. Whereas the overall prostate cancer risk in Asian-Americans appeared similar between those born in North America and those residing in North America for more than 25 years, the association with increased fat intake was clearly strongest in Asian-Americans born in North America. Prostate cancer risk showed no other significant association with food, alcohol, or vitamins. Nor was any association found with body mass, height, girth, or physical activity patterns.

Discussion.—Although prostate cancer is less common in Asian-Americans than in black and white North Americans, the risk for prostate cancer in Asian-Americans appears more closely tied to fat intake than it does for the other ethnic groups studied. However, fat intake, based on crude attributable risk calculations, may only explain a small percentage of the interethnic differences observed in prostate cancer incidence. As suggested by the similar rates of prostate cancer among Asian-Americans born in North America and those residing in North America for more than 25 years, factors in early male life may play a more important role.

▶ The association of dietary fat intake and prostate cancer has been found in a number of well-designed clinical studies. Further evidence of this association is found in the link between high-fat consumption in various countries correlating with higher rates of prostate cancer mortality. Whittemore and colleagues have refined this observation, noting that saturated fat may play the most significant role. The lack of correlation in dietary fat intake between African-Americans and whites, which would explain the 50% higher prostate cancer mortality in the former group, would seem a paradox. However, some evidence suggests that differences in diet may be measurable earlier—perhaps even in utero during prostatic development. With all the other salutary effects of a reduced fat diet, urologists should encourage their patients to consider this as one determinant of a healthy lifestyle.

I.M. Thompson, M.D.

Enhanced Reverse Transcriptase–Polymerase Chain Reaction for Prostate Specific Antigen as an Indicator of True Pathologic Stage in Patients With Prostate Cancer
Katz AE, de Vries GM, Begg MD, Raffo AJ, Cama C, O'Toole K, Buttyan R, Benson MC, Olsson CA (Columbia Univ, New York)
Cancer 75:1642–1648, 1995   21–9

Introduction.—Almost half the patients with prostate cancer are found to be understaged before radical surgery. The effectiveness of enhanced reverse transcriptase–polymerase chain reaction (RT-PCR) for its staging ability and prognostic value was evaluated in 94 consecutive patients with prostate cancer who underwent radical prostatectomy.

Methods.—Before surgery, patients underwent digital rectal examinations, serum prostate-specific antigen (PSA) determinations, and PSA RT-PCR. The sensitivity, specificity, and positive and negative predictive values of PT-PCR were compared with pathology results. Patients were followed up at 3-month intervals for up to 18 months after surgery.

Results.—Correlation of RT-PCR results and postoperative pathology indicated that RT-PCR was positive in 15 of 18 patients with positive surgical margins, 25 of 33 patients with capsular perforation, and 6 of 8 patients with tumor present in the seminal vesicle. Of 58 patients with organ-confined disease, 51 (88%) were PCR negative and 7 were PCR positive. Enhanced RT-PCR for PSA had a high positive predictive value (79%) and a high negative predictive value (84%). No other test had a higher predictive value. In patients with postoperative extraprostatic disease, RT-PCR sensitivity was 72% and specificity was 88%. As PSA levels increased, the percentage of patients who were PCR positive increased similarly. Patients (63%) with PSA values greater than 20 ng/mL were PCR-positive. The positive predictive value of the assay to detect extraprostatic disease in 14 patients with preoperative hormonal therapy was reduced from 88% to 56%.

Conclusion.—The diagnostic properties and positive and negative predictive values of the PCR assay were superior to other conventional modalities used. The coincidence of RT-PCR results with pathologic findings indicates that cancerous cells were escaping from the confines of the prostate gland.

▶ The RT-PCR test for circulating prostate tumor cells is now the focus of a major debate. The results presented by the authors in this and other recent publications from their institution indicate that the test has a high positive predictive value for extracapsular and extraprostatic extension. Unfortunately, other laboratories, including our own, have not confirmed these findings. The Molecular Biological Technology Committee of the American Urological Association is currently assessing the results from various institutions. A collaborative group has joined together to compare techniques and results to resolve the issues. The performance of RT-PCR is not simple and can be done with numerous modifications. Perhaps the results may vary because of differences in technique, which should be reconcilable through interinstitutional collaboration.

In the meantime, most people working in the field do not feel that this test is of sufficient clinical value to be used in the decision-making process. With new information, however, the test may indeed have an important role in staging in the future.

J.B. DeKernion, M.D.

Prostate-Specific Antigen Messenger RNA Is Expressed in Non-Prostate Cells: Implications for Detection of Micrometastases

Smith MR, Biggar S, Hussain M (Fox Chase Cancer Ctr, Philadelphia; VA Med Center, Allen Park, Mich; Wayne State Univ, Detroit)

Cancer Res 55:2640–2644, 1995   21–10

Introduction.—Non prostate cells were evaluated by polymerase chain reaction (PCR) for the presence of prostate specific antigen (PSA) RNA to determine whether this could be a suitable marker for prostate cancer metastases. As a traditional PCR technique was shown to have inadequate sensitivity for PSA RNA, a "nested primer" method was used to amplify the PCR signal for PSA RNA. Cell lines tested included PC-3, LNCaP, and DU145 prostate carcinoma, HCT-8 ileocecal adenocarcinoma, MCF-7 breast carcinoma, BG-1 ovarian carcinoma, A549 and SK-MES-1 lung carcinoma, and HL-60 myeloid leukemia. Blood and bone marrow samples were also analyzed.

Results.—In addition to the expected detection of PSA RNA in prostate cancer lines, PSA RNA was found in lung cancer cell lines, the ovarian carcinoma cell line, and in the myeloid leukemia cell line. Results were confirmed by ethidium staining and Southern analysis using a PSA-specific oligonucleotide probe. Samples in the absence of reverse transcriptase were negative, suggesting that there was no cross-reactivity with DNA. Kallikrein cross-reactivity was ruled out by hybridizing the amplified RNA fragments to an internal PSA oligonucleotide, by the RNA product's cleavage with an endonuclease, and by direct DNA sequencing. Additionally, all blood samples from 13 healthy donors were positive for PSA RNA by nested primer PCR, although none were positive by standard primary PCR reactions.

Discussion.—Although nested primer PCR appears to be a very sensitive method for PSA RNA detection, this gene lacks the specificity to be an adequate marker for prostate cancer metastasis.

▶ Using nested primers to increase the sensitivity of reverse transcriptase–PCR (RT-PCR) for the detection of prostatic micrometastasis, the authors unexpectedly found PSA expression in cells of nonprostatic origin. Pursuing this lead further, they detected circulating PSA-expressing cells in 13 "normal" male and female controls. These findings are extremely important. First, they suggest that PSA expression is not absolutely tissue specific, an important point as we develop "tissue specific" gene therapy delivery systems. Second, these results underscore the critical importance of negative controls in all studies of RT-PCR for the detection of micrometastatic disease. Finally, these results imply that there will be a limit to the sensitivity of RT-PCR assays for micrometastatic detection, in that increases in sensitivity will be hampered by decreases in specificity. Because the ultimate aim of RT-PCR presumably is to exclude patients with metastatic disease from local therapy (pending longer-term results following patients with positive RT-PCR results), any decrease in specificity will seriously compromise the utility of this test.

R.E. Reiter, M.D.

Are Transrectal Ultrasonically Guided Biopsies Required for the Accurate Diagnosis of Carcinoma of the Prostate? Can Digitally Guided Systematic Biopsies Offer an Acceptable Alternative?

Figueiredo AJC, Seeni K, Anson KM, Furtado AJL, Miller RA (Univ Hosp of Coimbra, Portugal; Whittington Hosp, London)
Br J Urol 76:187–191, 1995   21–11

Background.—Transrectal ultrasound (TRUS) has been suggested for use in guiding prostatic biopsy because cancers may produce a hypoechoic image, but a majority of such images do not correspond to neoplastic disease. As many as 40% of cancers arising in the peripheral part of the prostate go undetected by ultrasonography. Some have asked whether systematic digitally guided biopsies might be equally informative.

Objective and Methods.—The diagnostic yield of TRUS-guided systematic biopsies was compared prospectively with that of digitally guided biopsies in 52 patients with suspected prostatic cancer who had both studies at the same time. The patients, 54–88 years of age, had abnormal findings on digital rectal examination and/or an elevated serum prostate-

TABLE 1.—Patients With Carcinoma Diagnosed by Needle Biopsy

Patients	TRUS-guided		Digitally guided	
	Left	Right	Left	Right
1	Ca	Neg	Ca	Neg
2	Neg	Ca	Neg	Ca
3	Neg	Neg	Neg	Ca
4	Ca	Ca	Ca	Ca
5	Ca	Ca	Ca	Ca
6	Ca	Ca	Ca	Ca
7	Atypical	Ca	Atypical	Ca
8	Ca	Neg	Neg	Ca
9	Ca	Ca	Ca	Ca
10	Ca	Neg	Neg	Neg
11	Ca	Ca	Ca	Ca
12	Ca	Ca	Ca	Ca
13	Atypical	Ca	Atypical	Atypical
14	Ca	Neg	Ca	Neg
15	Ca	Ca	Ca	Ca
16	Neg	Ca	Neg	Ca
17	Ca	Ca	Ca	Ca
18	Ca	Neg	Ca	Neg
19	Ca	Neg	Ca	Neg

Abbreviations: Ca, carcinoma; *Neg*, negative.
(Courtesy of Figueiredo AJC, Seeni K, Anson KM, et al: Are transrectal ultrasonically guided biopsies required for the accurate diagnosis of carcinoma of the prostate? Can digitally guided systematic biopsies offer an acceptable alternative? *Br J Urol* 76:187–191, 1995.)

specific antigen (PSA) level. A spring-driven Biopty gun with an 18-G Tru-cut type needle was used in all cases. From 9 to 18 cores were taken in each case, the average number being 12.

Results.—Adequate tissue samples were obtained in all cases. Nineteen patients (36.5%) had cancers, 16 of which were detected by both methods. Two cancers were found only by TRUS-guided biopsy, and 1 only by digitally guided biopsy. Both methods detected the dysplastic foci present in 5 patients (Table 1). There were no postbiopsy infections, and a majority of patients did not express a preference for either technique.

Conclusions.—Digitally guided prostatic biopsy appears to be adequate for routine screening purposes. Transrectal ultrasound is indicated when biopsies of a normal-sized gland are negative but the PSA level is elevated. The TRUS technique also is helpful when staging cancers for surgical treatment.

▶ This paper demonstrates what most physicians suspect: skillfully done, finger-guided biopsies will have almost the same sensitivity in detecting prostate cancer as that of ultrasound. However, ultrasound gives a good estimate of volume (which may be important for PSA density) and local extension, especially to seminal vesicles. On the other hand, patients with a classic prostate cancer abnormality, especially with a typical, well-defined hard mass, can often be just as well served by finger-guided biopsy, avoiding the expense of TRUS.

J.B. DeKernion, M.D.

Antimicrobial Prophylaxis for Transrectal Prostatic Biopsy: A Prospective Randomized Trial of Cefuroxime Versus Piperacillin/Tazobactam
Brewster SF, MacGowan AP, Gingell JC (Bristol Urological Inst, England; Southmead Hosp, Bristol, England)
Br J Urol 76:351–354, 1995   21–12

Objective.—Two programs of antimicrobial prophylaxis were compared in 111 consecutive men who underwent transrectal prostatic core-biopsy (TPB) with ultrasound guidance.

Study Plan.—A prospective, randomized, open-label design was used to compare single-dose cefuroxime with a combination of piperacillin and tazobactam (PT). Fifty-six men received 1.5 g of cefuroxime intravenously 20 minutes before the procedure. The remaining 55 men received 4.5 g of PT. The anterior rectal wall was swabbed with an antiseptic before obtaining 4 biopsy samples.

Results.—Eight of the 109 evaluable men, 3 in the cefuroxime group and 5 given PT, were febrile (37.5°C) or had symptoms of urinary or systemic sepsis after TPB. Only 1 of these patients, a man who received cefuroxime, was bacteremic. Five men in all had bacteriuria or bacteremia after the procedure. Four failures were caused by an organism that was sensitive to the antimicrobial administered. In no case were anaerobic organisms cultured. Sixteen men given PT and 2 given cefuroxime had transient diarrhea.

Recommendation.—The additional use of oral prophylaxis may further reduce the risk of sepsis after TPB. At present the authors administer either 4.5 g of PT or 1.2 g of co-amoxyclav intravenously before TPB, and prescribe oral co-amoxyclav for 3 days afterwards.

▶ The authors conclude that a combination of intravenous antibiotics may further reduce the small risk of septicemia after prostate biopsy. In the United States, most of us use oral prophylaxis, and I doubt that our incidence of clinically significant infections is any greater than what the authors report in both of their groups. Oral medications are easier and usually less expensive to administer over the short-term and are more convenient for both the patient and physician. Unless intravenous regimens can prove superior, little enthusiasm for intravenous prophylaxis will be generated.

J.B. DeKernion, M.D.

PSA Assay of Dried Blood Samples From the Ear Lobe on a Filter Paper With Special Reference to Prostatic Mass Screening
Watanabe H, Ohe H, Saitoh M, Kojima M, Tanaka T, Ito S (Kyoto Prefectural Univ, Japan; SRL Inc, Tokyo)
Prostate 27:90–94, 1995   21–13

Objective.—As an alternative to conventional blood sampling for use in field studies of prostatic cancer, a method was developed for estimating prostate-specific antigen (PSA) in blood taken from the earlobe and air-dried on filter paper.

Method.—Prostate-specific antigen is measured using a DERFIA PSA KIT, a fluoroimmunoassay procedure that uses Eu^{2+} (europium) as a tracer. An 18-gauge syringe needle is placed in the inferior end of the ear lobe, and the sample is spread over a 1-cm-diameter area of filter paper. Four 4-mm sections are punched out for analysis.

Validation.—When venous blood and ear lobe estimates were compared in 25 patients with prostatic cancer, 14 with benign prostatic hyperplasia (BPH), and 24 normal individuals, the 2 values correlated at a level of 0.96. Ear lobe values averaged about half of those in venous blood. Ear lobe samples from 3 patients with prostate cancer who had very high PSA values remained nearly constant over 5 weeks when preserved at 4°C. When preserved at room temperature, however, the values declined starting 1 week after sample collection. Among 835 men who underwent mass screening, BPH was found in 6% of those whose ear lobe PSA values were less than 2 ng/mL. Nearly 60% of men with higher values had BPH, and 3 (4.3%) had prostatic cancer. The latter patients had values ranging from 2.3 to 15.6 ng/mL.

Conclusion.—Estimating PSA in blood from the ear lobe is a comparatively simple and inexpensive means of mass screening for prostate cancer.

▶ The only advantage of this technique is in situations of mass screening. It is faster and easier than setting up stations for venipuncture. Mass screenings using PSA alone (without digital rectal examination) are not currently planned, and the utility of the ear-lobe puncture method will have to await further study.

J.B. DeKernion, M.D.

Evaluation of Percentage of Free Serum Prostate-Specific Antigen to Improve Specificity of Prostate Cancer Screening

Catalona WJ, Smith DS, Wolfert RL, Wang TJ, Rittenhouse HG, Ratliff TL, Nadler RB (Washington Univ, St Louis, Mo; Hybritech Inc, San Diego, Calif)
JAMA 274:1214–1220, 1995   21–14

Background.—The use of relatively low serum prostate-specific antigen (PSA) cutoffs (4.0 ng/mL) for cancer screening purposes has led to high false-positive rates. Slightly elevated PSA levels can indicate prostate cancer in its curable stages but are also caused by benign prostatic hyperplasia and prostatitis. Total and free serum PSA levels in a large group of healthy men were retrospectively analyzed to improve the specificity of screening and reduce the rate of unnecessary biopsies.

Methods.—From July 1989 through March 1995, total serum PSA levels were measured in 10,249 men aged 50–90 years (mean 62.7 years); 99% of the men were white. None had a history of prostate cancer or prostatitis. Prostate cancer was suspected when PSA values were higher than 4.0 ng/mL. Those with 2 serum PSA concentrations above this level within a 1- to 2-week period underwent digital rectal examination and prostatic ultrasonography. A needle biopsy was performed when either procedure revealed abnormal or suspicious findings. Results of the biopsy, clinical and pathologic tumor stage, and tumor grade were recorded for these men, as were results of free PSA measurement.

Results.—Serum PSA concentrations of 4.1–10.0 ng/mL were found in 113 men, including 63 with histologically confirmed benign prostatic hyperplasia, 30 with prostate cancer with an enlarged gland, and 20 with cancer with a normal-sized gland. The median percentage of free PSA was 18.8% in men with benign prostatic hyperplasia, 15.9% in men with cancer and an enlarged gland, and 9.2% in men with cancer and a normal-sized gland. In contrast, total PSA did not differ across these groups (6.0%, 6.6%, and 5.3%, respectively). Thus measurement of the percentage of free PSA (Fig 1) yielded predictive information about the presence of prostate cancer above that provided by the total PSA level, the results of rectal examination, and prostate size. In men with an enlarged, palpably benign gland, at least 90% of cancers would have been detected with a free PSA cutoff of 23.4% or lower. About a third of negative

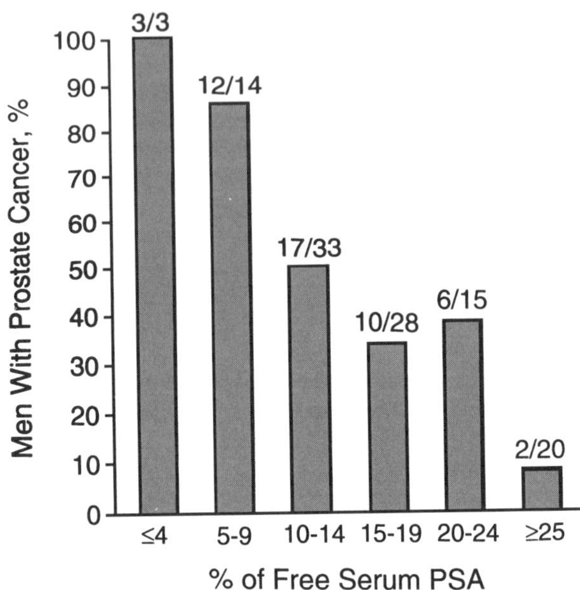

FIGURE 1.—Decreasing simple proportion of men in the combined study groups found to have prostate cancer on biopsy with each 5% increase in the percentage of free prostate-specific antigen (*PSA*) in serum (ratio of free PSA to total PSA multiplied by 100). (Courtesy of Catalona WJ, Smith DS, Wolfert RL, et al: Evaluation of percentage of free serum prostate-specific antigen to improve specificity of prostate cancer screening. *JAMA* 274:1214–1220, 1995. Copyright 1995, American Medical Association.)

biopsies would have been eliminated by using this cutoff. Because a relatively narrow range of cancer stages was represented, the percentage of PSA was not correlated with the Gleason score or the presence of pathologically advanced cancer.

Conclusion.—In selected men with elevated total serum PSA levels detected in prostate cancer screening, measurements of free PSA can reduce unnecessary biopsies. Appropriate cutoffs for men with slight elevations of total serum PSA and enlarged, palpably benign findings on digital rectal examination have yet to be determined.

▶ It seems clear that the ratio of free to total PSA will have clinical utility. The authors rightly point out the current deficits in our information before we can bring this test to appropriate clinical use. Its greatest use will be in patients with minimal PSA elevation and a normal-sized prostate gland. It also may be very helpful in patients with an elevated PSA and an enlarged prostate, whose first set of biopsy specimens show no cancer. The ratio may help decide who should or shouldn't have another biopsy performed. It is not clear, however, whether the initial level of PSA will require alteration of the breakpoint for the ratio.

J.B. DeKernion, M.D.

Free, Complexed and Total Serum Prostate Specific Antigen: The Establishment of Appropriate Reference Ranges for Their Concentrations and Ratios

Oesterling JE, Jacobsen SJ, Klee GG, Pettersson K, Piironen T, Abrahamsson P-A, Stenman U-H, Dowell B, Lövgren T, Lilja H (Univ of Michigan, Ann Arbor; Mayo Clinic and Mayo Found, Rochester, Minn; Univ of Turku, Finland; et al)

J Urol 154:1090–1095, 1995

21–15

Background.—Prostate-specific antigen (PSA) is the most useful tumor marker used to diagnose and treat prostatic cancer, but at present its sensitivity and specificity are less than ideal. Prostate-specific antigen exists in serum in a number of molecular forms that may be quantified by immune assays: free PSA; PSA complexed with α1-antichymotrypsin (so-called complexed PSA); and the sum of the free and complexed forms.

Objective and Methods.—A total of 422 healthy men aged 40–79 years were screened for prostate cancer to determine reference ratios for the various molecular forms of PSA, in the hope of making the test better able to distinguish between benign hyperplasia and potentially curable cancer. The individuals underwent digital rectal examination and transrectal ultrasonography. Immunofluorometric assays based on monoclonal antibodies were used to determine levels of free, complexed, and total PSA.

Findings.—All 3 forms of PSA correlated directly with age. Based on the 95th percentile, reference ranges for free, complexed, and total PSA were 0.5, 1.0, and 2.0 ng/mL for men 40–49 years of age; 0.7, 1.5, and 3.0 ng/mL for those aged 50–59 years; 1.0, 2.0, and 4.0 ng/mL for those aged 60–69 years; and 1.2, 3.0, and 5.5 ng/mL for those aged 70–79 years. None of the ratios correlated with age. The upper normal limit for men of all ages is 0.15 for the ratio of free-to-total PSA; less than 0.7 for complexed-to-total PSA; and more than 0.25 for free-to-complexed PSA. The free-to-total PSA ratio will be most helpful in men whose serum PSA levels range from 2 to 10 ng/mL.

Conclusion.—These reference ranges will allow urologists to use free, complexed, and total PSA when evaluating men at risk of early prostatic cancer.

▶ This paper is another of the recent papers studying the ratio of free-to-total PSA. The authors also looked at complexed PSA as another submarker. It is not clear how this will be used in the future. They used a cutoff of 0.15 for the free PSA ratio as a measure of cancer. This measure differs from others, and the assay used will influence the baseline in all the studies. Their reference range for total PSA also seems lower than other published reports. The authors suggest the ratio will be most useful in the lower PSA elevations, and I suspect that will be the case. More information will be needed before we know how to use this test.

J.B. DeKernion, M.D.

Measurement of the Proportion of Free to Total Prostate-Specific Antigen Improves Diagnostic Performance of Prostate-Specific Antigen in the Diagnostic Gray Zone of Total Prostate-Specific Antigen

Luderer AA, Chen Y-T, Soriano TF, Kramp WJ, Carlson G, Cuny C, Sharp T, Smith W, Petteway J, Brawer MK, Thiel R (Dianon Systems Inc, Stratford, Conn; Univ of Washington, Seattle; Southern Connecticut State Univ, New Haven)
Urology 46:187–194, 1995   21–16

Background.—Although estimates of prostate-specific antigen (PSA) have proved helpful in detecting prostatic cancer, they are not an ideal tumor marker for use in screening and early detection. Forms of PSA complexed with α_1-antichymotrypsin and α_2-macroglobulin have been identified. Levels of free (noncomplexed) PSA are much lower. The respective clinical importance of free and complexed PSA remains uncertain.

Objective.—Concentrations of free PSA and the ratio of free PSA to total PSA were determined in 55 newly diagnosed men aged 55–62 years of age with prostate cancer; 62 untreated men with benign prostatic disease; and 64 age-matched healthy men whose PSA values were less than 4 ng/mL.

Methods.—Total serum PSA was estimated using the PA immunoassay, and free serum PSA was estimated with an investigational double-antibody immunoradiometric assay.

Results.—Thirty-seven percent of patients with benign prostatic hyperplasia and only 7% of those with prostate cancer had a total PSA level less than 4 ng/mL. Significantly more patients with cancer had a free-to-total PSA less than 15%. The median free-to-total PSA differed significantly in

TABLE V.—Descriptive Statistics for Total PSA* and Proportion of Free to Total PSA for All Subjects by Patient Group

	Patient Group			
	Normal Control (n = 64)	Benign (n = 62)	Cancer (n = 55)	P Value†
Total PSA (ng/mL)				
Mean	1.24	5.52	13.64	
Median	1.07	4.89	9.60	<0.0001
Standard deviation	0.81	4.12	15.18	
95% CI for mean	1.03–1.44	4.47–6.75	9.54–17.75	
Free/Total PSA (%)				
Mean	26	23	13	
Median	23	21	13	<0.0001
Standard deviation	14	13	6	
95% CI for mean	23–30	20–27	11–14	

* TOSOH immunoassay.
† Wilcoxon test comparing median values between benign and cancer patients.
Abbreviations: PSA, prostate-specific antigen; *CI,* confidence interval.
(Reprinted by permission of the publisher. From Luderer AA, Chen Y-T, Soriano TF, et al: Measurement of the proportion of free to total prostate-specific antigen improves diagnostic performance of prostate-specific antigen in the diagnostic gray zone of total prostate-specific antigen. *Urology* 46:187–194. Copyright 1995 by Elsevier Science, Inc.)

Moving?

I'd like to receive my *Year Book of Urology* without interruption.
Please note the following change of address, effective:

Name: ____

New Address: ______________________________________

____

City: _______________________ State: _______ Zip: _______

Old Address: _______________________________________

____

City: _______________________ State: _______ Zip: _______

Reservation Card

Yes, I would like my own copy of *Year Book of Urology*. Please begin my subscription with the current edition according to the terms described below.* I understand that I will have 30 days to examine each annual edition. If satisfied, I will pay just $75.95 plus sales tax, postage and handling (price subject to change without notice).

Name: ____

Address: ____

City: _______________________ State: _______ Zip: _______

Method of Payment
O Visa   O Mastercard   O AmEx   O Bill me   O Check (in US dollars, payable to Mosby, Inc.)

Card number: _______________________ Exp date: _______________

Signature: ____

LS-0908

Your Year Book Service Guarantee:

When you subscribe to the *Year Book*, we'll send you an advance notice of future volumes about two months before they publish. This automatic notice system is designed to take up as little of your time as possible. If you do not want the *Year Book*, the advance notice makes it quick and easy for you to let us know your decision, and you will always have at least 20 days to decide. If we don't hear from you, we'll send you the new volume as soon as it's available. And, of course, the *Year Book* is yours to examine free of charge for 30 days (postage, handling and applicable sales tax are added to each shipment.).

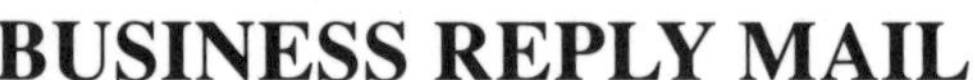

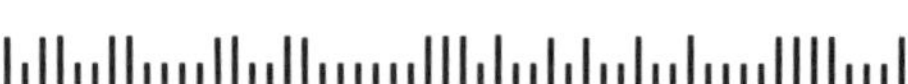

BUSINESS REPLY MAIL

FIRST CLASS MAIL   PERMIT No. 762   CHICAGO, IL

POSTAGE WILL BE PAID BY ADDRESSEE

Chris Hughes
Mosby-Year Book, Inc.
200 N. LaSalle Street
Suite 2600
Chicago, IL 60601-9981

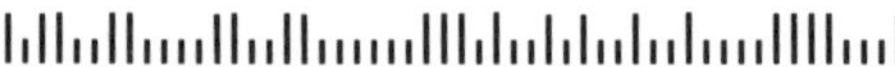

BUSINESS REPLY MAIL

FIRST CLASS MAIL   PERMIT No. 762   CHICAGO, IL

POSTAGE WILL BE PAID BY ADDRESSEE

Chris Hughes
Mosby-Year Book, Inc.
200 N. LaSalle Street
Suite 2600
Chicago, IL 60601-9981

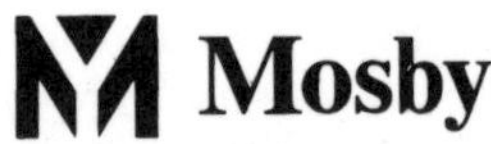

Dedicated to publishing excellence

the groups with cancer and benign disease (Table V). Total PSA and the free-to-total ratio were comparably diagnostic when all individuals were considered. For those with total PSA values in the "gray zone" of 4–10 ng/mL, however, the free-to-total PSA performed better than total PSA in that it was clearly more specific for nearly all levels of sensitivity.

Conclusion.—In addition to estimating free serum PSA, calculating the proportion of free PSA to total PSA makes it easier to distinguish between prostate cancer and benign prostatic hyperplasia.

▶ The free PSA, as one might expect, was most helpful in patients with total PSA of 4–10 ng/mL. The authors set the cutoff value at 0.15 ng/mL for cancer detection, similar to what others have done. Again, this may have to be adjusted based on the total PSA.

J.B. DeKernion, M.D.

Age-Specific Reference Ranges for Serum Prostate-Specific Antigen
Anderson JR, Strickland D, Corbin D, Byrnes JA, Zweiback E (Univ of Nebraska, Omaha; Health Fair of the Midlands, Inc, Omaha, Neb)
Urology 46:54–57, 1995   21–17

Background.—The incidence of prostate cancer, the second leading cause of death in men in the United States, has increased rapidly in recent years. Much of this increase is attributed to the widespread use of prostate-specific antigen (PSA) screening and of transurethral resection of the prostate for benign prostatic hyperplasia. Because serum PSA levels appear to increase with age, the current reference upper limit of normal of 4.0 ng/mL may not be appropriate for all age groups. Results from a group of men who underwent PSA screening at a health fair were examined to determine the relationship of the distribution of serum PSA levels to age.

Methods.—The 1,716 men who provided blood for serum PSA determination in March 1993 attended a health fair held at various sites in Iowa and Nebraska. Included in the predominantly white group were 376 men aged 40–49 years, 571 men aged 50–59 years, 532 men aged 60–69 years, and 237 men aged 70–79 years. Digital rectal examination (DRE) was offered as well, and 897 men had DRE in addition to the PSA test. For 8 consecutive 5-year age groups, descriptive statistics including the median, 25th, 75th, and 95th percentile of the distribution of serum PSA, were calculated.

Results.—A correlation was found between patient age and serum PSA concentration. The observed 95th percentile increased from 1.5 ng/mL for men 40–44 years of age to 7.7 ng/mL for those aged 75–79 years. In addition, variability in serum PSA concentrations increased with increasing age. The upper limits of normal (the 95th percentiles) for serum PSA were thus estimated to be 1.5 ng/mL for ages 40–49 years, 2.6 ng/mL for ages 50–59 years, 4.4 ng/mL for ages 60–69 years, and 7.5 ng/mL for ages

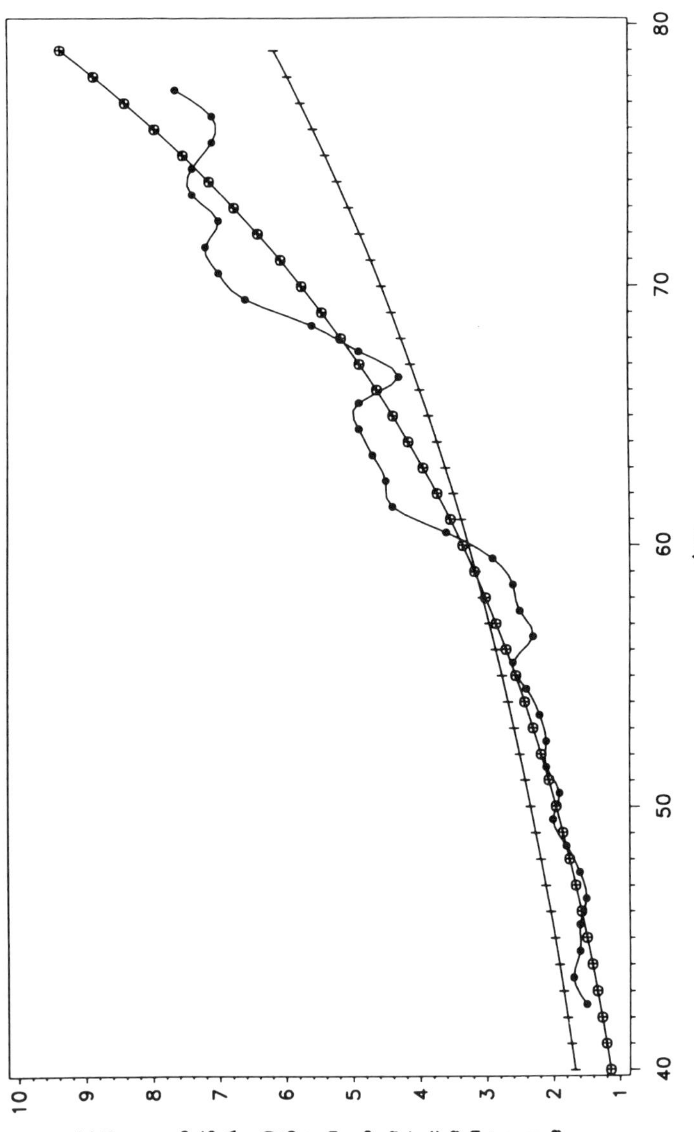

FIGURE 1.—Estimated 95th percentiles of prostate-specific antigen (*PSA*) by age (years). *Closed circles* denote observed 95th percentiles of distribution of serum PSA level estimated using 5-year moving averages. *Short vertical lines* denote model estimates of 95th percentile of distribution of serum PSA level obtained from constant variance regression model. *Circles with cross* denote model estimates of 95th percentile of distribution of serum PSA level obtained from the weighted regression model, which assumed that variance of PSA increased with increasing age. (Reprinted by permission of the publisher. From Anderson JR, Strickland D, Corbin D, et al: Age-specific reference ranges for serum prostate-specific antigen. *Urology* 46:54–57. Copyright 1995 Elsevier Science, Inc.)

70–79 years. These upper limits are substantially less that those previously proposed for men aged 40–59 years and greater for men aged 70–79 years (Fig 1).

Conclusion.—The increasing variability of PSA concentration with age was not considered in previously published, age-specific reference ranges. Thus, upper limits of normal may have been too high for men younger than 60 years and too low for those older than 70 years. The use of PSA for prostate cancer screening of the general population has been controversial, and there is a need for standardization of age-specific upper limits of normal.

▶ This study differs from others in that Anderson et al. showed that variability of PSA increases with increasing age. They make the argument that because of this, prior age-adjusted levels may have been too high for the younger population and too low for older men. The greatest significance of this and other age-adjusted PSA studies is the data which show that a "normal" level of PSA up to 4 ng/mL is extremely high for young men. Unfortunately, this message has not gotten to many family practitioners who will simply observe 50 year-old men with PSA levels of 3.5 or 4 ng/mL. This and other studies hopefully will bring the message home. I am not sure that the age adjustment is as important for the more elderly, except that it would give one comfort that the patient does not have prostate cancer when the first set of biopsy specimens are negative.

J.B. DeKernion, M.D.

The National Cancer Data Base Report on Prostate Cancer
Mettlin CJ, Murphy GP, McGinnis LS, Menck HR (American College of Surgeons, Chicago; American Cancer Society, Atlanta, Ga)
Cancer 76:1104–1112, 1995   21–18

Background.—Prostate cancer is the second most commonly diagnosed cancer in men in the United States. Advances in the technology to detect this cancer contribute to the increasing frequency of this diagnosis. There have also been changes in the patterns of care, including the use of radical prostatectomy. These and other trends in prostate cancer care have been documented by the Commission on Cancer using data from the National Cancer Data Base.

Methods.—Hospital cancer registries across the United States provided 52,597 prostate cancer reports for 1986–1987 and 101,903 for 1992. Data on a total of 154,500 patients with prostate cancer were analyzed.

Findings.—Prostate cancer is being detected more often at localized stages and in younger men. The pattern of diagnosis in African-American men is one of more advanced disease. Prostatectomy is increasingly selected as the primary treatment. The use of this treatment varies by region as well as patient and hospital characteristics. The choice of radiation therapy has increased to a lesser extent. Patients with prostate cancer diagnosed in 1986 and 1987 had a 5-year survival of 60%. Outcomes depended on disease stage, patient age, and race.

Conclusions.—The detection and treatment of prostate cancer have changed substantially in recent years. The increased use of early detection measures appears to be associated with these changes. However, the improvements in prostate cancer detection and treatment trends have not benefited everyone equally. African-American men continue to have more advanced disease at initial assessment and lower survival rates.

▶ This article points to the epidemiologic value of the National Cancer Data Base surveys of the American Cancer Society and the American College of Surgeons. Although some have claimed as high as a sixfold increase in radical prostatectomies in the Medicare population, this report confirms an increase of 2.5 times from 1987 to 1992.[1] However, during this period, the number of new cases of prostate cancer doubled, the number of cases of localized disease increased, and the expertise of urologists with the anatomic radical prostatectomy increased, which may explain this increase. What the article does confirm, and which cannot be easily explained, is the substantial regional variations in prostatectomies performed (20.7% in the Northeast to 35.5% in the West) or why we are performing this procedure in men in their late 70s or 80s. We (urologists) must be able to explain and defend this procedure, and I find this difficult in an 80-year-old man, even a "young 80-year-old."

B.J. Miles, M.D.

Reference

1. Lu-Yao GL, McLeman D, Wasson J, et al: An assessment of radical prostatectomy: Time trends, geographic variations, and outcomes. *JAMA* 269:2633–2636, 1993.

Long-Term Survival Among Men With Conservatively Treated Localized Prostate Cancer
Albertsen PC, Fryback DG, Storer BE, Kolon TF, Fine J (Univ of Connecticut Health Ctr, Farmington; Univ of Wisconsin, Madison; Yale Univ, New Haven, Conn)
JAMA 274:626–631, 1995   21–19

Purpose.—More men with localized prostate cancer are being treated with radiation therapy and radical surgery. However, there are insufficient data to document the therapeutic benefits of these treatments, compared with more conservative alternatives, for patients aged 65–75 years. The debate over the use of widespread screening and treatment for men in this age group depends on inferences about the natural history of conservatively managed localized prostate cancer. In a population-based study, mortality and life expectancy were analyzed retrospectively for 65- to 75-year-old men with newly diagnosed, clinically localized prostate cancer who were treated only with immediate or delayed hormonal therapy.

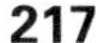

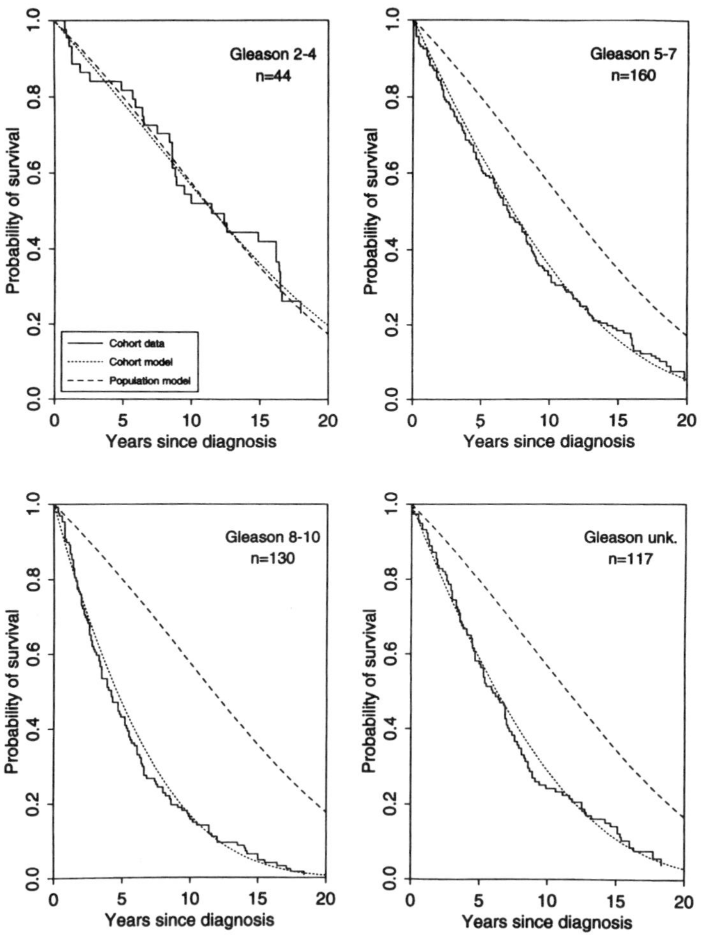

FIGURE 2.—Age-adjusted survival curves for low-, moderate-, and high-grade tumors. Observed cohort data are shown as Kaplan-Meier curves. *Smooth curves* are age-adjusted survival predicted for each group by the bivariate hazard model and by the general population model. **Top left graph** is for Gleason score 2 to 4 tumors ($n = 44$); **top right**, Gleason score 5 to 7 tumors ($n = 160$); **bottom left**, Gleason score 8 to 10 tumors ($n = 130$); and **bottom right**, Gleason score unknown ($n = 117$). (Courtesy of Albertsen PC, Fryback DG, Storer BE, et al: Long-term survival among men with conservatively treated localized prostate cancer. *JAMA* 274:626–631, Aug 23. Copyright 1995, American Medical Association.)

Methods.—Cases identified from the Connecticut Tumor Registry were reviewed. They included all men with clinically localized prostate cancer diagnosed in 1971–1976 who were aged 65–75 years at the time of diagnosis and were either untreated or treated with immediate or delayed hormonal therapy. The final cohort included 451 men who had a mean age of 71 years at the time of diagnosis. Patient data were abstracted from the records of 37 acute care hospitals and 2 VA medical centers in Connecticut. A pathologist evaluated the original pathology slides without knowledge of the patients' outcomes. The patients' survival was compared with that of men in the general population by parametric proportional hazards models that took into account the tumor histologic findings, comorbidity, and age at diagnosis.

Results.—At a mean follow-up of 15½ years, 9% of patients were alive at last contact, 34% had died of prostate cancer, 49% had died of other known causes, and 8% had died of unknown causes. Age-adjusted survival of patients with Gleason score 2 to 4 tumors was not significantly different from that of men in the general population. Men with Gleason score 5 to 7 tumors lost a maximum estimated life expectancy of 4–5 years, and those with Gleason score 8 to 10 tumors lost no more than 6–8 years (Fig 2). Survival was significantly and independently predicted by the tumor histologic findings and by the patients' comorbid illnesses.

Conclusions.—Men aged 65–75 years with conservatively treated, low-grade prostate cancer show no loss of life expectancy compared with the general population. As tumor grade increases, lost life expectancy increases progressively. Reports of survival and mortality for men with clinically localized prostate cancer must control for age, histologic findings, and comorbidity to avoid bias.

▶ In this article, the authors chose to focus on the fact that watchful waiting in well-differentiated, clinically localized prostate cancers resulted in no loss of life. Unfortunately, only 9% of their patients fall into this group. The other 91% had moderately to poorly differentiated cancers and lost from 4 to 8 years of life by being conservatively managed. The loss of life is even greater than predicted by a Markov model that was used by Beck et al. to predict the value (or lack of) of radical prostatectomy in the management of prostate cancer.[1] Although the authors presented this as further evidence supporting watchful waiting, I believe the results support the usefulness of treating almost all cases of clinically localized prostate cancer in appropriately selected men with low comorbidity and who are younger than 75 years.

B.J. Miles, M.D.

Reference

1. Beck JR, Kattan MW, Miles BJ: Critique of the decision analysis for clinically localized prostate cancer. *J Urol* 152:1894, 1994.

Early Detection of Prostate Cancer: Results of a Prostate Specific Antigen–Based Detection Program in Japan
Egawa S, Suyama K, Ohori M, Kawakami T, Kuwao S, Hirokado K, Hirano S, Yokoyama E, Uchida T, Koshiba K (Kitasato Univ, Sagamihara, Japan; Health Science Ctr, Sagamihara, Japan)
Cancer 76:463–472, 1995

21–20

Background.—Screening programs for prostate cancer seek to detect the cancer while it is confined to the gland, thus maximizing the chance for cure. Screening with serum prostate-specific antigen (PSA), along with digital rectal examination, has more than doubled the percentage of organ-confined cancers detected. The results of serum PSA screening in Japanese men were reported.

Methods.—During 1 year, 1,189 men aged 55 years or older took part in a program for early detection of prostate cancer. All underwent measurement of serum PSA, and those with a level of greater than 2.0 ng/mL—rather than the conventional cutoff point of 4 ng/mL—were referred for further evaluation.

Results.—Serum PSA values were elevated in 13% of men. About 3% had serum PSA values greater than 4 ng/mL. Ultrasound-guided biopsy was performed in 99 men, 16 of whom were found to have cancer, for a cancer detection rate of 1.3%. Eighty-one percent of the cancers detected were clinically localized. The serum PSA level was less than 4 ng/mL in 7 patients and less than 3 ng/mL in 5. Thirteen patients underwent radical prostatectomy. Clinically significant cancer was detected in all of these patients, and 69% had cancer pathologically confined within the gland.

Conclusions.—Serum PSA values may be lower in elderly Asian men than in Western men. Further studies are needed to define the optimal cutoff point for serum PSA in Asian populations. Previous studies may have overestimated ethnic differences in the incidence of prostate cancer.

▶ This is an interesting study in Japanese men which confirms that the "standard" upper normal limit of 4.0 ng/mL for serum PSA may not be valid for all nationalities and ethnic groups. Significantly, of the 16 positive biopsies, 7 occurred in men with PSA levels between 2.1 and 4.0 ng/mL, and 5 of these were in men in their 60s. Interestingly, in U.S. males, Gann et al. found that those with a PSA between 2 and 4 ng/mL have up to a fourfold risk of developing prostate cancer compared with men with PSA levels less than 2.0 ng/mL.[1] Despite such refinements as age-specific ranges for PSA, it is clear that our understanding of the most appropriate normative levels for different ethnic groups remains to be defined.

B.J. Miles, M.D.

Reference

1. Gann PH, Hennekens CH, Stampfer MJ: A prospective evaluation of plasma prostate-specific antigen for detection of prostatic cancer. *JAMA* 273:289–294, 1995.

A Prospective Evaluation of Plasma Prostate-Specific Antigen for Detection of Prostatic Cancer
Gann PH, Hennekens CH, Stampfer MJ (Brigham and Women's Hosp, Boston; Harvard Med School, Boston)
JAMA 273:289–294, 1995   21–21

Objective.—Prostate cancer, the second leading cause of cancer death among U.S. men, can be detected by measuring the level of prostate-specific antigen (PSA) in the serum. Because PSA levels are directly proportional to tumor volume and testing is relatively inexpensive, some

TABLE 3.—Relative Risk (RR) of Developing Prostate Cancer According to Baseline Prostate-Specific Antigen (PSA) Level: 10-Year Follow-Up, Physicians' Health Study*

PSA Level, ng/mL		All Cancers		Aggressive Cancers		Nonaggressive Cancers	
Polyclonal	Monoclonal	Cases/Controls, n	RR (95% CI)	Cases/Controls, n	RR (95% CI)	Cases/Controls, n	RR (95% CI)
≤1.60	≤1.00	29/386	1.0	15/203	1.0	13/161	1.0
1.61–2.50	1.01–1.50	40/259	2.2 (1.3–3.6)	13/126	1.9 (0.8–4.2)	24/112	2.5 (1.2–5.2)
2.51–3.50	1.51–2.00	33/139	3.4 (1.9–5.9)	8/64	1.7 (0.7–4.4)	24/72	4.5 (2.1–9.4)
3.51–5.50	2.01–3.00	57/148	5.5 (3.3–9.2)	28/73	6.8 (3.1–14.9)	24/64	4.7 (2.2–10.1)
5.51–7.30	3.01–4.00	37/70	8.6 (4.7–15.6)	17/31	10.2 (4.1–25.4)	16/34	7.3 (3.0–17.9)
7.31–18.4	4.01–10.0	102/84	22.2 (12.9–38.2)	53/45	31.0 (13.4–71.5)	42/33	21.0 (9.4–46.9)
>18.40	>10.00	68/12	145.3 (59.1–357.0)	49/7	461.4 (93.9–2271.0)	17/4	91.6 (22.5–372.4)

* Relative risks estimated by odds ratios obtained from conditional logistic regression models with matching on age and follow-up time. Eight cases also selected as controls were excluded from the control set.

Abbreviation: CI, confidence interval.

(Courtesy of Gann PH, Hennekens CH, Stampfer MJ: A prospective evaluation of plasma prostate-specific antigen for detection of prostatic cancer. *JAMA* 273:289–294, Jan. 25. Copyright 1995, American Medical Association.)

advocate routine screening of men for prostate cancer. Others argue that because PSA does not measure severity of the disease, routine screening is not cost-effective. The specificity and sensitivity of the PSA test, as well as lead time, cutoff levels, and relative risks associated with PSA levels, were evaluated prospectively.

Methods.—A total of 366 men with prostate cancer and 1,098 randomly selected controls participated in the 10-year study. Titers of PSA were compared, and sensitivity and specificity were determined for each year of follow-up. There were 183 aggressive (stage C or D) tumors, 160 nonaggressive (stage A or B) tumors, and 23 intermediately aggressive tumors.

Results.—Overall sensitivity at the standard cutoff of 4.0 ng/mL was 46%, but decreased significantly with time since last blood collection, particularly for younger men. Sensitivity was 87% for aggressive tumors and 53% for nonaggressive tumors. The overall specificity was 91% and changed little from year to year. Maximum validity was achieved at a cutoff of 3.3 ng/mL. The diagnostic lead time was estimated at 5.5 years. Only 40% of cancers detected after 5 years were nonaggressive. Men with PSA levels between 2.0 and 3.0 ng/mL had a relative risk of 5.5 compared with men whose PSA values were less than 1.0 ng/mL (Table 3).

Conclusion.—One PSA test had a high specificity and sensitivity for detecting prostate cancer within 4 years. Values of PSA below the standard cutoff were associated with a significantly increased risk of prostate cancer. The value of routine screening must be assessed in terms of cost and prognosis for prostate cancer patients.

▶ An extremely important article for urologists and for our understanding of the clinical value of PSA. The authors found a single PSA test to be extremely valuable, detecting up to 80% of aggressive cancers within 5 years and, importantly, that the cancers diagnosed in men younger than 70 years were a significant health problem, being responsible for three quarters of the deaths in these men. This paper strongly underscores the value of PSA in the clinical arena and calls for the development of screening protocols that incorporate this important test. Amen.

B.J. Miles, M.D.

Acute Normovolemic Hemodilution is a Cost-Effective Alternative to Preoperative Autologous Blood Donation by Patients Undergoing Radical Retropubic Prostatectomy

Monk TG, Goodnough LT, Birkmeyer JD, Brecher ME, Catalona WJ (Washington Univ, St Louis, Mo; Dartmouth-Hitchcock Med Ctr, Lebanon, NH; Univ of North Carolina Hosps, Chapel Hill)

Transfusion 35:559–565, 1995   21–22

Introduction.—Preoperative autologous blood donation (PABD) has become an accepted standard of care for patients undergoing radical prostatectomy. However, there are concerns about the expense associated with PABD. In acute normovolemic hemodilution (ANH), autologous blood is obtained immediately before the onset of surgical blood loss. The 2 autologous blood collection techniques were compared for their costs and benefits.

Methods.—Thirty consecutive patients scheduled for radical prostatectomy were studied. All underwent ANH to a target hematocrit of 28% and received blood transfusions in the perioperative period to maintain hematocrit at greater than 25%. The patients' hematocrit values, transfusion outcomes and costs, and perioperative outcomes were compared with those of a matched cohort of 30 prostatectomy patients who had previously been managed with PABD.

Results.—In the ANH group, the mean hematocrit value was 29% and the mean volume of blood collected was 1,740 mL. Allogeneic blood was needed by 10% of patients in each group. Transfusion costs were $330 for the PABD group vs. $191 for the ANH group. There were no differences in postoperative outcomes.

Conclusions.—Acute normovolemic hemodilution is a well-tolerated, simple, and cost-effective alternative to PABD for patients undergoing radical prostatectomy. The use of an integrated blood conservation program with hemodilution and a defined transfusion trigger can reduce the need for PABD.

▶ Acute normovolemic hemodilution may indeed be more cost-effective than usual PABD. The cost savings were significant but not enormous. In California, the Gann Act requires that patients be offered the opportunity to store blood preoperatively. This study would suggest that the risk of needing allogeneic blood is the same with either the ANH or PABD method. However, some or all patients in the PABD group stored 3 units of blood and were probably anemic. We also do not know how results would compare with other practices such as ours in which patients store 2 units of blood only and wait at least 1 week or longer before surgery while taking oral iron. Our need for autologous allogeneic transfusion is significantly less than reported in this article, and one would have to demonstrate the equivalent of that to the ANH method. This comparison should be done because cost containment is increasingly important.

J.B. DeKernion, M.D.

Clinical Outcomes Associated With the Implementation of a Cost-Efficient Programme for Radical Retropubic Prostatectomy
Kock MO, Smith JA Jr (Vanderbilt Univ Med Ctr, Nashville, Tenn)
Br J Urol 76:28–33, 1995   21–23

Background.—A broad-based cost-containment program for patients undergoing radical retropubic prostatectomy for carcinoma of the prostate was developed after all aspects of perioperative care were reviewed. Standardized procedures for operative and perioperative care based on medically valid information were implemented and replaced prior procedures based on anecdotal experience or tradition. Experience with this new program was reported.

Methods.—Hospital charges from the first 50 patients to undergo radical retropubic prostatectomy after the cost-containment program was implemented were analyzed in detail. Also, clinical outcome was determined. Data were compared to data from control patients who underwent the same procedure before the program was implemented.

Results.—After the cost-containment program was implemented, overall hospital charges per patient and length of hospital stay decreased by 44%. The greatest savings were in operating room and routine care costs. Length of surgery, intraoperative blood loss, and need for transfusion were also reduced. There were no adverse effects on incidence of major or minor complications, or hospital readmissions. All patients accepted the new program well.

Conclusions.—The cost-containment program resulted in significant savings, reduced hospital stay, and excellent acceptance by patients without adversely affecting outcome. This system also provides a means of implementing and monitoring further refinements in management as they are needed.

▶ This important study demonstrates how appropriate cost-containment efforts can be applied to radical prostatectomy. The authors essentially developed a "care-path" as defined in a number of other institutions, including our own. By carefully using only essential laboratory tests, eliminating other unnecessary diagnostic and imaging tests, improving efficiency of nursing care, restricting medications to only those essential, almost totally eliminating narcotic medications, and decreasing hospital stay, costs can be markedly reduced. They also minimized the use of autologous blood storage. In California, the law requires that patients be informed of the option for autologous blood storage, and most patients opt for it. It is, however, wasteful because the transfusion is seldom needed. Kock and Smith also dispensed with the use of pulsatile stockings in favor of heparin. Many of us are unwilling to do this because of the demonstrated efficacy of the pulsatile stockings. In addition, because we and others use ketoralac, a known platelet inhibitor, the addition of heparin might be hazardous.

It is unclear why their operating time was decreased, unless they refined their surgical technique. This is a worthwhile effort because operating costs at many institutions constitute the major portion of the hospital bill.

Every large hospital should attempt to adopt similar standardized care paths. As these authors and others have demonstrated,[1] the care paths ultimately translate into cost savings and improved patient care.

J.B. DeKernion, M.D.

Reference

1. Litwin MS, Smith RB, Thind A, et al: Cost-efficient radical prostatectomy with a clinical care path. *J Urol* 155:989–993, 1996.

Progression in Untreated Carcinoma of the Prostate Metastatic to Regional Lymph Nodes (Stage T0 to 4,N1 to 3,M0,D1)

Davidson PJT, and the European Organization for Research and Treatment of Cancer Genitourinary Group (Erasmus Univ, Rotterdam, The Netherlands; Univ of Amsterdam; Norwegian Radium Hosp, Oslo, Norway)

J Urol 154:2118–2122, 1995   21–24

Background.—The best treatment for patients with prostate cancer who have nodal disease but no other obvious metastases at initial assessment is debatable. The natural history of the disease needs to be considered when evaluating the various options. One series of patients whose disease remained untreated until progression was studied prospectively.

Methods and Findings.—Sixty-one patients with node-positive prostate cancer were followed up for a mean of 41 months. All patients were observed for at least 1 year. Patients' ages ranged from 50 to 80 years. Univariate and multivariate analyses were performed to determine the effect of T and P categories, grade, tumor volume, and prostate-specific antigen (PSA) change on the interval to progression. The median interval to disease progression was 18 months. Twenty-three percent of the patients had local subjective, 23% had local objective, and 54% had metastatic progression. Mean follow-up in patients without progression was 31 months. Time to progression was associated with grade and PSA-doubling time (Fig 1). Changes in prostatic volume with time did not predict progression.

Conclusions.—Disease progresses rapidly in most men with untreated stages T0 to T4, N1 to N3, M0 prostate carcinoma. The cancer remains stable for a prolonged time in a small number of such patients. These 2 groups can be differentiated by initial grade and T stage and percentage of increase in PSA over time.

▶ This study is interesting because few groups have ever followed such a large number of untreated patients with node-positive prostate cancer. Hopefully, the authors will be able to provide survival data after another 3 or 4 years of follow-up, which can then be compared with some of the surgically treated series.

It is not surprising that grade is an extremely important determinant of progression. It is surprising, however, that tumor volume, both in the primary and in the lymph nodes, was not significantly predictive, although there was a difference. As we and others have shown, PSA-doubling time is simply an expression of the growth of the tumor in all cases and predicts progression in node-positive patients. Perhaps those patients should be treated early with endocrine therapy.

Because most of us do not feel that local or regional therapies are effective in patients with detectable nodal metastases, this paper may give us some guidelines for predicting behavior and thus deciding when to institute therapy. The ultimate value will be the long-term follow-up, which I suspect will demonstrate that the survival of these patients, when separated accord-

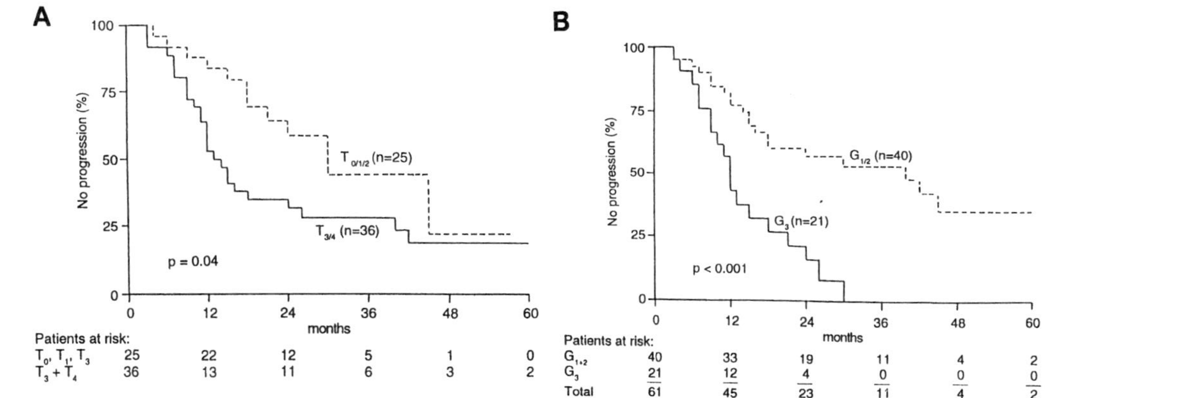

FIGURE 1.—Kaplan-Meier projections for interval to progression in 61 patients with stages T0 to 4,N1 to 3,M0 prostate cancer. **A,** according to T category. **B,** according to grade (**G**) of prostatic biopsy. (Courtesy of Davidson PJT, and the European Organization for Research and Treatment of Cancer Genitourinary Group: Progression in untreated carcinoma of the prostate metastatic to regional lymph nodes [stage T0 to 4,N1 to 3,M0, D1]. *J Urol* 154:2118–2122, 1995.)

ing to grade, stage, and PSA progression, is similar to that achieved in surgical series of node-positive patients.

J.B. DeKernion, M.D.

Morbidity and Mortality Following Radical Prostatectomy: A National Analysis of Civilian Health and Medical Program of the Uniformed Services Beneficiaries
Optenberg SA, Wojcik BE, Thompson IM (Army Med Ctr, San Antonio, Tex; Brooke Army Med Ctr, San Antonio, Tex)
J Urol 153:1870–1872, 1995   21–25

Background.—A recent study found that Medicare patients undergoing radical prostatectomy may have substantially greater perioperative mortality than has been reported in institutional series. The mortality and morbidity of men 40–65 years of age after radical prostatectomy were determined using a 100% national sample from the Civilian Health and Medical Program of the Uniformed Services (CHAMPUS) database.

Methods.—Claims data from Oct. 1, 1987, to Jan. 1, 1993, were analyzed. One thousand fifty-nine patients were included. All were younger than 65 years, with a mean age of 60 years.

Findings.—Postoperative mortality was 0.28% at 30 and 90 days, 1.02% at 1 year, 1.95% at 2 years, 3.14% at 3 years, and 4.64% at 4 years, according to Kaplan-Meier estimates. Compared with the general population, observed 1 to 5 mortality rates ranged from 0.36 to 0.49 of that expected. The differences were significant. Rehospitalization was needed in 3.1% of the patients 30 days after surgery and in 4.6% of the patients 90 days after surgery.

Conclusions.—The mortality and morbidity associated with radical prostatectomy were low. Outcomes analyses of prostate carcinoma treatment should include the entire age range of patients undergoing this procedure in the United States.

▶ The authors used the CHAMPUS database to study a population of younger men undergoing radical prostatectomy. They compared this with the Medicare database. This generally represents a population of patients with prostate cancer, many of whom probably had their surgery outside of major centers. The point of the study is well made—acute morbidity after radical prostatectomy in young patients is markedly less than that seen in the Medicare database. Analyses by health outcomes experts, based on Medicare data, can never be construed as representative of the entire population of patients, and extrapolating such data to all prostatectomies is inappropriate.

J.B. DeKernion, M.D.

Nerve Sparing Radical Prostatectomy: A Different View
Geary ES, Dendinger TE, Freiha FS, Stamey TA (Stanford Univ, Calif)
J Urol 154:145–149, 1995   21–26

Introduction.—Several studies have described the recovery of erectile function after nerve-sparing radical prostatectomy for prostate cancer. However, patient-reported potency rates after this procedure tend to be much lower. There are few data on preoperative sexual function in patients who are potent postoperatively. The rates and quality of postoperative potency were evaluated in men who underwent radical prostatectomy.

Methods.—Erectile dysfunction and preoperative and postoperative sexual function were evaluated in 459 men who had undergone radical prostatectomy. One hundred eighty-seven patients had a non–nerve-sparing procedure, 201 had a unilateral nerve-sparing procedure, and 69 had a bilateral nerve-sparing procedure. Postoperative potency—defined as the ability to perform unassisted intercourse with vaginal penetration—was analyzed in terms of type of operation, preoperative sexual function, and age.

Results.—Fifty-one patients were potent postoperatively. Potency rates were 1% in patients who had non–nerve-sparing surgery, 13% in those who had a unilateral nerve-sparing procedure, and 32% in those who had bilateral nerve-sparing surgery. However, less than half of patients who were sexually active postoperatively expressed satisfaction with their erections or reported intercourse at least once monthly. Factors associated with postoperative potency included the number of neurovascular bundles spared, preoperative frequency of intercourse, absence of seminal vesicle or lymph node involvement, absence of postoperative incontinence or strictures, patient age, and cancer volume.

Conclusions.—Potency rates after nerve-sparing radical prostatectomy may be lower than reported in previous studies. For the average patient, it is misleading to expect a 50% or better chance of recovering sexual potency. Many factors influence postoperative potency rate, including the number of neurovascular bundles spared and preoperative frequency of intercourse. Radical prostatectomy does not appear to change the patients' ability to achieve intercourse, thus making them good candidates for interventions to aid erectile function.

▶ Surprisingly few patients in this large series had bilateral nerve-sparing. This almost certainly reflects the patient population as well as the preference and philosophy of the surgeon. The implication is that results are not as good as we thought.

Other series have much higher reports of potency. This is, in part, because of the definition of potency. Most studies have not looked at the quality of erection or the frequency and satisfaction of sexual function. Undoubtedly, many men who can have erections sufficient for intercourse after surgery do not have the quality of erections they once had. Also, they may not have sexual activity very often. Nonetheless, most of these patients, properly questioned, would feel strongly that they prefer "some to none."

The major concern with this study is the method of collecting data. These types of data are supportable only when done by a carefully constructed and validated questionnaire that covers all aspects of, in this case, sexual function. It is my view that nerve sparing for many patients is important and worthwhile for their quality of life.

J.B. DeKernion, M.D.

Anterior Bladder Neck Tube Reconstruction at Radical Prostatectomy Preserves Functional Urethral Length: A Comparative Urodynamic Study

Connolly JA, Presti JC Jr, Carroll PR (Univ of California, San Francisco)
Br J Urol 75:766–770, 1995   21–27

Objective.—The exact role of anterior bladder neck reconstruction in achieving urinary continence after radical prostatectomy is not clear. To elucidate further, urodynamic studies were prospectively performed before and after radical prostatectomy with or without anterior bladder neck tube reconstruction.

Methods.—Seventeen patients with clinically localized prostate cancer were studied. Eight control patients underwent conventional "racket handle" closure of the bladder neck, and the other 9 underwent anterior bladder neck reconstruction by constructing 2-cm anterior bladder neck tubes over 22F catheters.

Outcome.—All patients in both groups were fully continent at 3 months after surgery. Patients who underwent anterior bladder neck reconstruction had significantly longer functional urethral length (4.6 cm) than the control group (3.4 cm). When preoperative and postoperative urodynamics were compared, functional urethral length was preserved in patients who underwent bladder neck tube reconstruction but was significantly shorter in control patients. The longer functional urethral length in patients with anterior bladder neck reconstructions was confirmed by the finding of a long tubularized bladder outlet on postoperative voiding cystourethrograms. No other urodynamic parameters differed significantly between groups after surgery.

Implication.—In patients undergoing radical prostatectomy, anterior bladder neck tube reconstruction may promote urinary continence by preservation of functional urethral length. A randomized trial should be conducted to assess the relative efficacy of bladder neck tube reconstruction on urinary continence.

▶ Construction of the bladder neck tube increased urethral length. However, the group that did not have the tube also regained their urinary control in the same manner. It is therefore difficult to argue that construction of the tube really made a difference. Also, the authors did not include a third group in which a good portion of the bladder neck was preserved, and no closure was required. I have not found that bladder tubes make any difference in continence, although certainly if a surgeon is convinced that it is a helpful technical modification, then it should be used.

J.B. DeKernion, M.D.

Bladder Neck Preservation Following Radical Prostatectomy: Continence and Margins

Braslis KG, Petsch M, Lim A, Civantos F, Soloway MS (Univ of Miami, Fla)
Eur Urol 28:202–208, 1995   21–28

Background.—The most common malignancy in males in the United States is prostate cancer. Major side effects of radical prostatectomy include incontinence and impotence, although new meticulous surgical techniques have resulted in a lower incidence of both. Preservation of bladder neck fibers and adjacent proximal prostatic urethra may improve postoperative continence, but there is concern that tumor may be left behind. The effect of bladder neck preservation on patient incontinence and surgical margins was reported.

Methods.—Radical retropubic prostatectomy with bladder neck preservation was performed in 134 patients. One month preoperatively and 3 months postoperatively, 36 patients completed a questionnaire regarding continence.

Results.—Of the 134 patients, 49 had a positive margin. In 10 patients, a tumor was identified at the bladder neck. In these 10 patients, a tumor was also identified at multiple other sites. This indicates that bladder neck preservation may not compromise the efficacy of radical prostatectomy. At 3 months, 67% of the 36 patients who completed the questionnaire did not wear any pads, 19% wore pads occasionally, and 14% wore pads daily. An anastomotic stricture developed in only 1 patient.

Conclusions.—Bladder neck preservation during radical prostatectomy does not result in a higher rate of positive margins. This method may improve continence or contribute to earlier return of continence. Bladder neck preservation during radical prostatectomy for stage T_{1c}, T_2, and some T_3 tumors is supported.

▶ We do not really know whether bladder neck preservation had anything to do with the continence. This can only be established by a comparative study in which the bladder neck was not preserved. The incidence of bladder neck involvement seems rather high, and perhaps this was a matter of patient selection. I assiduously preserved the bladder neck for approximately 5 or 6 years. Now, I do not preserve the entire bladder neck, although I usually do not remove enough to require bladder neck closure. I have not noticed any difference at all in rapidity of continence return or long-term continence. With due respect to the authors, I and others feel rather strongly that the bladder neck has little to do with continence, and we are unwilling to risk a positive bladder neck margin by preserving it.

J.B. DeKernion, M.D.

Endoscopic Evaluation and Treatment of Anastomotic Strictures After Radical Retropubic Prostatectomy
Dalkin BL (Arizona Health Sciences Ctr, Tucson)
J Urol 155:206–208, 1996
21–29

Introduction.—Stricture at the vesicourethral anastomosis occurring as a complication of radical retropubic prostatectomy has been treated by a variety of methods. In 17 patients with anastomotic strictures, endoscopic findings were examined and outcome was assessed after treatment by cold-knife urethrotomy and/or urethral dilation.

Methods.—The complication occurred in 12.6% of patients operated by a single surgeon between July 1991 and April 1995. All had undergone radical retropubic prostatectomy for clinically localized adenocarcinoma of the prostate. The vesicourethral anastomosis was performed over a 20F Teflon-coated catheter using 2-zero chromic interrupted sutures. No patient had gross or microscopic evidence of extraprostatic extension of the tumor, either intraoperatively or histopathologically at final evaluation of the specimen. Symptoms of stricture were a markedly weakened urinary stream or almost total urinary retention. Dilation and subsequent cold-knife urethrotomy were performed in 6 men with an immature stricture at endoscopic evaluation; those with a mature stricture underwent cold-knife urethrotomy or dilation followed by urethrotomy.

Results.—The immature strictures were observed in patients in whom symptoms appeared less than 8 weeks after prostatectomy. Endoscopy revealed poorly defined margins and an unhealed appearance. The mature strictures showed characteristic white scarification at the anastomotic area. Treatment was successful in 15 of 17 cases. Two patients with immature strictures failed multiple attempts at dilation and/or cold-knife incision and required periodic dilation. The various treatment procedures did not have a significant long-term impact on urinary continence, and all patients are now continent.

Conclusion.—Patients with an immature anastomotic stricture at endoscopic evaluation present a technical challenge, but most have good long-term results with initial filiform and follower dilation. Cold-knife optical internal urethrotomy may be performed when the stricture matures. In patients initially seen with mature strictures, a cold-knife incision is safe and efficacious.

▶ The author describes the appearance of the "immature" strictures. It is my opinion that this ragged inflammatory appearance at the anastomosis can be partially attributed to the chromic suture. We have changed to a monofilament suture, and our stricture problem has been markedly reduced. These strictures are mainly acutely inflamed and edematous and do respond to soft dilation and catheter drainage. We agree that optical internal urethrotomy should be performed only once the scar tissue forms. Two of their patients required long-term dilations, which is surprising because with repeat visual internal urethrotomy (VIU), virtually all patients can be sufficiently cured of the stricture and urinate without chronic dilation. We also now use an 18 Foley that is silicone-coated, and our impression is that it is less bothersome for patients, causing less reaction at the meatus and throughout the urethra and bladder neck.

J.B. DeKernion, M.D.

Ultrasound Guided Seminal Vesicle Biopsies in Men With Suspected Prostate Cancer

Pandey P, Fowler JE Jr, Seaver LE, Feliz TP, Brooks JP (Univ of Mississippi, Jackson)
J Urol 154:1798–1801, 1995   21–30

Background.—Many authorities do not recommend radical prostatectomy in patients with prostate cancer when there is seminal vesicle invasion, which is often microscopic and often missed on digital rectal examination. Transrectal ultrasonography can be used for imaging the prostate and adjacent structures using automated biopsy needles. This technique may improve tumor staging in patients who may be eligible for radical prostatectomy. The histology of ultrasound-guided seminal vesicle biopsies was evaluated.

Methods.—Ultrasound-guided sextant biopsy of the prostate and biopsy of the base of both or 1 of the seminal vesicles were performed in 517 male patients. The mean age of the patients was 69 years. Results were correlated with the clinical or pathologic stage of cancer.

Results.—Of 1,032 biopsy specimens, seminal vesicle epithelium and muscularis were identified in 490 specimens. Smooth muscle consistent with seminal vesicle muscularis was detected in 393 specimens. The biopsy specimens were positive for cancer in 7 of 123 patients with stage T1c or T2 tumors, 27 of 60 patients with stages T3 to 4 tumors, and 9 of 13 patients with metastatic cancer. Radical prostatectomy was performed in 39 patients, and seminal vesicle biopsies were positive in 1 of 36 patients without seminal vesicle invasion and in 0 of 3 patients with seminal vesicle invasion.

Discussion.—Seminal vesicle muscularis or smooth muscle consistent with seminal vesicle muscularis can be obtained with ultrasound-guided biopsy techniques in most patients. False-negative biopsies can be common, however, and the contribution of seminal vesicle biopsies to the staging of T1c and T2 tumors is negligible.

▶ This analysis is of great practical significance. In this large series of patients, it appears that routine seminal vesicle biopsy will not help in making treatment decisions. However, one can also infer that patients with large tumors and those with suspected seminal vesicle involvement would almost certainly be benefited by preoperative biopsy when a positive result would preclude a surgical cure. Until more accurate staging methods are available, we will have to rely on ultrasound for local staging, buttressed with biopsies in selected circumstances.

J.B. DeKernion, M.D.

Critical Evaluation of Salvage Surgery for Radio-Recurrent/Resistant Prostate Cancer

Lerner SE, Blute ML, Zincke H (Mayo Clinic and Mayo Found, Rochester, Minn)
J Urol 154:1103–1109, 1995   21–31

Rationale.—The advent of ultrasound-guided transrectal biopsy and serial serum prostate-specific antigen (PSA) testing has resulted in the more frequent discovery of recurrent and radiation-resistant cancers, possibly at an earlier stage. It is possible that a positive postradiation biopsy associated with a rising PSA identifies a group of patients who may be cured by salvage surgery, even in the absence of evident local progression.

Objective.—The outcome of salvage surgery afer local radiotherapy had failed was examined in 132 patients who underwent surgery in 1967–1992. Radical retropubic prostatectomy was the most common procedure, used in 79 cases. Thirty-eight patients underwent anterior

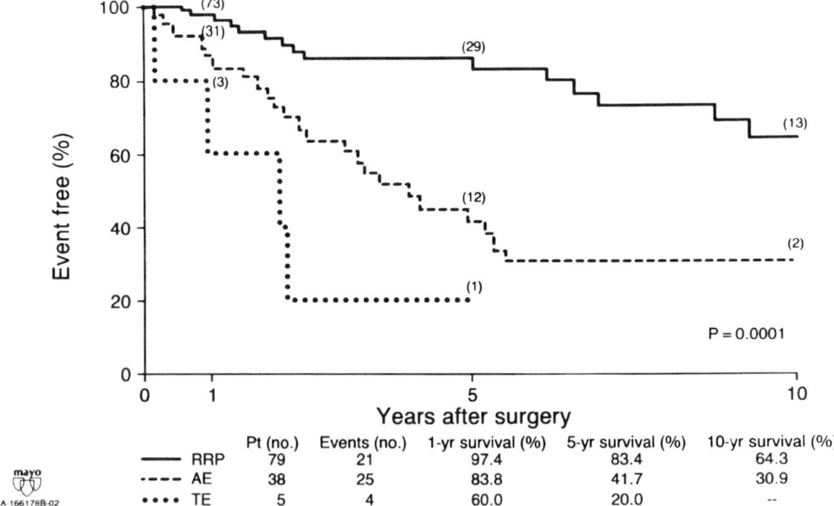

	Pt (no.)	Events (no.)	1-yr survival (%)	5-yr survival (%)	10-yr survival (%)
—— RRP	79	21	97.4	83.4	64.3
- - - - AE	38	25	83.8	41.7	30.9
•••• TE	5	4	60.0	20.0	--

FIGURE 2.—Overall survival of prostate cancer patients undergoing salvage surgery for local radiation failure according to procedure. *Abbreviations: RRP*, radical retropubic prostatectomy; *AE*, anterior exenteration; *TE*, total exenteration. (Courtesy of Lerner SE, Blute ML, Zincke H: Critical evaluation of salvage surgery for radio-recurrent/resistant prostate cancer. *J Urol* 154:1103–1109, 1995.)

exenteration, 5 had total exenteration, and 10 had bilateral pelvic adenectomy alone. The median interval from radiotherapy to radical surgery was 38 months.

Results.—Forty of 56 deaths were ascribed to prostatic cancer. The 76 surviving patients have been followed for 5½ years on average. Cause-specific survival rates were 70% at 5 years and 53% at 10 years. Patients who underwent radical retropubic prostatectomy had a significant survival advantage (Fig 2). Both overall survival and survival without recurrent disease were superior in these patients, but they gained no further advantage from adjuvant hormonal treatment. There were no treatment-related deaths.

Conclusion.—Serial estimates of serum PSA and ultrasound-guided biopsies are able to identify those patients with recurrent or radioresistant prostatic cancer who may be cured by radical retropubic prostatectomy, done as a salvage procedure.

▶ The authors studied a group of patients selected for salvage prostatectomy after radiotherapy. They indeed were very selective. During the period of study, approximately 4 or 5 patients per year had this operation at an institution that performs hundreds of standard radical prostatectomies. Yet, in spite of this careful selection, only 30% of the patients who had radical prostatectomy had organ-confined disease. Furthermore, approximately a third of the patients during the whole study died of prostate cancer. Finally, the complications were significant as one would expect in this population of patients.

The authors' point is an important one, however—we should now be able to select patients for salvage surgery who have early radiation recurrence and who have a reasonable probability of still having organ-confined tumor. The patient, however, must accept significant risks.

J.B. DeKernion, M.D.

Salvage Radical Prostatectomy After Failed Transperineal Cryotherapy: Histologic Findings From Prostate Whole-Mount Specimens Correlated With Intraoperative Transrectal Ultrasound Images

Grampsas SA, Miller GJ, Crawford ED (Univ of Colorado Health Sciences Ctr, Denver)

Urology 45:936–941, 1995

21–32

Background.—Because of certain unique advantages, including minimal bleeding, low morbidity, and the lack of limitation of treatment options after failure, cryosurgery has gained in acceptance as an initial therapy for prostate cancer. Transperineal cryotherapy will fail in a certain number of patients, but there is currently no established management approach to these patients. The results of salvage radical prostatectomy after failed cryosurgical prostatectomy were evaluated.

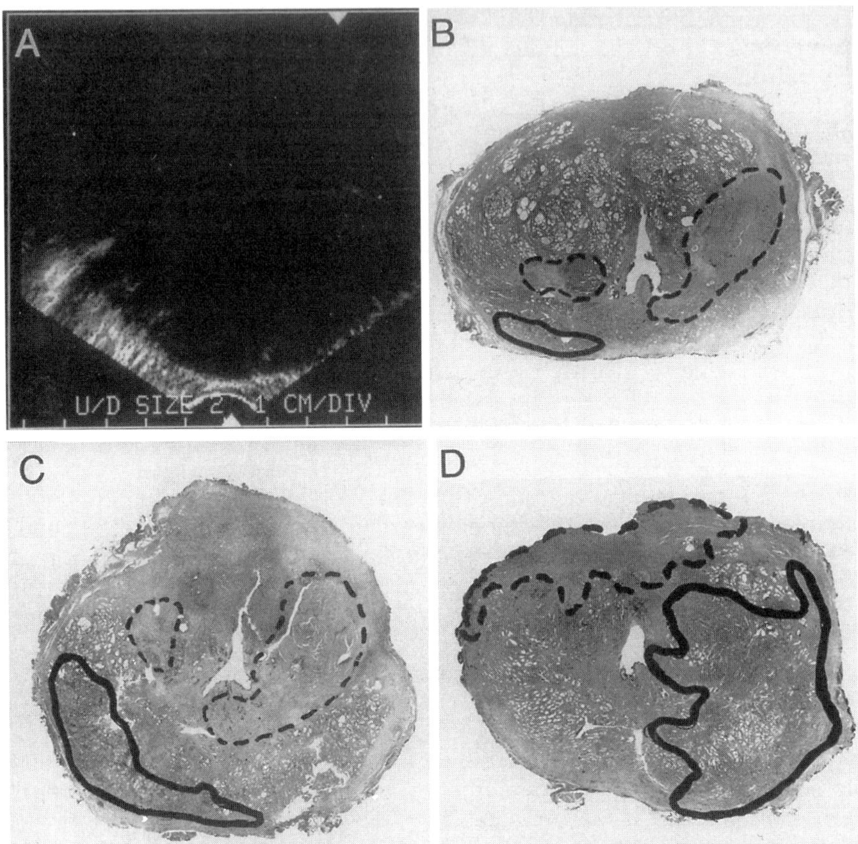

FIGURE 1.—**A,** transverse transrectal ultrasonography image showing cryotherapy ice ball filling entire prostate. **B,** transverse whole-mount section of the prostate seen in **A.** *Dotted lines* represent area of necrosis resulting from cryodestruction. *Solid lines* demarcate area of persistent carcinoma. **C and D,** representative whole-mount sections of 2 other salvage prostatectomy specimens showing the extent of cryoablation and residual carcinoma as described in **B.** Note the separation between areas of necrosis and foci of residual adenocarcinoma. (Reprinted by permission of the publisher. From Grampsas SA, Miller GJ, Crawford ED: Salvage radical prostatectomy after failed transperineal cryotherapy: Histologic findings from prostate whole-mount specimens correlated with intraoperative transrectal ultrasound images. *Urology* 45:936–941. Copyright 1995 by Elsevier Sciences, Inc.)

Methods.—Six patients with confirmed clinical stage T3 carcinoma of the prostate, all of whom had undergone transrectal ultrasound-guided transperineal cryotherapy of the prostate, were studied. All 6 patients had documented persistence of prostate cancer, for which they underwent salvage radical perineal prostatectomy. The procedures were performed in a standard manner by a single surgeon, without pelvic lymphadenectomy. Whole-mount sections were prepared, and zones of freeze destruction and residual adenocarcinoma were mapped. The zones of freeze destruction, which represented successfully treated prostate tissue, were then compared with the hypoechoic ice ball treatment zones observed and intraoperative transrectal ultrasound (TRUS).

Results.—The whole-mount sections included necrotic areas of cryodestruction that were much smaller than they appeared on intraoperative ultrasound. Areas of residual, viable adenocarcinoma were found in every case (Fig 1). At 0.5–12 months' follow-up after salvage surgery, all patients were alive and clinically free of localized disease.

Conclusions.—For patients in whom transperineal cryosurgery of the prostate fails, salvage radical prostatectomy is a feasible and effective treatment option. During cryotherapy, TRUS appears to overestimate the area of prostatic tissue destroyed. The findings suggest that the entire prostate is not necessarily lethally frozen when it is encompassed by the hypoechoic ice ball seen on TRUS.

▶ The authors had surprisingly little trouble performing radical prostatectomy as salvage after cryoablation. It seems probable that the ease of surgery was related to the limited freezing of the prostate gland that left viable tumor in all 6 patients. In patients whose prostates have been virtually eradicated by the freezing, considerable periprostatic scarring occurs and prostatectomy may be difficult or impossible. It still seems that complete eradication of large tumors is difficult to achieve with cryoablation alone. Their 6 patients remain clinically free of recurrence after short follow-up. However, there is no reason to believe that these patients with T3 tumors will fare any better than other patients treated primarily with surgery or radiotherapy for the same stage of disease.

J.B. DeKernion, M.D.

Significance of Normal Serum Prostate-Specific Antigen in the Follow-Up Period After Definitive Radiation Therapy for Prostatic Cancer
Zelefsky MJ, Leibel SA, Wallner KE, Whitmore WF Jr, Fuks Z (Mem Sloan-Kettering Cancer Ctr, New York)
J Clin Oncol 13:459–463, 1995   21–33

Introduction.—A documented increase in prostate-specific antigen (PSA) serum levels after definitive therapy is a sensitive marker of prostate cancer recurrence. For patients having previously undergone radiotherapy, further definition is needed of the upper limit of an apparent recurrence-free state, and the significance of multiple years of such a state. Long-term follow-up with PSA determination was conducted for 403 patients whose prostate cancer was treated with pelvic lymph node dissection and retropubic radioactive iodine-125 implantation.

Methods and Findings.—Serum PSA levels were normal (less than or equal to 4.0 ng/mL) upon the first testing (PSA-1) for 182 of these patients. Of these patients, those with initial values less than or equal to 1.0 ng/mL showed a 5-year PSA relapse-free survival rate of 85%, whereas those

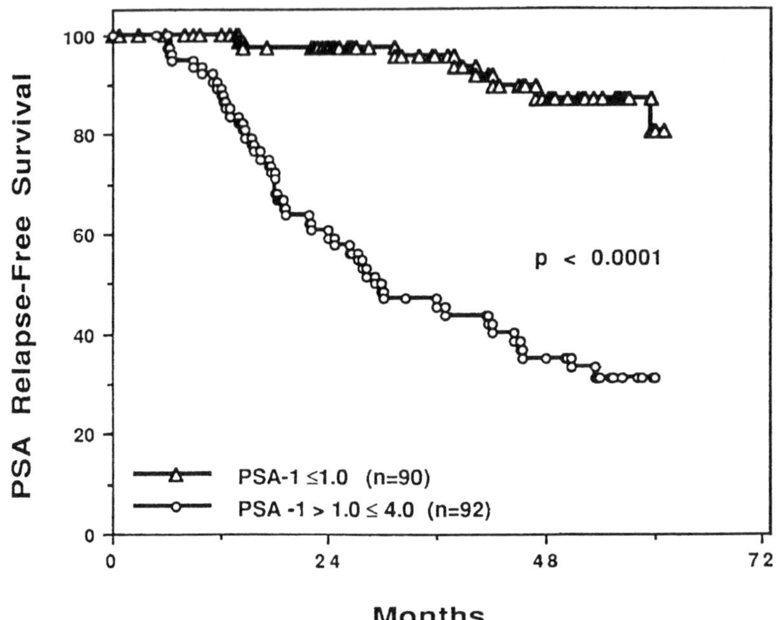

Months

FIGURE 1.—Prostate-specific antigen (*PSA*) relapse-free survival calculated from the date of PSA-1 for patients with PSA-1 values ≤1.0 vs. patients with values in the upper ranges of normal. (Courtesy of Zelefsky MJ, Leibel SA, Wallner KE, et al: Significance of normal serum prostate-specific antigen in the follow-up period after definitive radiation therapy for prostatic cancer. *J Clin Oncol* 13:459–463, 1995.)

with higher (but still normal) PSA levels showed a relapse-free survival rate of 27% (Fig 1). Multivariate analyses showed that a negative impact on continued PSA relapse-free survival was imparted only by a PSA-1 level from over 1.0 through 4.0 ng/mL combined with grade II/III histologic character. Local relapse-free survival was independently affected only by PSA-1 level from over 1.0 through 4.0 ng/mL; distant metastases-free survival was affected by high-grade histologic character and local failure.

Conclusions.—A high likelihood of long-term survival is indicated for patients previously treated for prostate cancer when a serum PSA level of less than or equal to 1.0 ng/mL is obtained years later. A serum PSA level of less than or equal to 1.0 ng/mL (as opposed to less than or equal to 4.0 ng/mL) may be the expected normal value after prostatic irradiation. Serum PSA determinations can be used to predict postradiotherapy probability of cure vs. a higher risk of recurrence. A serum PSA value of less than or equal to 1.0 ng/mL has potential use as an end point for early efficacy evaluation of experimental prostate cancer therapy protocols.

▶ Zelefsky et al. in their study (although not prospective) might have put to rest which level of PSA should be considered as negative after radiation therapy. In this elegant study, the Memorial group identified that there is a significant (*p* <0.0001) difference in PSA relapse-free survival between those patients who are found after radiation therapy to have a level of 1.0 ng/mL or less as compared with those patients who have a level of more than 1.0 ng/mL and up to 4.0 ng/mL. The difference in PSA relapse-free survival between these 2 groups is highly significant (p <0.0001). It is hoped that other radiotherapy groups adhere to this level of definitive treatment success.

H. Zincke, M.D., Ph.D.

The Treatment of Prostate Cancer by Conventional Radiation Therapy: An Analysis of Long-Term Outcome
Zietman AL, Coen JJ, Dallow KC, Shipley WU (Massachusetts Gen Hosp, Boston; Harvard Med School, Boston)
Int J Radiat Oncol Biol Phys 32:287–292, 1995   21–34

Background.—Recently the use of external-beam radiotherapy as primary treatment for prostate cancer has been challenged for 2 reasons. A number of reports indicate high failure rates even in relatively early-stage cases. In addition, many patients may actually be worse off than if they had not been treated at all, apparently because of very rapid progression of disease.

Objective.—The results of conventional external-beam treatment were examined in 1,041 men who were treated for T1–4NxM0 prostate cancer between 1977 and 1991 and who were followed for a median of 49 months.

Methods.—Patients received 10- to 25-MV megavoltage treatment using a 4-field technique. The lymph nodes were treated electively unless bowel pathology had been documented or an early-stage lesion was present. The primary tumor was boosted to a total tumor dose of 68.4 Gy. Treatment was considered to have failed if the prostate-specific antigen (PSA) level increased by more than 1 ng/mL 2 years or longer after treatment, or if clinical failure emerged.

Results.—Patients with T1–2NxM0 tumors had a clinical 10-year disease-free survival rate of 65%, but including the PSA criterion lowered the rate to 40%. Only 29% of patients with T2b–c disease were biochemically free of disease after 10 years. Tumor grade was a major factor influencing the outcome. Only 18% of T3–4 patients were biochemically free of disease at 10 years. In no group did treatment appear to be disadvantageous, and men with high-grade tumors exhibited a survival advantage when compared with observation-only reports from the literature.

Conclusions.—Conventional external-beam radiotherapy has cured fewer than 40% of men with early prostate cancers and fewer than 20% of those with advanced-grade disease. Nevertheless even patients who are not cured may have a reduced risk of locally progressive disease and better disease-specific survival compared with those who are merely observed.

▶ This is a straightforward report from Massachusetts General Hospital on more than 1,000 patients, followed for a median of 4 years, who underwent external-beam radiation of 10 to 25-MV treatment using a 4-field technique for clinical T1–4, NxM0 adenocarcinoma of the prostate from 1977 to 1991. These results are credible because strict criteria were used. A level of 1.0 ng/mL or greater at 2 years was considered a treatment failure. Of patients with T2b–c and T3–4 disease, 29% and 18%, respectively, were PSA negative at 10 years. Dismal PSA-negative rates were achieved with patients having a Gleason score of 8 or greater,—20% and 10% only at 10 years for those patients in the T1–2 group and T3–4 group, respectively. An interesting finding was that the median doubling time on progression was twice as fast for high-grade disease (9.6 months) as for low-grade disease (18.8 months).

In this sobering report, the authors conclude that their "conventional external beam radiation cured less than 40% of the men with T1–2, Nx tumors and fewer than 20% of those with T3–4, Nx tumors." Furthermore, rather than comparing their data with surgical results, they compared them with that of an observation study by Chodak et al. which showed no difference at 10 years between patients with low or moderately differentiated cancer and only demonstrated an advantage for radiation for the undifferentiated cancer group in regard to metastasis-free and cause-specific survival.[1]

Recently reported data in a series of more than 3,000 patients with clinically localized disease ($\leq$T2), as well as a report on clinical T3 cancer by Lerner et al., seem to indicate that surgery, with or without adjuvant treatment, is a more effective treatment for cancer of the prostate.[2, 3] However, prospective randomized studies are needed to confirm this statement.

H. Zincke, M.D., Ph.D.

References

1. Chodak GW, Thirsted RA, Gerber GS, et al: Results of conservative management of clinically localized prostate cancer. *N Engl J Med* 330:242–248, 1994.
2. Zincke H, Oesterling JE, Blute ML, et al: Long-term (15 years) results after radical prostatectomy for clinically localized (stage T2c or lower) prostate cancer. *J Urol Suppl* 152:1850–1857, 1994.
3. Lerner SE, Blute ML, Zincke H: Extended experience for clinical stage T3 prostate cancer: Outcome and contemporary morbidity. *J Urol* 154:1447–1452, 1995.

Carcinoma of the Prostate: Race as a Prognostic Indicator in Definitive Radiation Therapy
Kim JA, Kuban DA, El-Mahdi AM, Schellhammer PF (Eastern Virginia Med School, Norfolk, Va)
Radiology 194:545–549, 1995   21–35

Background.—Possible causes of the higher mortality rate of black men with prostate cancer, compared with that of white men, are the presence of more advanced or more aggressive tumors at diagnosis, occupational exposures, and socioeconomic barriers to receipt of medical care. The outcome of definitive radiation therapy for prostate cancer in black and white men was compared retrospectively.

Methods.—During 15 years, 646 men, 489 white and 157 black, underwent definitive radiation therapy for prostate cancer. The same therapeutic dose using the same equipment was given to all. Serum prostate-specific antigen (PSA) levels were available, beginning in 1987, for 120 white and 26 black patients.

Results.—Median age at diagnosis and tumor stage did not vary between black and white patients, except that significantly more blacks (23%) than whites (13%) had stage A2 when first seen. Significantly fewer blacks had well-differentiated tumors and significantly more had poorly differentiated ones. Both before and after treatment, serum PSA levels were higher among blacks. After treatment, PSA levels were significantly more likely to be above 10 ng/mL in blacks (48%) than whites (27%). Overall survival was significantly lower for blacks at 5 and 10 years, as was survival with stage C and poorly differentiated tumors. Cause-specific survival was also significantly worse for blacks, especially with stage C tumors, but was no different when compared by tumor grade. Treatment of distant disease yielded significantly higher failure at 5 years for blacks (68%) than for whites (40%), with stage C tumors.

Conclusion.—Poorly differentiated prostate tumors and higher PSA levels before and after treatment were found among black, compared with white, patients. Treatment failure for distant disease and poorer overall, cause-specific, and disease-free survival were found for black patients, especially those with stage C tumors.

▶ This large retrospective study of radiation therapy for clinically localized prostate cancer by the Eastern Virginia Medical School group adds to the debate regarding the etiology for racial differences in prostate cancer outcome. The authors found 40% of blacks had poorly differentiated tumors compared with 26% of whites ($P < 0.001$). Few patients had pretreatment PSA values available, but of the ones that did, 73% of blacks and 58% of whites had PSA levels greater than 10 ng/mL. Overall survival was less for black patients, and even when stratified by clinical stage C and poorly differentiated disease, blacks had significantly lower overall, cause-specific, disease-free, and distant failure-free survival. The investigators concluded that black men have more aggressive prostate tumors and implied racial differences in intrinsic tumor aggressiveness.

Although this may be true, other factors should be considered. The authors did not perform multivariate analysis, and even though stratification by clinical stage C and poor grade showed a racial difference, a formal Cox analysis is needed. This point was demonstrated in a recent similar study we did.[1] In 366 white and 107 black patients who underwent radical prostatectomy, race remained as an important prognostic factor, along with PSA and acid phosphatase values, and tumor stage and grade. However, when we included margin positivity in the Cox model, race was no longer significant.[1] Furthermore, our group has also recently shown that within clinical stages e.g., (stage C), black patients with prostate cancer have higher tumor volume and higher tumor volume is associated with Gleason 8–10 poorly differentiated disease.[2] The findings of Kim, et al., may result from greater within-stage tumor volume for black patients. The "64-thousand-dollar question," however, that remains is: What is the tumor-volume disparity due to? Is it simply caused by a delay in diagnosis because of problems with access, ignorance, and fear, or do the tumors "get bigger quicker" because of biological differences as Kim et al. imply?

J.W. Moul, M.D.

References

1. Moul JW, Douglas TH, McCarthy WF, et al: Black race is an adverse prognostic factor for prostate cancer recurrence following radical prostatectomy in an equal-access health care system. *J Urol* 155:1667–1673, 1996.
2. Moul JW, Sesterhenn IA, Connelly RR, et al: Prostate-specific antigen values at the time of prostate cancer diagnosis are higher in African-American men. *JAMA* 274:1277–1281, 1995.

Androgen Deprivation With Radiation Therapy Compared With Radiation Therapy Alone for Locally Advanced Prostatic Carcinoma: A Randomized Comparative Trial of the Radiation Therapy Oncology Group
Pilepich MV, Sause WT, Shipley WU, Krall JM, Lawton CA, Grignon D, Al-Sarraf M, Abrams RA, Caplan R, John MJ, Rotman M, Cox JD, Scotte Doggett RL, Rubin P (C McAuley Health System, Ann Arbor, Mich; Radiation Therapy Oncology Group Statistical Unit, Philadelphia; Wayne State Univ, Detroit; et al)
Urology 45:616–623, 1995

21–36

Background.—In patients undergoing radiation therapy for carcinoma of the prostate, the probability of locoregional recurrence rises with increasing size of the primary tumor. For patients with disseminated carcinoma of the prostate, androgen deprivation therapy has a high response rate. Adjuvant androgen deprivation therapy, by reducing tumor volume, might lead to better outcomes of radiation therapy. The effects of androgen deprivation therapy before and during radiation therapy were assessed in patients with locally advanced carcinomas of the prostate.

Methods.—The phase III trial included 471 patients with large T2, T3, or T4 prostatic carcinomas but no evidence of bony metastasis. The patients were randomly assigned to 1 of 2 treatment arms: those in arm I received goserelin, 3.6 mg subcutaneously every 4 weeks, and flutamide, 250 mg orally 3 times daily, 2 months before and during radiation therapy; and those in arm II received radiation therapy only. Radiation dosage to the pelvis was 1.8–2.0 Gy/day to a total of 45 Gy. This was followed by a radiation boost to the prostate target volume, for a total dose of 65–70 Gy. The 2 groups were compared for local tumor control, disease-free survival, and overall survival.

Results.—Four hundred fifty-six patients were evaluable, with a median potential follow-up of 4½ years. The cumulative incidence of local progression at this time was 46% in arm I vs. 71% in arm II. The incidence of distant metastasis was 34% in arm I and 41% in arm II (Fig 2). Five-year progression-free survival—including normal levels of prostate-

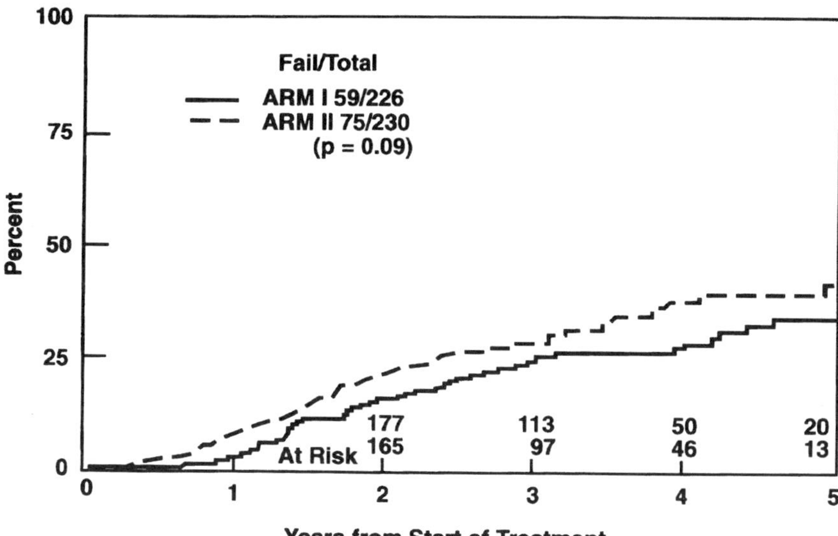

FIGURE 2.—Cumulative incidence of distant metastasis by treatment group. *Arm I* is goserelin and flutamide plus radiation therapy. *Arm II* is radiation therapy alone. (Reprinted by permission of the publisher. From Pilepich MV, Sause WT, Shipley WU, et al: Androgen deprivation with radiation therapy compared with radiation therapy alone for locally advanced prostatic carcinoma: A randomized comparative trial of the Radiation Therapy Oncology Group. *Urology* 45:616–623. Copyright 1995 by Elsevier Sciences, Inc.)

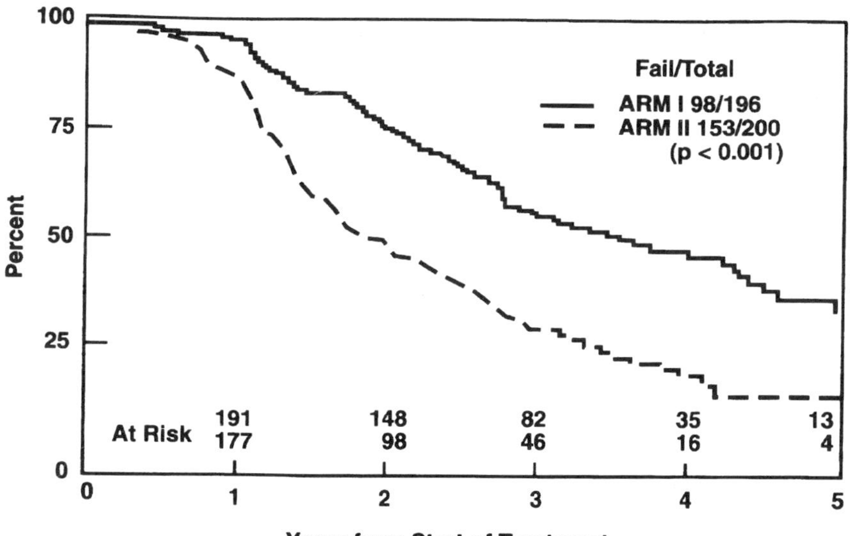

FIGURE 3.—Progression-free survival by treatment group. *Arm I* is goserelin and flutamide plus radiation therapy. *Arm II* is radiation therapy alone. (Reprinted by permission of the publisher. From Pilepich MV, Sause WT, Shipley WU, et al: Androgen deprivation with radiation therapy compared with radiation therapy alone for locally advanced prostatic carcinoma: A randomized comparative trial of the Radiation Therapy Oncology Group. *Urology* 45:616–623. Copyright 1995 by Elsevier Sciences, Inc.)

specific antigen, measured at least once in 396 patients—was 36% in arm I vs. 15% in arm II (Fig 3). There was no significant difference in overall survival at 5 years, however.

Conclusions.—In patients with locally advanced carcinoma of the prostate, the addition of short-term androgen deprivation to radiation therapy yields significant increases in local control and disease-free survival. There is no associated increase in major toxicity. Longer follow-up is needed to determine the effects of androgen deprivation on overall survival.

▶ More than a decade ago, Dr. Malcolm Bagshaw made the comment that radiation therapy alone for clinical stage C adenocarcinoma of the prostate is inadequate. This has been the opinion of some surgeons who have shied away from radiation therapy for early clinical stage T3 cancer, and they have treated select patients with this stage of the disease with radical prostatectomy with or without adjuvant radiation or hormonal treatment. In one of these retrospective studies of 812 patients, 5- and 10-year prostate-specific antigen (PSA) progression-free ($\leq$ 0.2 ng/mL) survival rates were 58% and 41%, respectively.[1] These surgical results seem to be superior to the timely Radiation Therapy Oncology Group (RTOG) data of 396 patients whose progression-free survival, including PSA ($\leq$ 4.0 ng/mL), were 36% and 15% in those patients undergoing concomitant hormonal treatment ($\leq$ 4 months) and no concomitant hormonal treatment, respectively. The RTOG local control at 5 years was only 54% and 29%, respectively, for these groups. This compares with an 80% and 71% local control rate at 5 and 10 years, respectively, in the surgery with or without adjuvant treatment group; however, these 2 studies may not be comparable.[1] The radiation study considered only tumors of at least 25 cm³ or more (a soft measurement!) and also used a soft PSA end point of 4.0 ng/mL rather than that suggested by Willard et al. who recommend that PSA levels be less than 1.0 ng/mL.[2] These and other studies have shown that adjuvant therapy in combination with the primary treatment, be it surgery or radiation, does not seem to provide an improved survival, although it undoubtedly provides a better local control rate and thus possibly an improved quality of life.

H. Zincke, M.D.

References

1. Lerner SE, Blute, ML, Zincke H: Extended experience with radical prostatectomy for clinical stage T3 prostate cancer: Outcome and contemporary morbidity. *J Urol* 154:1447–1452, 1995.
2. Willard ZG, Zietman AL, Shipley WU, et al: The effect of pelvic radiation therapy on serum levels of prostatic specific antigen. *J Urol* 151:1579–1581, 1994.

Adjuvant Radiotherapy for Pathologic Stage T3/4 Adenocarcinoma of the Prostate: Ten-Year Update

Anscher MS, Robertson CN, Prosnitz LR (Duke Univ, Durham, NC)
Int J Radiat Oncol Biol Phys 33:37–43, 1995   21–37

Introduction.—Although postoperative radiotherapy (RT) after radical prostatectomy (RP) would be expected to improve local control and possibly survival in patients with advanced stage adenocarcinoma of the prostate, these benefits have not been proved in clinical trials, mainly because the trials generally have had short follow-up. The potential benefits of postoperative RT were studied in a large series followed for a median of 10 years.

Methods.—A total of 159 patients who underwent RP between 1970 and 1983 for the treatment of newly diagnosed pathologic stage T3/4 adenocarcinoma of the prostate were studied. Adjuvant RT was given, at the discretion of the attending urologist, to 46 of the 159 patients. These patients typically received 45–50 Gy to the whole pelvis plus boost doses of 10–15 Gy to the prostate bed. The patients treated with (RT group) and without (RP group) adjuvant RT were compared for survival, disease-free survival, local control, and distant failure.

Results.—Both groups were followed for a median of 10 years. Actuarial survival was 62% in the RT group and 52% in the RP group at 10 years and 62% in the RT group and 37% in the RP group at 15 years. The actuarial disease-free survival rates were 55% in the RT group and 37% in the RP group at 10 years and 48% in the RT group and 33% in the RP group at 15 years. Failure occurred at a median time of 12.4 years in the RT group and 7.5 years in the RP group. The actuarial rate of metastasis-free survival was 67% in the RT group and 65% in the RP group at 10 years and 57% in both groups at 15 years. In contrast, 92% of the RT group and 60% of the RP group were free of local disease at 10 years, and 82% of the RT group and 53% of the RP group had local control at 15 years.

Conclusions.—Compared with surgical treatment alone, adjuvant radiotherapy results in highly significantly better local control in patients treated for stage T3/4 adenocarcinoma of the prostate. However, adjuvant RT does not influence the development of probable occult metastatic disease in these patients and thus does not significantly improve survival and disease-free survival.

▶ This study by Anscher et al. is actually the second report of a paper that appeared in 1987 in which the authors claimed a 15-year, 90% actuarial survival for the same 46 patients receiving adjuvant RT after RP, as compared with only 21% for patients undergoing RP alone.[1] The former paper was misleading because at 15 years, there was only 1 patient under observation for each arm. Hence, statements in regard to 15-year survival were then invalid.

In this study, with satisfactory follow-up (median, 10 years), the 10-year survival rates for the adjuvant and surgical-only groups were 62% and 52%, respectively. No difference was found in regard to outcome except for significantly improved local control using adjuvant radiation. This paper is not only lacking from small numbers; more disturbing is that an unknown number of patients received postoperative hormonal treatment—"used at the discretion of the urologist." Hence, the data cannot be taken seriously as being consistent with an adjuvant radiation effect only.

However, more carefully performed studies, although also retrospective, have shown that adjuvant RT is beneficial in preventing local recurrence.[2, 3] In the paper by Hawkins et al., adjuvant orchiectomy rather than adjuvant RT was more effective treatment in preventing local recurrence; and indeed, adjuvant radiation was without benefit in patients with nondiploid tumors, suggesting that patients with unfavorable tumors (nondiploid) will need systemic rather than local adjuvant treatment because most of these tumors have already settled outside of the pelvis.[3]

H. Zincke, M.D., Ph.D.

References

1. Anscher MS, Prosnitz LR: Postoperative radiotherapy for patients with carcinoma of the prostate undergoing radical prostatectomy with positive surgical margins, seminal vesicle involvement and/or penetration through the capsule. *J Urol* 138:1407–1412, 1987.
2. Syndikus I, Pickles T, Kostashuk E, et al: Postoperative radiotherapy for stage pT3 carcinoma of the prostate: Improved local control. *J Urol* 155:1983–1986, 1996.
3. Hawkins CA, Bergstralh EJ, Lieber MM, et al: Influence of DNA ploidy and adjuvant treatment on progression and survival in patients with pathologic stage T3 (pT3) prostate cancer after radical retropubic prostatectomy. *Urology* 46:356–364, 1995.

Advanced Prostate Cancer: The Results of a Randomized Comparative Trial of High Dose Irradiation Boosting With Conformal Protons Compared With Conventional Dose Irradiation Using Photons Alone

Shipley WU, Verhey LJ, Munzenrider JE, Suit HD, Urie MM, McManus PL, Young RH, Shipley JW, Zietman AL, Biggs PJ, Heney NM, Goitein M (Massachusetts Gen Hosp, Boston; Harvard Med School, Boston)

Int J Radiat Oncol Biol Phys 32:3–12, 1995   21–38

Purpose.—For men with advanced prostate adenocarcinoma extending beyond the gland, long-term local recurrence is a common problem. As in tumors at many other sites, local prostate tumor control rates have been improved with higher total radiation doses. In a previous phase I/II study, the authors established the feasibility of conformal external beam therapy delivered perineally by protons for men with advanced prostate cancer. The results of a phase III trial of high- vs. conventional-dose external beam irradiation as monotherapy for patients with stage T3–T4 prostate cancer were reported.

Methods.—A total of 202 patients with stage T3–T4, Nx, N0–2, M0 prostate cancer were studied. All received 50.4 Gy of radiation by 4-field photons. The patients were then randomly selected to receive either an additional 25.2 cobalt gray equivalent (CGE) by conformational protons (arm 1); or an additional 16.8 Gy by photons (arm 2). Total dose was 75.6 CGE in arm 1 and 67.2 Gy in arm 2. The 2 groups were compared for overall survival (OS), disease-specific survival (DSS), total recurrence-free survival (TRFS), and local control. Total recurrence-free survival was defined as clinical freedom from tumor; a prostate-specific antigen level of less than 4 ng/mL; and a negative prostate biopsy, done in 38 patients without evidence of disease. Local control was assessed by digital rectal examination and by rebiopsy.

Results.—Ninety percent of patients and 97% of those in arm 2 completed their respective protocols. At a median follow-up of 61 months, 135 were alive, 47 had died of prostate cancer, and 20 had died of other causes. Grade 1 and 2 rectal bleeding and urethral stricture were more common in arm 1. There were no significant differences in OS, DSS, TRFS, or local control. For patients who completed their randomized treatment, the local control rate at 5 and 8 years was 92% and 77%, respectively, in arm 1, and 80% and 60%, respectively in arm 2. Local control for poorly differentiated tumors—i.e., Gleason 4 or 5—at 5 and 8 years was 94% and 84%, respectively, in arm 1 vs. 64% and 19%, respectively, in arm 2. The positive biopsy rate for patients whose digital examination normalized after treatment was lower in arm 1 vs. arm 2 (28% vs. 45%), and was lower for patients with well- and moderately differentiated tumors vs. those with poorly differentiated tumors (32% vs. 50%). These differences were not significant.

Conclusions.—Among patients with advanced prostate cancer, increasing the total tumor dose by 12.5% by a conformal proton boost significantly improves local control only for patients with poorly differentiated tumors. The photon boost technique increases late radiation sequelae and, so far, has failed to improve OS, DSS, or TRFS in any patient subgroup. The authors are conducting another phase III trial of the same proton boost technique in patients with T1, T2a, and T2b prostate tumors.

▶ This study is basically a consequence of the previous Massachusetts General Hospital study, which showed that conventional radiation therapy by photon therapy alone is associated with poor results for T3–4 prostate cancer.[1] An attempt has been made in a randomized study to test the feasibility of conformable external beam radiation therapy delivered perineally by protons (total of 75.6 CGE) as compared with photon therapy only (total of 67.2 Gy). The authors decided to use a PSA level of less than 4.0 ng/mL as indicating freedom from tumor.

For 189 patients who have completed the study, there was no difference in outcome in regard to crude and cause-specific survival as well as overall progression-free and local recurrence-free survival. However, local control was significantly ($P = 0.0014$) superior in 52 patients with an undifferentiated cancer (n = 57) receiving high-dose rather than conventional-dose therapy. Furthermore, in those patients who had biopsies performed (not all patients had biopsies), there seemed to be a better control rate in the high-dose than the conventional-dose control (28% and 45% with a positive prostate biopsy rate during follow-up, respectively). This advantage of better control in patients with high-grade disease was achieved at the cost of a significantly ($P = 0.002$) higher complication rate in patients who had high-dose therapy, particularly in regard to rectal bleeding. The authors will also test this approach in patients with small tumor volume ($\leq$ T2b disease). Again, this study shows that radiation therapy alone is insufficient treatment for large-volume cancer.

H. Zincke, M.D., Ph.D.

Reference

1. Zietman AL, Coen JJ, Dallow KC, et al: The treatment of prostate cancer by conventional radiation therapy: an analysis of long-term outcome. *Int J Radiat Oncol Biol Phys* 32:287–292, 1995.

Longitudinal Evaluation of Serum Androgen Levels in Men With and Without Prostate Cancer
Carter HB, Pearson JD, Metter EJ, Chan DW, Andres R, Fozard JL, Rosner W, Walsh PC (Johns Hopkins Univ, Baltimore, Md; Natl Inst on Aging, Baltimore, Md; Roosevelt Hosp, New York)
Prostate 27:25–31, 1995

21–39

Background.—Although the precise role of androgens in the development of prostatic cancer remains unclear, responses to androgen withdrawal do suggest that there is at least a permissive role.

Objective.—Androgen levels were monitored prospectively in 20 men older than 60 years who had a histologic diagnosis of prostate cancer while being followed in the Baltimore Longitudinal Study of Aging. Twenty age-matched men with benign prostatic hyperplasia who underwent simple prostatectomy also were studied, along with 16 men without prostatic disease. Four of the men with cancer had metastatic disease. Sex steroid levels were estimated 6–9 times over a period of 7–25 years before prostatic disease was diagnosed.

Findings.—There were no significant differences between the 3 groups of men in age-adjusted levels of luteinizing hormone, total testosterone, or sex hormone–binding globulin up to 15 years before diagnosis. Men in whom cancer developed had higher average free testosterone levels, as determined by radioimmunoassay, 10–15 years before diagnosis, but free testosterone levels calculated from measured concentrations of total testosterone and sex hormone–binding globulin did not differ significantly. The ratio of estimated to calculated free testosterone correlated with the length of time the serum was stored.

Conclusion.—The circulating level of testosterone is not a useful predictor of the later development of prostatic cancer.

▶ This study suggests that factors other than the absolute level of circulating androgens are necessary for the development of prostate cancer. Given that the presence of androgens is a necessary but not sufficient condition for prostate cancer to develop, it seems likely that individual differences in sensitivity to androgens may explain differences in cancer risk. Evidence in support of this hypothesis is growing. For example, recent genetic epidemiologic studies have defined men at risk for the hereditary form of prostate cancer, which appears to be related to an inherited genetic susceptibility.[1] Another study has demonstrated individual and ethnic differences in the molecular structure of the androgen receptor gene that may account for differences in tumor aggressiveness.[2] These sorts of studies are likely to improve the understanding of biological progression of prostate cancer, as well as yield new strategies for screening, prevention, and therapy.

E.A. Klein, M.D.

References

1. Carter BS, Bova GS, Beaty TH, et al: Hereditary prostate cancer: Epidemiologic and clinical features. *J Urol* 150:797–802, 1993.
2. Giovannucci E, Stampfer M, Krithivas K, et al: The CAG repeat contained within the androgen receptor is a heritable factor that influences the clinical behavior of prostate cancer. *Proceedings of the American Society of Clinical Oncology* 15:646A, 1996.

The Final Analysis of the EORTC Genito-Urinary Tract Cancer Co-Operative Group Phase III Clinical Trial (Protocol 30805) Comparing Orchidectomy, Orchidectomy Plus Cyproterone Acetate and Low Dose Stilboestrol in the Management of Metastatic Carcinoma of the Prostate

Robinson MRG, Smith PH, Richards B, Newling DWW, de Pauw M, Sylvester R (Pontefract Gen Infirmary, England; St James's Univ Hosp, Leeds, England; District Hosp, York, England; et al)

Eur Urol 28:273–283, 1995

21–40

Introduction.—Reported is the third and final analysis of the European Organization for Research and Treatment of Cancer (EORTC) clinical trial that evaluated response to hormonal therapy in patients with advanced carcinoma of the prostate gland. Because of concern about cardiovascular complications and prognostic factors in phases I and II, the presence or absence of chronic disease, especially cardiovascular disease, at the time of entry into the trial was emphasized.

Methods.—Patients in phase III of this trial were randomly assigned to 1 of 3 groups: orchidectomy; orchidectomy plus treatment with cyproterone acetate (CPA), 50 mg 3 times a day; or treatment with diethylstilbestrol (DES), 1 mg once a day. Patients underwent extensive evaluation before treatment. Follow-up evaluations were done every 3 months in the first year after surgery, then every 6 months thereafter.

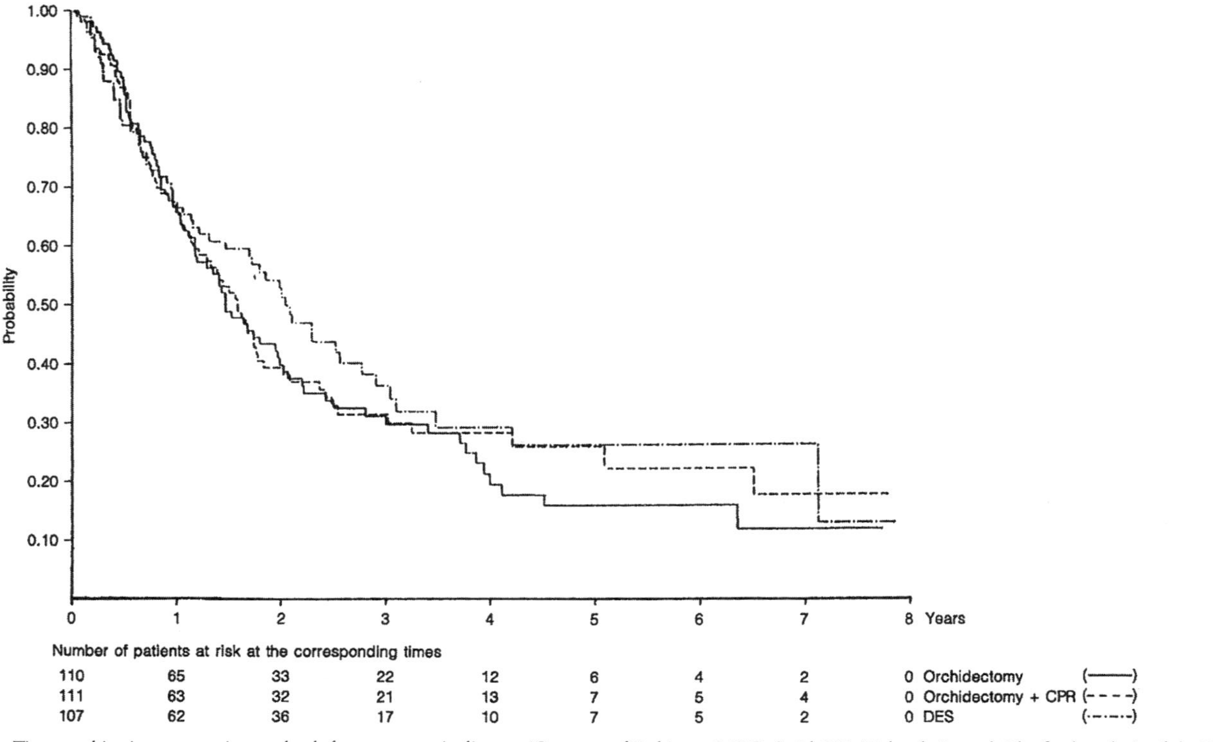

FIGURE 1.—Time to objective progression or death from metastatic disease. (Courtesy of Robinson MRG, Smith PH, Richards B, et al: The final analysis of the EORTC Genito-Urinary Tract Cancer Co-Operative Group Phase III Clinical Trial (protocol 30805) comparing orchidectomy, orchidectomy plus cyproterone acetate and low dose stilboestrol in the management of metastatic carcinoma of the prostate. *Eur Urol* 28:273–283. Copyright 1995 S. Karger AG, Basel, publisher.)

Results.—The median duration of follow-up for 351 patients from 16 European institutions was 4 years. A total of 328 patients were eligible for follow-up. Analysis of patient and disease characteristics at time of trial entry indicated that patients receiving DES had a better performance status and the highest percentage of cardiovascular abnormalities. No significant between-group differences in time to objective progression or death from metastatic disease were observed (Fig 1). At the time of last available information, 63% of patients had died of malignant disease and 20% were still alive. There were no significant between-group differences in the time to death or cause of death. In the DES arm, there was a tendency for slightly fewer malignant deaths and slightly more cardiovascular deaths. The incidence of angina, ischemic heart disease, cerebrovascular accidents, and hypertension were comparable for the 3 treatment arms. There was a higher incidence of edema, deep vein thrombosis of the lower limb, cramps, and dyspnea in the DES group, compared with the other 2 groups. Patients in the DES group had the lowest incidence of hot flashes and the highest incidence of painless and painful gynecomastia. Treatment was discontinued in 13, 3, and 0 patients, respectively, in the DES, orchidectomy plus CPA, and orchidectomy-only groups because of cardiovascular complications. Further analysis indicated that the increased incidence of cardiovascular side effects in patients in the DES treatment group was not because of the larger number of patients with cardiovascular disease upon trial entry. Patients with the lowest risk scores at trial entry had a median survival of approximately 3 years, compared with a median survival of about 6 months for patients with the highest risk scores.

Conclusions.—There were no significant differences in time to metastatic progression and overall survival between the 3 treatment groups. Allowing for the fact that more patients in the DES arm had pre-existing cardiovascular disease, there remained an unacceptable higher risk of cardiovascular disease for this treatment group. There was no treatment advantage for orchidectomy plus CPA, compared with orchidectomy alone. The major prognostic factor was performance at the time of trial entry in patients with metastatic disease, irrespective of the type of hormonal therapy used.

▶ This trial compared 3 treatment regimens for metastatic prostate cancer: DES, 1 mg daily; orchiectomy alone; and orchiectomy plus CPA, 50 mg 3 times daily. There was no significant advantage in any of the regimens with regard to time to progression or survival. Overall, DES, 1 mg a day, was associated with an increased number of cardiovascular events, withdrawals because of cardiovascular toxicity, and cardiovascular-related deaths. Even the patients who had no adverse cardiovascular risk profile on trial entry manifested cardiovascular toxicity. Although DES, 1 mg a day, was demonstrated effective treatment for metastatic prostate cancer, cardiovascular side effects were not avoided at this low dose. Similar to the Veterans research trial results, the DES arm had fewer deaths from malignant disease but more deaths related to cardiovascular toxicity. As has been noted in numerous trials treating men with metastatic prostate cancer, performance status at entry is the strongest prognosticator for favorable outcome.

P.F. Schellhammer, M.D.

Maximum Androgen Blockade in Advanced Prostate Cancer: An Overview of 22 Randomised Trials With 3283 Deaths in 5710 Patients
Prostate Cancer Trialists' Collaborative Group (The Netherlands Cancer Inst, Amsterdam; Middelheim Gen Hosp, Antwerp, Belgium; Erasmus Univ, Rotterdam, The Netherlands; et al)
Lancet 346:265–269, 1995   21–41

Introduction.—Maximum androgen blockade (MAB) is the combination of castration, either by operative orchiectomy or by a luteinizing hormone–releasing hormone agonist, with an antiandrogen in patients having locally advanced or metastatic prostate cancer.

Objective.—A meta-analysis was undertaken of 25 randomized clinical trials comparing conventional surgical or medical castration with MAB in patients with advanced prostate cancer. Data were collected on 5,710 patients in 22 of the trials, 3,283 of whom died during a median follow-up of 40 months. Maximum androgen blockade entailed the prolonged use of an antiandrogen such as flutamide, nilutamide, or cyproterone acetate.

Results.—Crude mortality was 58% for patients undergoing castration alone and 56% for those managed by MAB. Life-table estimates of 5-year survival were 22.8% and 26.2%, respectively, an insignificant difference (Fig 3). There was no indication that the various trials differed significantly or that different forms of MAB made a difference. Stratifying patients for age at the time of randomization made little difference in the overall results.

Conclusion.—These findings fail to demonstrate that MAB significantly lengthens the survival of patients with advanced prostatic cancer compared with castration alone.

▶ This large meta-analysis demonstrates a small advantage to complete androgen blockade that is not statistically significant. As illustrated in Figure 3, there appears to be a divergence of the 2 survival curves at 2 years. As pointed out in the article, this is consistent with no advantage of complete androgen blockade among patients with extensive disease whose survival is limited, but it hints at a potential survival difference for those patients surviving beyond 2 years—the minimal disease group. The reanalysis with longer follow-up and inclusion of the large intergroup trial, promised in 1997, will test this possibility.

In regards to issues of quality of life, the trialist group makes the observation that a treatment may be beneficial if it improves quality of survival even if there is no advantage in quantity. A critical analysis of this meta-

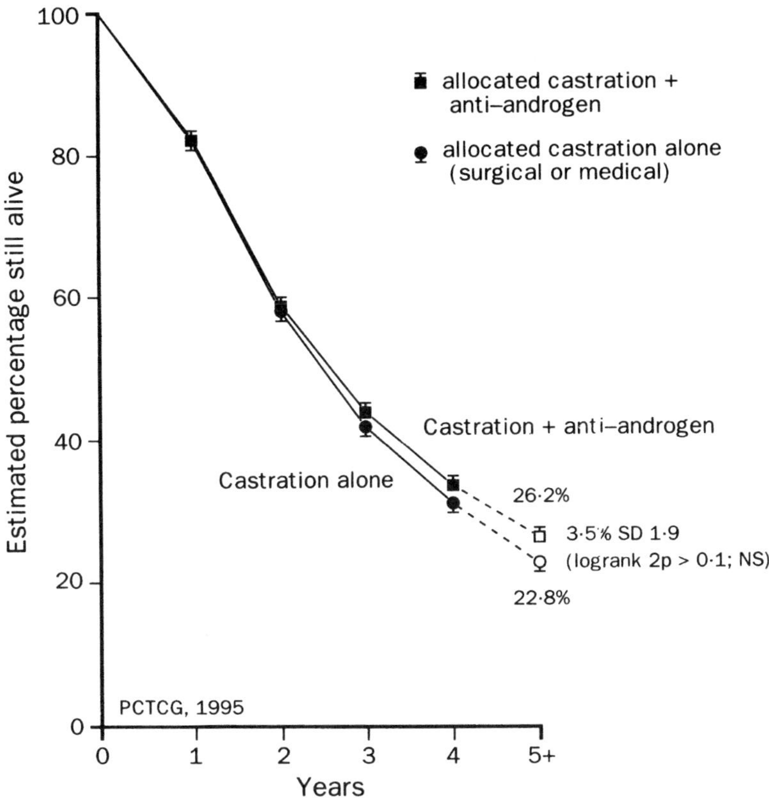

FIGURE 3.—Survival in 22 randomized prostate cancer trials: maximum androgen blockade (MAB) vs. castration alone (5,710 patients, 3,283 deaths). In the first year there were 475 deaths out of 2,512 person-years in the MAB group (logrank O-E = − 6.0, variance −196.1 NS) vs. 498/2,561 in the controls. In the second year there were 594/1,778 (−0.5, 212.5, NS) vs. 606/1,787. After year 2 there were 525/1,911 (−34.1, 206.5, 2 P < 0.02) vs. 587/1,774. *Abbreviations: NS,* not significant; *PCTCG,* Prostate Cancer Trialists' Collaborative Group. (Courtesy of Prostate Cancer Trialists' Collaborative Group: Maximum androgen blockade in advanced prostate cancer: An overview of 22 randomised trials with 3,283 deaths in 5,710 patients. *Lancet* 346:265–269. Copyright 1995, The Lancet Ltd.)

analysis by Dr. Brent Blumenstein points out nuances that will help the urologist through the perils and pitfalls of statistical analysis.[1]

P.F. Schellhammer, M.D.

Reference

1. Blumenstein B: Overview analysis issues using combined androgen deprivation overview analysis as an example. *Urol Oncol* 1:95–100, 1995.

Goserelin Versus Orchiectomy in the Treatment of Advanced Prostate Cancer: Final Results of a Randomized Trial

Vogelzang NJ, for the Zoladex Prostate Study Group (Univ of Chicago; Univ of Miami, Fla; Eastern Virginia Med School, Norfolk, Va; et al)
Urology 46:220–226, 1995

21–42

Objective.—A randomized multicenter study compared orchiectomy with the luteinizing hormone–releasing hormone (LHRH) agonist goserelin in 283 previously untreated adult men with stage D2 prostatic cancer. All tumors were histologically confirmed. All the patients were expected to live for at least 3 months.

Management.—A total of 145 patients were assigned to undergo orchiectomy, whereas 138 were to receive goserelin, administered subcutaneously in a dosage of 3.6 mg every 28 days. Patients in both groups were followed for a minimum of 4 years.

Results.—Eleven goserelin-treated patients and 17 who underwent orchiectomy had no documented tumor response. The respective objective response rates were 82% and 77%. Survival times were similar in the 2 treatment groups after adjusting for stratification factors (Fig 2). Both treatments were well tolerated.

Conclusion.—The LHRH agonist goserelin is as effective a treatment as orchiectomy for men with stage D2 prostatic cancer, and is equally well tolerated.

▶ Medical and surgical castration produced equivalent results with regard to time to treatment failure, overall survival, and adverse events. As reported in this article, mean testosterone levels were virtually identical in the 2 groups. This does not mean, however, that every patient treated with an LHRH

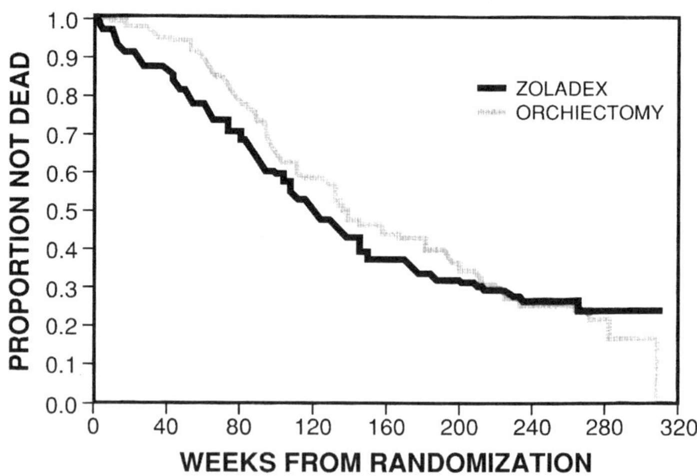

FIGURE 2.—Overall survival. (Reprinted by permission of the publisher. From Vogelzang NJ, for the Zoladex Prostate Study Group: Goserelin versus orchiectomy in the treatment of advanced prostate cancer: Final results of a randomized trial. *Urology* 46:220–226. Copyright 1995 by Elsevier Sciences, Inc.)

analogue had a serum testosterone in the castrate range. Before declaring a patient androgen insensitive after medical castration, it is probably prudent to document a castrate level of serum testosterone.

P.F. Schellhammer, M.D.

Improved Subjective Responses to Orchiectomy Plus Nilutamide (Anandron) in Comparison to Orchiectomy Plus Placebo in Metastatic Prostate Cancer
Dijkman GA, for the International Anandron Study Group (Ignatius Hospital, Breda, The Netherlands; Univ Hospital, Nijmegen, The Netherlands; Univ Hospital, Maastricht, The Netherlands)
Eur Urol 27:196–201, 1995   21–43

Objective.—When it is not possible to prolong life for a patient with metastatic prostate cancer, the goal of treatment shifts to improving the patient's subjective parameters until death. This is done by combining testicular hormone deprivation—either by orchiectomy or administration of a luteinizing hormone–releasing hormone agonist—with a nonsteroidal antiandrogen to produce maximum androgen blockade (MAB). Although several studies have suggested that MAB, as opposed to castration, lengthens the time to subjective and objective progression and increases survival time, few studies have considered the patient's comfort. The results of one such study were reassessed in an attempt to analyze the patients' subjective improvement.

Methods.—The randomized, placebo-controlled study included 423 patients with stage D-II metastatic prostate cancer. In the study, complete androgen blockade with orchiectomy plus nilutamide had clear benefits in terms of objective delay of disease progression. However, the study included no validated tool to assess subjective improvement. The current analysis examined the symptoms of advanced prostate cancer that interfere the most with patient well-being: pain, performance status, disease-related weight loss, urinary impairment, and subjective progression. The gains in quality of life were weighed against any drug-related adverse events.

Findings.—Both treatments—orchiectomy plus nilutamide and orchiectomy plus placebo—produced significant improvements in performance status and urinary obstruction. Median time to subjective progression was consistently and significantly longer in the nilutamide group than in the placebo group. This difference paralleled the improvement in time to objective progression and death (Fig 2). Side effects were reported by about 80% of each group. Adverse events caused 16% of the nilutamide group vs. 9% of the placebo group to withdraw from the study prematurely. Although some side effects were more common with nilutamide, all were reversible on discontinuation of treatment. In contrast, adverse events deemed likely to be related to disease progression were more common with placebo, including anemia, 11% vs. 5%; peripheral edema, 7% vs. 4%; and urinary signs or symptoms, 16% vs. 10%.

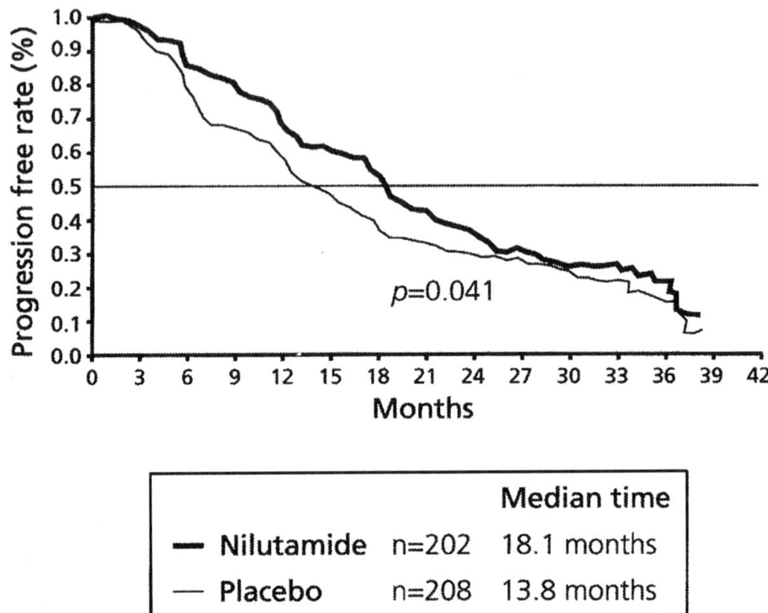

FIGURE 2.—Time to first objective or subjective progression rates (evaluable patients) with orchiectomy plus nilutamide (202 patients at risk, 133 with progression, median time 18.1 months) and orchiectomy plus placebo (208 patients at risk, 153 with progression, median time 13.8 months; $P = 0.011$). (Courtesy of Dijkman GA, for the International Anandron Study Group: Improved subjective responses to orchiectomy plus nilutamide (Anandron) in comparison to orchiectomy plus placebo in metastatic prostate cancer. *Eur Urol* 27:196–201. Copyright 1995, S. Karger AG, Basel, publisher.)

Conclusions.—For patients with metastatic prostate cancer, orchiectomy plus nilutamide appears to improve quality of life. Although no validated quality-of-life questionnaire has been used to study this issue, significant improvement or delayed deterioration in key subjective parameters outweighs the adverse events of nilutamide therapy in most cases.

▶ Quality-of-life assessment is entering into the evaluation process of most treatments. It is not sufficient to say that a treatment works without quantitating morbidity in the patient's own estimation. Androgen deprivation can significantly reduce quality of life in the asymptomatic patient with metastatic prostate cancer. Quality-of-life instruments were not available at the initiation of this study. As a substitute, subjective responses were assessed as reflective of quality of life. Patients receiving MAB enjoyed better subjective outcome. Sixty-four percent of patients had pain, and a better relief was noted with MAB. However, of those patients who were pain free at the institution of therapy, there was no difference in the time to reappearance of pain on progression. Treatment trials are being prospectively evaluated with quality-of-life instruments, and necessarily so.

P.F. Schellhammer, M.D.

Intermittent Androgen Suppression in the Treatment of Prostate Cancer: A Preliminary Report
Goldenberg SL, Bruchovsky N, Gleave ME, Sullivan LD, Akakura K (Univ of British Columbia, Vancouver, Canada; British Columbia Cancer Agency, Vancouver, Canada; Chiba Univ, Japan)
Urology 45:839–845, 1995
21–44

Background.—A previous study showed that consecutive cycles of androgen withdrawal and replacement delayed progression to androgen independence in the androgen-dependent Shionogi carcinoma tumor model and in a small group of men with prostate cancer. The feasibility of using intermittent androgen suppression in the treatment of prostate cancer was investigated in a larger group of men with prostate cancer.

Treatment.—Forty-seven patients with prostate cancer received treatment with a combined androgen blockade consisting of either cyproterone acetate and low-dose diethylstilbestrol or a luteinizing hormone–releasing hormone agonist plus an antiandrogen. Treatment was continued for at least 6 months until a serum prostate-specific antigen (PSA) nadir was observed. Treatment was then withheld until the serum PSA increased to a level between 10 and 20 ng/mL. This cycle of treatment and no treatment was repeated until the regulation of serum PSA became androgen independent. Twenty-four patients had metastatic cancer (clinical stage D2, 14; D1, 10), and 23 had locally advanced cancer (stage C, 11; B2, 2; A2, 2). The mean follow-up was 125 weeks (range, 22–310 weeks).

Outcome.—The first 2 treatment cycles lasted for a mean of 73 and 75 weeks, with a mean time off therapy of 30 and 33 weeks, and a percentage time off therapy of 41% and 45%, respectively. The time to reach a serum PSA nadir was 20 weeks in the first cycle and 18 weeks in the second cycle. Within 8 weeks (range, 1–26 weeks) of stopping treatment, serum testosterone levels returned to the normal range. This was associated with an improved sense of well-being and a recovery of libido and potency in men with previously normal or near-normal sexual function. In 7 patients with stage D2 disease, the cancer progressed to an androgen-independent state at a mean of 128 weeks (median, 108 weeks). Seven patients died, including 1 from an unrelated cause, with a mean survival time of 210 weeks (median, 166 weeks).

Summary.—Intermittent androgen suppression is clinically tenable for the treatment of prostate cancer. Only patients whose serum PSA has reached a stable or decreasing value in the normal range at 24 and 32 weeks of induction should be considered eligible for intermittent androgen suppression. Although it is not known whether intermittent androgen suppression alters survival, this approach affords an improved quality of life, possibly delays tumor progression, reduces toxicity and cost of treatment, and provides the potential for alternating with other treatment modalities.

▶ One of the least understood areas in oncology is the chronic biological and psychological effects of prolonged androgen deprivation in men with advanced prostate cancer. In addition to hot flashes, breast tenderness, and loss of libido, a syndrome of weight gain, lassitude, and dulled mentation while on therapy is not uncommon. This syndrome can be debilitating, and for the initially asymptomatic patient treated only for a rising PSA, the effects of treatment can truly be worse than the disease. Intermittent androgen deprivation may ameliorate some of these symptoms and improve a patient's sense of well-being, although it may also increase psychological distress while waiting for monthly PSA values to be reported. Although laboratory data suggest that intermittent therapy has the potential to prolong survival, this has not been demonstrated in humans and it is possible that survival may be worse with this form of therapy. The optimum PSA at which therapy should be reinstated after a period of withdrawal is not defined, nor is the issue of whether the promise of this approach should preclude the routine use of orchiectomy until further studies are completed.

E.A. Klein, M.D.

A Controlled Trial of Bicalutamide Versus Flutamide, Each in Combination With Luteinizing Hormone–Releasing Hormone Analogue Therapy, In Patients With Advanced Prostate Cancer
Schellhammer P, for the Casodex Combination Study Group (Eastern Virginia Med School, Norfolk)
Urology 45:745–752, 1995

21–45

Background.—Combination treatment with a luteinizing hormone–releasing hormone analogue (LHRH-A) and an antiandrogen have been found to be superior to monotherapy in prolonging time to treatment failure or to disease progression and in improving survival in patients with advanced prostate cancer. The efficacy and safety of bicalutamide and flutamide, each combined with LHRH-A therapy, were investigated in patients with untreated metastatic prostate cancer.

Methods.—Eight hundred thirteen patients were enrolled in the randomized, double-blind, multicenter trial. The patients were assigned in a 1:1 ratio to bicalutamide, 50 mg once a day, and flutamide, 250 mg 3 times a day, and in a 2:1 ratio to goserelin acetate, 3.6 mg every 28 days, and leuprolide acetate, 7.5 mg every 28 days. Median follow-up was 49 weeks.

Findings.—Patients receiving bicalutamide plus LHRH-A had a significantly better time to treatment failure than those receiving flutamide plus LHRH-A (Fig 1). Patients in the latter group were 34% more likely to fail therapy during the given period. The 2 treatment groups had similar survival rates, quality of life, and subjective responses. Twenty-four percent of the patients in the flutamide plus LHRH-A group and 10% of those in the bicalutamide plus LHRH-A group had diarrhea.

Conclusions.—The time to treatment failure resulting from therapy with bicalutamide plus LHRH-A is better than that associated with flutamide plus LHRH-A in patients with metastatic prostate cancer. Patient tolerance

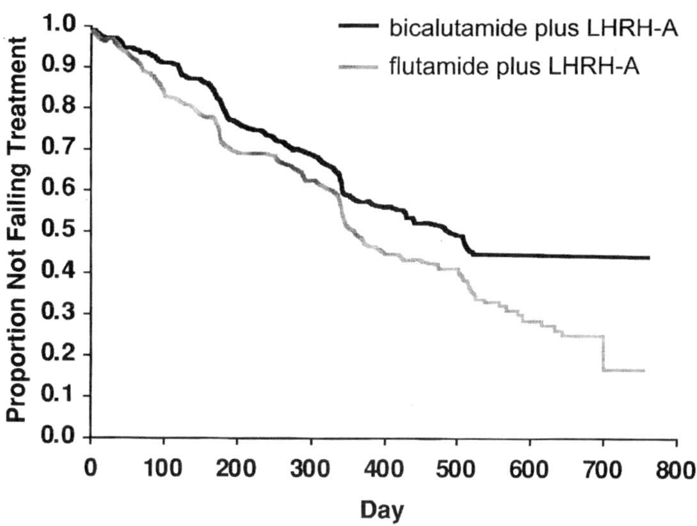

FIGURE 1.—Time to treatment failure. (Reprinted by permission of the publisher. From Schellhammer P, for the Casodex Combination Study Group: A controlled trial of bicalutamide versus flutamide, each in combination with luteinizing hormone–releasing hormone analogue therapy, in patients with advanced prostate cancer. *Urology* 45:745–752. Copyright 1995 by Elsevier Science, Inc.)

of the former treatment regimen is also better. The effects of these regimens on long-term survival need to be investigated in studies with longer follow-up periods.

▶ Despite the use of an unusual end point (time to treatment failure instead of objective progression), this study suggests that bicalutamide is therapeutically equivalent to flutamide when used with an LHRH agonist for treatment of advanced prostate cancer. Longer observation of this cohort of patients has demonstrated no differences in survival between treatment arms at 95 weeks of follow-up. Bicalutamide has the convenience of once-a-day dosing and may cause less diarrhea, but currently is more expensive than flutamide.

E.A. Klein, M.D.

Randomized Prospective Study Comparing Radical Prostatectomy Alone Versus Radical Prostatectomy Preceded by Androgen Blockade in Clinical Stage B2 (T2bNxM0) Prostate Cancer
Soloway MS, for the Lupron Depot Neoadjuvant Prostate Cancer Study Group (Univ of Miami Fla; Univ of Florida, Gainesville; Univ of Illinois, Chicago; et al)
J Urol 154:424–428, 1995   21–46

Objective.—For men undergoing radical prostatectomy, a positive surgical margin is a negative prognostic factor. It has been suggested that giving androgen deprivation therapy before surgery might decrease the chances of positive surgical margins in patients with clinically localized prostate cancer. However, the only evidence for this has come from non-randomized clinical trials. The ability of preoperative androgen deprivation to decrease the incidence of postoperative margins at radical prostatectomy was examined.

Methods.—The randomized trial included 303 patients with stage cT2bNxM0 prostate cancer from 27 participating centers. One hundred forty-nine were assigned to receive 3 months of androgen deprivation therapy with leuprolide acetate depot plus the antiandrogen flutamide, and 154 were assigned to surgery alone. Of 144 patients who underwent surgery, all had pelvic node dissection and 138 had prostatectomy.

Results.—The 2 groups were similar in terms of operating time, blood loss, need for transfusion, postoperative morbidity, and length of hospital stay. Prostate-specific antigen (PSA) level decreased to at least 2 ng/mL or less in all pretreated patients. In the surgery-only group, 4 patients had rectal injuries and 2 had ureteral injuries; these complications did not occur in the pretreatment group. The rate of capsule penetration by tumor was 47% in the patients who received preoperative androgen deprivation, compared with 78% in the surgery-only group. The incidence of positive surgical margins was 18% vs. 48%, respectively. Six percent of the pretreated patients had tumor at the urethral margin, compared with 17% of those who had surgery only.

Conclusions.—In men with clinical stage B2 prostate cancer, preoperative androgen deprivation therapy can reduce the rate of positive surgery margins, normalize PSA levels, and reduce prostate size. The ultimate value of preoperative androgen deprivation will depend on its impact on interval to relapse, clinical progression, and survival.

▶ This study is 1 of 3 that have shown that preoperative hormones will decrease the incidence of positive margins. The authors must be congratulated for doing a randomized trial. However, those of us who do not believe in preoperative therapy would argue that the ultimate PSA-free survival will be no different between the 2 groups. In fact, data will soon be reported showing that at least at 1 year, that is the case.

Until a clear PSA/disease-free survival advantage is demonstrated for hormones, they should not be used. They are costly, not without toxicity, and confuse the pathologic analysis.

J.B. DeKernion, M.D.

The Antiandrogen Withdrawal Syndrome: Experience in a Large Cohort of Unselected Patients With Advanced Prostate Cancer
Small EJ, Srinivas S (Univ of California, San Francisco)
Cancer 76:1428–1434, 1995

21–47

Objective.—Discontinuing flutamide has proved effective in some patients with hormone-resistant prostatic cancer. The results of withdrawing flutamide were examined in 107 consecutive men with metastatic prostatic cancer who had progressive disease while receiving the drug. In addition to antiandrogen therapy, the patients had undergone orchiectomy or received a luteinizing hormone–releasing hormone agonist.

Observations.—Three of the 82 evaluable patients had at least an 80% decrease in serum prostate-specific antigen (PSA) and 9 others had a 50% or greater decrease in PSA, for an overall response rate of 15%. The median duration of response was 3½ months, although some patients responded for longer than a year. Whether concomitant treatment was given did not influence the response to flutamide withdrawal. Patients who responded had received flutamide for a longer time than nonresponders (21.5 months vs. 12 months), but the difference was not statistically significant. Patients who responded to drug withdrawal lived longer after the start of treatment of metastatic disease (44.5 months vs. 35 months), but this difference also was not significant.

Implication.—Antiandrogen withdrawal should be tried before starting treatment for hormone-resistant prostatic cancer.

▶ The observed syndrome of antiandrogen withdrawal has important biological, clinical, and psychological implications. Molecular biological studies have suggested that mutations in the androgen receptor gene in a subset of prostate cancer cells may be responsible for this phenomenon, paradoxically causing antiandrogens to become growth stimulators. It is not yet clear whether this process represents selection of cells with pre-existing mutations or whether antiandrogen therapy causes new mutations. In any event, it seems prudent to stop antiandrogen therapy at the first sign of disease progression in patients treated with combined androgen blockade and observe for a reduction in PSA values before proceeding with additional therapy. This is especially important for patients entering clinical trials for hormone-refractory disease so that a PSA decline is not falsely attributed to the antitumor effect of the new therapeutic agent. At present, there is no convincing data to suggest a survival advantage for those patients who exhibit an antiandrogen withdrawal response.

E.A. Klein, M.D.

N,N-Diethyl-2-[4-(Phenylmethyl)Phenoxy]Ethanamine in Combination With Cyclophosphamide: An Active, Low-Toxicity Regimen for Metastatic Hormonally Unresponsive Prostate Cancer

Brandes LJ, Bracken SP, Ramsey EW (Manitoba Cancer Treatment and Research Found, Winnipeg, Canada; Univ of Manitoba, Winnipeg, Canada)
J Clin Oncol 13:1398–1403, 1995
21–48

Background.—Attempts to treat hormonally unresponsive prostate cancer with cytotoxic agents have been largely unsuccessful. The tamoxifen analogue N,N-diethyl-2-[4-(phenylmethyl)phenoxy]ethanamine. HCl (DPPE) has been reported to improve tumor response to chemotherapeutic agents (including cyclophosphamide) in some patients with advanced refractory cancer. The response to and clinical toxicity of DPPE in combination with cyclophosphamide were studied in patients with hormonally nonresponsive metastatic prostate cancer.

Methods.—Twenty patients with advanced, hormonally unresponsive prostate cancer, 19 of whom were symptomatic, received a maximally tolerated dose of DPPE (6 mg/kg) IV over 80 minutes. During the last 20 minutes of this infusion, cyclophosphamide was also administered at a dose of 600–800 mg/m^2 (maximum 1,500 mg). Treatment was administered once weekly for 4 weeks, then after a 1-week rest period, treatments were administered for 2 of every 3 weeks. Treatment continued as long as the patients benefitted.

Findings.—Partial remission occurred in 5 of 7 patients with measurable soft tissue disease and in 2 of 16 patients with assessable bone disease. One patient with assessable bone disease had complete remission. More than a 50% decrease in serum level of prostate-specific antigen (PSA) occurred in 9 of 18 patients with previously elevated PSA levels. Of 13 patients with bone pain, 11 reported partial or complete resolution of this symptom; 6 had improved PSA levels and 2 had an improved bone scan. All patients had acute ataxia correlating with peak levels of serum DPPE, and 6 also had acute nausea and vomiting. Tiredness and mild nausea occurred in some patients 1 or 2 days after treatment, and hemorrhagic cystitis developed in 1 patient. Toxicity to bone marrow was negligible in 14 patients and toxicity to hair follicles was negligible in 15.

Discussion.—Given the historically poor therapeutic response of this form of cancer and the relatively low systemic toxicity reported for this protocol, the 35% combined tumor response rate of patients treated with DPPE/cyclophosphamide is promising, even though this trial is uncontrolled and still includes a relatively small number of patients. DPPE is an intracellular histamine antagonist that potentiates chemotherapy cytotoxicity to malignant cells while protecting normal bone marrow, gut, and hair. A randomized clinical trial is currently planned to compare DPPE/cyclophosphamide therapy with cyclophosphamide therapy alone.

▶ Although reductions in serum PSA values have been reported in response to many new chemotherapy regimens for hormone-refractory prostate cancer, little data exist to suggest that chemotherapy in this setting prolongs survival for the average patient. It is not clear, therefore, whether chemotherapy should be used outside a clinical protocol, what the optimum regimen is, or whether the optimum time to begin treatment is in the asymptomatic patient with a rising PSA ("better to get it as early as possible when the tumor burden is lowest") or to wait until the patient is symptomatic ("avoid toxicity until treatment is really necessary").

In the absence of data suggesting improved survival with treatment, many chemotherapy trials now focus on quality of life rather than survival as the main therapeutic goal and include such end points as reduction in bone pain or amelioration of other symptoms, reduced need for analgesics, and patient-reported sense of well-being in response to treatment. This study suggests that DPPE in combination with cyclophosphamide holds some promise both in improving quality of life and in improved antitumor effect, but the results are preliminary.

E.A. Klein, M.D.

The Incidence of High Grade Prostatic Intraepithelial Neoplasia in Needle Biopsies
Bostwick DG, Qian J, Frankel K (Mayo Clinic, Rochester, Minn; Glendale Mem Hosp and Health Ctr, Calif)
J Urol 154:1791–1794, 1995   21–49

Background.—High-grade prostatic intraepithelial neoplasia has a high predictive value for invasive prostate cancer. Diagnostic criteria for high-grade prostatic intraepithelial neoplasia have been defined for whole-mount autopsy and radical prostatectomy specimens, but it is unclear whether these criteria can be applied to contemporary 18-gauge needle biopsies because of the small amount of available tissue. The incidence of high-grade prostatic intraepithelial neoplasia in needle biopsies was determined.

Methods.—The pathologic findings from 400 prostatic needle biopsies from 2 geographically diverse medical centers were evaluated by 3 pathologists and compared. Biopsy specimens were classified as benign, high-grade prostatic intraepithelial neoplasia, or foci suspicious for cancer.

Results.—Diagnostic agreement was reached by the 3 observers in all cases. For the 2 medical centers, biopsy specimens revealed benign prostatic tissue in 41.5% and 50% of cases; prostatic intraepithelial neoplasia in 16.5% and 9.5% of cases; foci suspicious for but not diagnostic of malignancy in 1.5% and 2.5% of cases; and cancer in 40.5% and 38% of cases. There was no difference in distribution of findings by digital rectal examination or transrectal ultrasound for 200 patients from 1 of the medical centers. The median serum prostate-specific antigen concentration was higher in patients with prostatic intraepithelial neoplasia and cancer than in patients with benign biopsy specimens.

Discussion.—Up to 18% of needle biopsies are abnormal histopathologically and warrant repeating the biopsy. The incidence of prostatic intraepithelial neoplasia and cancer was similar in these 2 geographically and demographically diverse medical centers.

▶ I was at the podium session of the United States and Canadian Academy of Pathology a couple of years ago when this paper was presented. Many experienced prostate pathologists who were in attendance felt that an 18% incidence of isolated high-grade prostatic intraepithelial neoplasia (PIN) was much too high. Most were of the opinion that an incidence of 4% to 5% would be reasonable based on experience in their own laboratory. On the other hand, it was difficult to argue that perhaps different diagnostic criteria could account for the seemingly increased incidence, because Dr. Bostwick was an author in the original study defining the diagnostic criteria. That this paper is a retrospective study with the express purpose of finding high-grade PIN probably accounts for the higher-than-expected incidence.

Most pathologists scan needle biopsy specimens from a medium magnification, which is adequate for identifying the architectural derangements of adenocarcinoma but which may not identify all cases of high-grade PIN. This study should cause all pathologists who interpret prostate biopsy specimens to look carefully at their own experience in this regard, because it has been well demonstrated that patients with isolated high-grade PIN have a twofold to threefold greater risk of having adenocarcinoma upon repeat biopsy than those without atypical findings.

T. Wheeler, M.D.

Minimal or No Cancer in Radical Prostatectomy Specimens: Report of 13 Cases of the "Vanishing Cancer Phenomenon"
Goldstein NS, Bégin LR, Grody WW, Novak JM, Qian J, Bostwick DG (Cedars-Sinai Med Ctr, Los Angeles; McGill Univ, Montreal; Univ of California, Los Angeles; et al)
Am J Surg Pathol 19:1002–1009, 1995   21–50

Introduction.—Efforts at detecting prostate cancer early in its course often means that a smaller tumor volume will be present in the radical prostatectomy specimen. In some instances, thorough sampling will fail to demonstrate residual cancer. This is known as the "vanishing cancer" phenomenon. The questions arise of whether biopsy eliminated the tumor and whether the initial diagnosis was accurate.

Objective.—The clinical and histologic findings were reviewed in 13 patients with biopsy-confirmed prostate cancer, in whose prostatectomy specimens it was difficult or impossible to identify residual cancer.

Patients.—The 13 men had an average age of 67 years. Digital rectal examination was suggestive of cancer in 2 instances, equivocal in 9, and negative in 2. In no case had transurethral resection been done previously. Serum prostate-specific antigen (PSA) levels ranged from 3 to 18 ng/mL and averaged 8 ng/mL.

Findings.—A single focus of carcinoma was found in 8 cases. Three samples contained 2 foci, but 2 others were negative for cancer. An average of 79 slides were examined, not counting the seminal vesicles and pelvic nodes. In patients with residual cancer the mean tumor volume was 0.019 cc. The largest focus measured less than 3 mm in extent. All tumors were well differentiated or moderately differentiated. Genotype analysis made it extremely unlikely that the biopsy and prostatectomy specimens were from different patients.

Implications.—The inability to identify prostatic cancer in an operative specimen despite biopsy confirmation does not necessarily indicate technical failure. "Vanishing cancer" may become more prevalent as more patients with low-stage cancer undergo prostatectomy.

▶ The authors have done us a great service in publishing this paper because they highlight an increasingly prevalent problem in surgical pathology and clinical urology. Indeed, as I write these comments, I am in the process of cutting deeper into the paraffin blocks of a radical prostatectomy specimen that I diagnosed as less than 1 mm of well-differentiated prostate cancer in 1 of 6 cores. Although I have faced this problem 3 or 4 times during the last few years, this problem was virtually unheard of in the pre-PSA era, when patients were treated for cancer because the tumor was palpable. Pathologists have found that the tables have turned; whereas in the past we lamented that a patient with a particularly aggressive, probably incurable cancer had been subjected to radical surgery, now we see much more commonly that a patient with a clinically insignificant cancer has been overtreated. There is a clear need for better markers to select appropriate patients for "watchful waiting."

T. Wheeler, M.D.

Pathology of Androgen Deprivation Therapy in Prostate Carcinoma: A Comparative Study of 173 Patients
Civantos F, Marcial MA, Banks ER, Ho CK, Speights VO, Drew PA, Murphy WM, Soloway MS (Univ of Miami, Fla; Universidad Central Del Caribe, Bayamon, Puerto Rico; Veterans Affairs Med Ctr, Lexington, Ky; et al)
Cancer 75:1634–1641, 1995   21–51

Introduction.—Two small trials reporting the pathologic alterations associated with androgen deprivation give conflicting results. The pathologic changes associated with androgen deprivation with leuprolide (plus flutamide) were evaluated in 113 patients who underwent radical prostatectomy for clinical stage T2 adenocarcinoma.

Methods.—Sixty patients not treated with androgen deprivation before radical prostatectomy acted as controls. Prostatectomy specimens were processed to produce 26–40 blocks per patient. Hematoxylin and eosin stains were performed and distinctive histologic findings were tabulated.

Results.—Tumor involvement at the specimen margin was recorded in 19% and 43% of treated and untreated prostates, respectively. The incidence of high-grade prostatic intraepithelial neoplasia (PIN) was 35% and 82% in treated and untreated prostates, respectively. Histologic changes in non-neoplastic tumor areas of treated prostates included atrophy, basal cell prominence, vacuolated luminal cell layer, and squamous transitional cell metaplasia. Histologic changes in treated prostate tumors included reduction in the sizes of individual neoplastic cells, presence of cytoplasmic clearing, and vacuolization. The most frequently noted effect of androgen deprivation was the presence of small tumor glands separated by stroma. Other histologic patterns were pykinosis and branching empty spaces, and large clear tumor cells within an inflammatory response. Unaffected areas of prostate cancer were observed in 43% of treated prostates.

Conclusion.—Androgen deprivation was associated with significant reductions in the frequency of high-grade PIN and tumor involvement at specimen margins. Changes in treated prostates may resemble those of poor differentiation in untreated glands, resulting in overgrading a treated prostate cancer.

▶ This is one of several recent studies to clarify the pathologic changes in the benign and neoplastic prostate of patients who have undergone androgen deprivation therapy before radical prostatectomy. All of these studies have demonstrated a decrease in the incidence of high-grade PIN (the most likely precursor of prostatic adenocarcinoma) but a paradoxical increase in the Gleason grade. The latter is clearly an artifact of gland collapse as a response to therapy; the nuclear grade of the tumor actually improves.

Improvement in surgical margin status in this study is more problematic; although the authors show a statistically significant decrease in positive margins from 43% to 19% in untreated and treated patients, respectively, the low incidence of positive margins is still higher than that reported in series from centers where androgen deprivation before surgery is not used routinely (such as my own institution). Of course, the final answer will not be known until differences in recurrence rates or better yet, survival can be demonstrated.

T. Wheeler, M.D.

Castration Therapy Rapidly Induces Apoptosis in a Minority and Decreases Cell Proliferation in a Majority of Human Prostatic Tumors

Westin P, Stattin P, Damber J-E, Bergh A (Univ of Umeå, Sweden)
Am J Pathol 146:1368–1375, 1995
21–52

Background.—Castration therapy is initially effective in prostatic cancers, reducing pain and other symptoms. Most of these tumors relapse, however, growing independent of androgen and with tumor cell morphology unaffected. The short-term response of prostatic tumors to castration was examined to distinguish patients who eventually will have positive outcome from those who require additional treatment.

Methods.—One day before and 7 days after castration, at least 3 ultrasound-guided core biopsies were taken in 18 patients with prostatic cancer. Seven of 16 patients for whom bone scans were available had distant metastasis. Three patients were staged to T2, 11 to T3, and 4 to T4. Tumors were classified into high (G1), moderate (G2), and low (G3) differentiation. Morphometry, monoclonal antibodies against *Bcl-2, c-myc,* Ki-67, and p53 proteins, and an in situ method were used to visualize apoptotic cells.

Results.—Four tumors were classified as G1, 9 as G2, and 5 as G3. Histologic grade was not influenced by castration, but biopsy sections from 15 patients exhibited changes in morphology. The epithelial tumor cell cytoplasm was often filled with vacuoles, and the glands and the individual tumor cells appeared smaller. The magnitude of these responses appeared to be related to histologic grade. Treatment significantly reduced the average tumor cell nuclear area and the Ki-67 index. Grade 2 and 3 tumors had a slightly lower response to castration, but the magnitude of response did not appear to be related to p53, *Bcl-2 ,* or *c-myc* staining. The apoptotic index was significantly increased in 6 of these 15 tumors, decreased in 3, and largely unaffected in 6. Tumors responding with an increase in apoptotic index were G1 or G2 and negative or weakly positive for p53, *c-myc,* and *Bcl-2* before therapy. Tumors with a decreased or unaffected apoptotic index were G2 or G3 and immunopositive for one or more of p53, *Bcl-2,* or *c-myc* proteins before castration therapy. Ten patients demonstrated a significant change in the *Bcl-2* index.

Conclusion.—Castration therapy is thought to induce an increased apoptotic index and a decreased cell proliferation index in prostatic tumors. Yet findings in these patients revealed the apoptotic index to be decreased or unaffected in 9 of 15 cases 7 days after castration. Prostatic tumors appear to respond to therapy in a variety of ways, and these initial responses may be related to long-term prognosis.

▶ Apoptosis, also known as programmed cell death, has recently received much attention in cancer research, primarily because clinical growth of cancer must reflect a greater degree of cell proliferation than cell death, both of which are known to occur to a variable extent in all human cancers. Factors influencing either of these would therefore be important in defining the growth characteristics of a given tumor.

The authors show that even in the majority of the patients whose tumors show degenerative changes secondary to castration 1 week previously, the apoptotic rate in each individual tumor varied according to precastration grade, p53, *Bcl-2,* and *c-myc* expression. Thus the authors conclude that the classification of prostate cancer as either androgen dependent or independent may be an oversimplification. However, it is difficult to draw firm conclusions from a study with only 2 data points—1 day before and 7 days after castration. A similar study with many sequential biopsies would be more informative but probably not possible today because of ethical considerations. An appropriate animal model would be invaluable.

T. Wheeler, M.D.

Application of a Tumor Suppressor (C-CAM1)-Expressing Recombinant Adenovirus in Androgen-Independent Human Prostate Cancer Therapy: A Preclinical Study
Kleinerman DI, Zhang W-W, Lin S-H, Van NT, von Eschenbach AC, Hsieh J-T
(Univ of Texas MD Anderson Cancer Ctr, Houston)
Cancer Res 55:2831–2836, 1995

21–53

Background.—The cell adhesion molecules (CAMs) are important factors in regulating normal cellular growth and differentiation. Altered expression of these molecules has been implicated in tumorigenesis. Recent observations show that C-CAM, an androgen-regulated member of this family, acts as a tumor suppressor in prostatic cancer, raising the possibility that it might prove helpful in developing gene therapy for this malignancy.

Objective and Methods.—An expression vector for C-CAM1, a C-CAM isoform, was transfected into PC-3, a tumorigenic prostate cancer cell line. A recombinant adenovirus carrying the C-CAM1 gene was constructed and, along with its antisense construct, examined for tumor-suppressing ability in vivo. Viral infectivity of PC-3 cells was estimated by fluorescent-activated cell scanning.

Observations.—The prostate cancer cells proved sensitive to adenoviral infection. The C-CAM1 protein was demonstrated in cells infected by C-CAM1 adenovirus but not in those infected by the antisense control virus. Expression was evident 24 hours after infection; its level was a function of the amount of virus delivered. A single dose of C-CAM adenovirus suppressed the growth of PC-3–induced tumors in nude mice for at least 3 weeks, but the tumors had regained the ability to grow by week 6.

Conclusions.—The C-CAM1 adenovirus inhibits the growth of prostatic cancer cells without causing significant host toxicity. This agent is highly infective but, unlike retrovirus, is not integrated into the host chromosome.

▶ The use of various forms of gene therapy for prostate cancer is now under serious consideration. Recent experimental work by Kleinerman et al. demonstrate the efficacy of direct injection gene therapy for suppressing the growth of human prostate cancer cells in vivo. In this study, recombinant adenoviral vectors were used to transduce the C-CAM1 gene, an androgen-regulated cell adhesion molecule, into established tumors initiated by the subcutaneous injection of PC-3 cells into nude mice. The results clearly demonstrated that repeated transduction of the C-CAM1 gene results in significant growth suppression in the PC-3–nude mouse model system.

Through these studies, the notion of modulating the adhesive properties of tumor cells through gene therapy approaches gained considerable support. In addition to demonstrating the therapeutic potential of the C-CAM1 gene in a human gene therapy protocol, this study also raised significant questions regarding the titers necessary for therapeutic activity, the dosing regimen, as well as potential toxicities. Further studies will better define a role for recombinant adenovirus-mediated transduction of genes that both suppress tumor growth as well as induce cytotoxic effects.[1]

T.C. Thompson, Ph.D.

Reference

1. Eastham JA, Chen S-H, Sehgal I, et al: Prostate cancer gene therapy: Herpes simplex virus thymidine kinase gene transduction followed by ganciclovir in mouse and human prostate models. *Hum Gene Ther* 7:515–523, 1996.

Mutation of the Androgen-Receptor Gene in Metastatic Androgen-Independent Prostate Cancer
Taplin M-E, Bubley GJ, Shuster TD, Frantz ME, Spooner AE, Ogata GK, Keer HN, Balk SP (Univ of Massachusetts, Worcester; Beth Israel Hosp, Boston; Harvard Med School, Boston)
N Engl J Med 332:1393–1398, 1995   21–54

Background.—Prostate cancer is the second leading cause of cancer-related death among men in the United States. Metastases are common at diagnosis, and most patients relapse after androgen ablation because of tumor cells that become independent of the need for androgen. Ten patients with metastatic androgen-independent prostate cancer were studied to determine whether mutations in the androgen-receptor genes have a role in androgen independence.

Methods.—Prostate tumor tissue was obtained from the patients who were in relapse after androgen ablation by either orchiectomy or the administration of a luteinizing hormone–releasing hormone agonist. Complementary DNA was synthesized from the samples and the expression of the androgen-receptor gene estimated by amplification with the polymerase chain reaction (PCR). Exons B through H of the androgen-receptor gene were cloned and mutations identified by DNA sequencing. Cells transfected with mutant genes were used to assess the functional effects of the mutations.

Results.—Metastatic androgen-independent prostate cancers were confirmed to contain high levels of androgen-receptor gene transcripts, in contrast to cells in normal bone marrow that have relatively little. Tumor cells were obtained from bone marrow in 8 patients, pleural fluid in 1, and a skin nodule in 1. From 10–14 isolates from each patient were sequenced. Androgen-receptor gene mutations were identified and confirmed by independent PCR amplifications in 5 of the 10 patients. One mutation was in the same codon as the mutation previously detected in the androgen-independent prostate cancer cell line. In 2 cases the mutations were not detected in the primary tumors. The mutant androgen receptors from 2 patients were stimulated by estrogen and progesterone.

Conclusion.—Semiquantitative amplification with reverse transcription PCR was able to detect transcripts of the androgen-receptor gene in metastatic androgen-independent prostate cancer cells. Most of these cancers express high levels of androgen-receptor gene transcripts. Mutations of the androgen-receptor gene appear to promote growth after androgen ablation and may be useful targets of new drugs for the treatment of prostate cancer.

▶ Despite decades of research, the mechanisms that underlie androgen action in normal and malignant prostate cells remain poorly understood. As the use of antiandrogens are being considered for expanded therapeutic roles, it is imperative to increase our understanding of the role of the androgen receptor and the genes under androgenic control in normal and malignant prostatic growth. In this paper by Taplin et al., experimental results that support a role for the androgen receptor in prostate cancer progression were provided.

In this study, specimens obtained from metastatic deposits were analyzed for androgen-receptor expression and androgen-receptor gene mutations. Polymerase chain reaction–based amplification, cloning, and sequencing protocols revealed that 50% of the metastatic, androgen-independent prostate cancers analyzed contained mutations. Further studies indicated that these mutations could impart transcriptional activation in response to progesterone or estradiol in vitro. Interestingly, one of the detected mutations was in the same codon as the previously described mutation in the LNCaP prostate cancer cell line.[1]

Overall, these results serve to further focus future studies regarding the specificity of androgen-receptor point mutations and their possible functional significance. Additional studies that will examine the occurrence and functional significance of androgen-receptor mutations both within the primary tumor and its corresponding metastatic lesion are now clearly indicated.

T.C. Thompson, Ph.D.

Reference

1. Veltlscholte J, Ris-Stalpers C, Kuiper GGJM, et al: A mutation in the ligand binding domain of the androgen receptor of human LNCaP cells affects steroid binding characteristics and response to anti-androgens. *Biochem Biophys Res Commun* 173:534–540, 1990.

Chromosomal Anomalies in Prostatic Intraepithelial Neoplasia and Carcinoma by Fluorescence *In Situ* Hybridization
Qian J, Bostwick DG, Takahashi S, Borell TJ, Herath JF, Lieber MM, Jenkins RB (Mayo Clinic, Rochester, Minn)
Cancer Res 55:5408–5414, 1995   21–55

Introduction.—Among men, the most prevalent malignancy and second leading cause of death is prostate cancer. Prevention, early detection, and treatment can be aided by further understanding the genetic events that occur with the progression of precursor lesions. The most likely precursor is high-grade prostatic intraepithelial neoplasia (PIN), but the genetic changes in PIN and the relationship of these changes to malignancy are not well understood. Fluorescence in situ hybridization (FISH) was used to determine whether there is a genetic linkage between PIN and eventual carcinoma, to assess the genetic heterogeneity of the foci of PIN and carcinoma, and to evaluate the association between multiple primary foci of carcinoma and metastases to lymph nodes.

Methods.—Three years of surgical pathology files were reviewed for patients who had undergone radical retropubic prostatectomy with bilateral pelvic lymphadenectomy. No patient had prior hormone or radiation therapy. Specimens of PIN, prostatic carcinoma, and lymph node metastases from a total of 40 patients were selected. Prostate specimens from patients with benign prostatic hypertrophy were also examined as controls. All sections were analyzed for chromosomal abnormalities using FISH with centromere-specific probes for chromosomes 7, 8, 10, 12 and Y.

Results.—Prostatic intraepithelial neoplasia, prostatic carcinomas, and metastases showed chromosomal abnormalities 50%, 51% and 100% of the time, respectively, with the average number of abnormal foci being 0.66, 1.09, and 3.75, respectively. The most common abnormalities of PIN, in descending order, were found on chromosomes 8, 10, 7, 12, and Y. For the carcinoma specimens, the abnormalities were found on chromosomes 7, 8, 10, 12, and Y. The greater the gain on chromosome 8, the greater the pathologic stage and Gleason score.

Conclusion.—Similar proportions of anomalies were found in PIN and carcinomas. Carcinoma chromosomes had more alterations. These data suggest that PIN is frequently a precursor of prostatic carcinoma even though some foci have few chromosomal alterations. The most common alteration was a gain of chromosome 8. This chromosome appears to be involved with the initiation and progression of prostatic cancer. Chromosomal abnormalities were shared with 1 or more foci of the primary tumor and subsequent metastases, indicating that a single focus of the cancer can lead to metastases.

▶ A persistent dilemma that faces urologists involved with the treatment of prostate cancer involves the uncertain biological and clinical potential of early disease. It has thus far proved exceedingly difficult to predict the clinical course of prostate cancer using conventional pathologic criteria.

Qian et al. provide information that significantly increases our understanding of the pattern of progression of prostate cancer and enlightens clinical decisions related to prostate cancer diagnosis and therapy.

Using FISH technology, the research group from Mayo Clinic demonstrated that the overall frequencies of numeric chromosomal anomalies in PIN and malignant foci were remarkably similar. These data, obtained through the use of molecular biology techniques, support the opinion that PIN can be a precursor of prostatic carcinoma.[1, 2] Finally, this study revealed that metastases do not necessarily seed from the largest primary or index cancer. Analysis with FISH detected shared chromosomal anomalies between a small low-grade tumor and a lymph node metastasis, whereas larger and higher grade tumors in the same specimen showed no abnormalities. These data are in agreement with previous experimental work, as well as clinical analyses, suggesting that loss of p53 function may trigger changes that can rapidly lead to prostate cancer metastases from relatively small cohorts of malignant cells present either in small focal areas or admixed with larger, less malignant-appearing lesions.[3] Overall, the results of this study have increased our understanding of the natural course of prostate cancer progression.

T.C. Thompson, Ph.D.

References

1. Bostwick DG, Brawer MK: Prostatic intra-epithelial neoplasia and early invasion in prostate cancer. *Cancer* 159:788–794, 1987.
2. Davidson D, Bostwick DG, Qian J, et al: Prostatic intraepithelial neoplasia is predictive of adenocarcinoma. *J Urol* 154:1295–1299, 1995.
3. Thompson TC, Park SH, Timme TL, et al: Loss of p53 function leads to metastasis in *ras+myc*-initiated mouse prostate cancer. *Oncogene* 10:869–879, 1995.

High Expression of a CD38-Like Molecule in Normal Prostatic Epithelium and Its Differential Loss in Benign and Malignant Disease
Kramer G, Steiner G, Födinger D, Fiebiger E, Rappersberger C, Binder S, Hofbauer J, Marberger M (Univ of Vienna; Vienna Internatl Research Ctr)
J Urol 154:1636–1641, 1995   21–56

Introduction.—Prostatic epithelial cells react with 2 distinct monoclonal antibodies specific for CD38. The extent to which prostatic epithelial cells from normal males express CD38 as described for leukocytes was examined. Whether this expression changes in benign prostatic hyperplasia and prostatic carcinoma was also determined.

Methods.—Ten benign prostatic hyperplasia resection specimens, 3 normal prostatic specimens, and 10 cancerous prostatic specimens were analyzed using immuno-electron microscopy, immunohistochemistry, and the Western blot test.

Results.—Prostatic and lymphatic CD38 antigen were compared. Identical bands at 45 kD were observed. Using electron microscopy, anti-CD38 reactivity on the cytoplasmic membrane and in secretory vacuoles was noted. Double labeling with anti-cytokeratin types 5/15 and 8/18, verified that basal and secretory normal prostatic epithelial cells express CD38. A complete loss was noted in some malignant, tumor-surrounding nonmalignant, and benign prostatic hyperplasia derived glands.

Discussion.—CD38 is a novel prostatic antigen. Insights into the physiologic function of prostatic epithelial cells and their secretory products in the human prostate may be gained by these findings.

▶ The authors suggest that CD38, a well-known cell surface marker of lymphocytic differentiation, is expressed on normal prostatic epithelium. Although it is not clear from this study whether the prostatic molecule recognized by anti-CD38 monoclonal antibody is equivalent to CD38, its size on Western blot analysis would suggest this to be the case. Further analysis, in any case, is needed. Regardless, this is an intriguing study, in that it raises the possibility that an antigen thought to be specific for hematopoietic cells is also expressed by prostate. Although multiple functions have been ascribed to CD38, its true role in lymphocytic differentiation is still not known. One possible role of CD38 is in differentiation. Retinoic acid, a well-known differentiation agent, induces CD38 expression, leading one to speculate that the loss of CD38 expression seen in 50% of cancers in this study reflects dedifferentiation. CD38, therefore, might be a useful marker for therapies involving differentiation agents. The presence of CD38 on prostatic cells also leads to speculation about the similarities in prostatic and hematopoietic development and about the propensity of prostate cells to metastasize specifically to bone marrow. Clearly this study represents the tip of the iceberg. It will be interesting to see where these results lead.

R.E. Reiter, M.D.

22 Infertility

Vasectomy in the United States, 1991
Marquette CM, Koonin LM, Antarsh L, Gargiullo PM, Smith JC (Assoc for
Voluntary Surgical Contraception, New York; Natl Ctr for Chronic Disease
Prevention and Health Promotion, Atlanta, Ga)
Am J Public Health 85:644–649, 1995   22–1

Introduction.—Although vasectomy is a common procedure in the
United States, little is known about the annual number of vasectomies
performed and the methods used. A national survey of urology, general
surgery, and family physician practices was conducted to determine the
number of vasectomies performed and the methods used in the United
States during 1991.

Methods.—Data for the 3 sampled specialties were stratified by the 4
census regions of the United States. The resulting sample consisted of
1,685 practices: 42% were urology practices; 39%, general surgery; and
19%, family physician practices. Because family physicians perform fewer
vasectomies than do urologists and general surgeons, the smallest portion
of the sample was allocated to their practices. The overall response rate to
the survey was 82%.

Results.—In 1991, an estimated 493,487 vasectomies were performed
in the United States, for a rate of 10.3 procedures per 1,000 men aged
25–49 years. Seventy-two percent of vasectomies were performed by
urologists, and the Midwest had the highest number and rate of procedures among the 4 geographic regions. Whereas 94% of sampled urology
practices performed vasectomies, only 29% of general surgery and 18% of
family physician practices reported the procedure. Nearly all vasectomies
were performed in physicians' offices (77%) or hospital outpatient settings
(19%); fewer than 1% were inpatient procedures. Local anesthesia was
used in 99% of cases. Occlusion methods included ligation (39%), ligation
and cautery (22%), cautery alone (20%), clips alone (11%), and cautery
and clips (7%).

Conclusion.—Approximately half a million vasectomies are performed
each year in the United States. Most are performed by urologists in an
office setting with local anesthesia. The ratio of female-to-male steriliza-
tions is 1.3:1. Some regional variations were noted, perhaps the result of
attitudes toward sterilization, demographic differences, and political or

religious environments. Vasectomy rates and numbers should continue to be monitored, and the effectiveness of ligation should be compared with that of other occlusion methods.

▶ This survey documents useful information. The fact that approximately a half million vasectomies are performed each year in the United States becomes important periodically when false alarms, such as those regarding atherosclerotic disease or prostatic cancer, are raised. The most surprising finding in this study is that 29% of general surgeons perform vasectomies.

S.S. Howards, M.D.

Potential of Testosterone Buciclate for Male Contraception: Endocrine Differences Between Responders and Nonresponders

Behre HM, Baus S, Kliesch S, Keck C, Simoni M, Nieschlag E (Inst of Reproductive Medicine of the Univ, Münster, Germany)
J Clin Endocrinol Metab 80:2394–2403, 1995
22–2

Objective.—The use of testosterone (T), alone or in combination with other agents, to suppress serum levels of luteinizing hormone (LH) and follicle-stimulating hormone (FSH) offers a promising approach to male contraception. The only androgen preparation tested for this purpose so far is T enanthanate, which must be injected every week and is associated with supraphysiologic serum levels of T. Testosterone buciclate (TB) is a new T ester that has a favorable pharmacokinetic profile and a terminal half-life of 29.5 days. The effectiveness of TB for male contraception was investigated in a clinical trial.

Methods.—Twelve healthy men received a single IM injection of TB. Group 1 (4 men) received a dose of 600 mg, and group 2 (8 men) received 1,200 mg. The participants were assessed every 2 weeks thereafter for up to 32 weeks.

Results.—Serum levels of T remained in the range of normal throughout the study. In group 2, serum levels of dihydrotestosteone were slightly above normal for several weeks, with a maximal concentration of 3.8 nmol/L at week 6. Three of 8 men in group 2 had suppression of spermatogenesis to azoospermia in week 10 that persisted up to week 22. These 3 men also had suppressed levels of LH and FSH to the assay detection limits; in the other 5 men in this group, levels of LH and FSH decreased only to or near the lower normal limit. Suppression of spermatogenesis was not observed in group 1.

Mean serum level of sex hormone–binding globulin was 21–26 nmol/L for responders vs. 36–46 nmol/L for nonresponders. Responders also had lower serum levels of LH and total and free T at baseline and after injection of TB. After gonadotropin-releasing hormone (GnRH) stimulation, the 2 subgroups showed similar increases in serum levels of LH and FSH. A new GnRH antagonist suppression test showed that serum levels of LH and T decreased to significantly lower levels in responders.

Conclusions.—In 3 of 8 normal men studied, a single IM injection of 1,200 mg TB results in azoospermia with normal serum levels of T. The difference between responders and nonresponders probably reflects a different hormonal equilibrium and different susceptibility to feedback regulation. Testosterone buciclate, alone or combined with gestagens or GnRH antagonists, appears to be a promising agent for male contraception.

▶ The search for an effective male contraceptive has been frustrating. It has long been apparent that T is a potential male contraceptive agent. Several published studies have reviewed trials of parenteral T for this purpose. However, not all men become azoospermic, and many individuals object to the frequent IM injections. This paper presents preliminary data on an agent that has the advantage of a longer half-life and, thus, less frequent administration than standard T preparations. At the dosage used, however, it was not dependable in rendering the men azoospermic.

S.S. Howards, M.D.

Decline in Semen Quality Among Fertile Men in Paris During the Past 20 Years
Auger J, Kunstmann JM, Czyglik F, Jouannet P (Université Paris Sud, Le Kremlin Bicêtre, France)
N Engl J Med 332:281–285, 1995   22–3

Objective.—Whether there has been a decline in the quality of semen in normal men during the past 20 years was studied retrospectively.

Methods.—Semen quality data collected from 1,351 healthy, fertile men from 1973 to 1992 at 1 sperm bank in Paris were analyzed. The data included volume of seminal fluid, sperm concentration, and percentages of motile and morphologically normal spermatozoa. The data from each calendar year were analyzed as a function of the age of the patient, the year of the donation, the year of birth, and the duration of sexual abstinence before semen collection.

Results.—The seminal fluid volume remained the same (3.8 mL) throughout the study. During the same time period, however, significant decreases were noted in mean concentration of sperm (2.1%; from 89 × 10^6/mL to 60 × 10^6), motile spermatozoa (0.6%), and normal spermatozoa (0.5%). When the data were adjusted for age and duration of sexual abstinence and analyzed by multiple regression, 2.6%, 0.3%, and 0.7% of the yearly declines in concentration of sperm, motility, and normal morphology, respectively, were found to be associated with each successive calendar year of birth. The concentration of sperm decreased by 3.7% in a group of 382 men who were matched for age and duration of sexual abstinence. The decline in percentage of normal spermatozoa per year in this subgroup (0.7%) was also more pronounced than in the entire study population.

Conclusions.—Unexplainable declines in concentration of sperm and in the percentages of motile and normal spermatozoa with each successive year of birth were documented in 1,351 men. There was no concomitant decline in seminal volume. Increased age of the donor and the duration of sexual abstinence before collection of semen correlate with more pronounced declines in concentration of sperm, motility, and normal morphology.

▶ Whether sperm counts are declining has become a very hot topic of discussion, in both the scientific and lay press. Although this debate is not new, it was brought to the forefront after the publication of a meta-analysis by Carlsen et al.[1] in 1992. The results suggested that there had been a dramatic decline in semen quality worldwide during the past 50 years. That analysis is subject to many criticisms, particularly because most of the decrease relates to the results of 4 very early studies from New York City. Except for these results, no statistically significant alterations in semen quality have been observed. The above paper by Auger et al. provides the strongest evidence yet of a decrease over time in semen quality. Nevertheless, the consensus, but by no means the universal opinion, of experts is that there is no documentation of such a decline. Several recently published papers do not show any decline in semen quality. One study was from a Wisconsin sperm bank; 1 reviewed data from sperm banks in New York City, Minneapolis, and California; and 1 summarized research data from Seattle. The alleged decline may be real, but the data are inclusive, and the best guess is that there is no significant decline.

S.S. Howards, M.D.

Reference

1. Carlsen E, Giwercman A, Keiding N, et al: Evidence for decreasing quality of semen during past 50 years. *BMJ* 305:609–613, 1992.

Effects of Smoking on Testicular Function, Semen Quality and Sperm Fertilizing Capacity
Sofikitis N, Miyagawa I, Dimitriadis D, Zavos P, Sikka S, Hellstrom W (Tottori Univ, Yonago, Japan; Japanese-Greek Fertility Inst, Franzi, Neos Kosmos, Athens, Greece; Univ of Kentucky, Lexington; et al)
J Urol 154:1030–1034, 1995   22–4

Introduction.—Many men of reproductive age still smoke, and there is considerable evidence that smoking has adverse effects on the concentration and motility of spermatozoa. Although the effect of smoking on human Leydig-cell function remains uncertain, the results of animal studies suggest that function may be compromised. A number of assays known to correlate with sperm-fertilizing potential and the outcome of in vitro fertilization were performed.

Methods.—Forty-nine men, aged 21–38 years, who had smoked more than a pack of cigarettes a day for longer than 3 years were included. Twenty-eight men of similar age who had never smoked were also included. The acrosin assay, zona-free hamster oocyte sperm penetration assay, and hypoosmotic swelling test were done, and Sertoli-cell secretion was evaluated. Semen samples were collected by intercourse a month before hernia repair, and a testicular biopsy was obtained at the time of surgery. Semen and blood were again collected 6 months after surgery.

Findings.—Smokers had lower proportions of morphologically normal spermatozoa, poorer morphometric parameters, and less motile sperm than did nonsmokers. Sperm function tests demonstrated significantly poorer function in the smokers. In addition, they had significantly lower levels of testosterone in the left testicular vein than did nonsmoking men and lower in vitro androgen-binding protein secretion rates.

Conclusions.—Sperm-fertilizing potential is reduced in men who smoke, possibly because of alterations in the sperm cytoskeleton during either spermatogenesis or sperm maturation in the epididymis. The primary defect may be deficient secretory function of the Leydig and Sertoli cells.

▶ This paper adds to the evidence that smoking has a significant, but small, negative effect on semen quality and perhaps fertility. There is evidence that smoking and varicocele combined may have a much greater negative effect than would be predicted by either factor alone.

S.S. Howards, M.D.

Vibratory Stimulation and Rectal Probe Electroejaculation as Therapy for Patients With Spinal Cord Injury: Semen Parameters and Pregnancy Rates

Nehra A, Werner MA, Bastuba M, Title C, Oates RD (Boston Univ)
J Urol 155:554–559, 1996   22–5

Background.—In the United States, there are approximately 8,000 new cases of spinal cord injury in men every year. These men, who are typically younger than 25 years of age, have erectile and ejaculatory dysfunction. In patients who have anejaculate spinal cord injuries, penile vibratory stimulation and rectal probe electroejaculation are the most common methods of obtaining semen. There is little information, however, regarding conception rates. The success rates of penile vibratory stimulation and rectal probe electroejaculation, as well as the pregnancy rates from self-insemination, intrauterine insemination, and assisted reproductive techniques, were determined.

Methods.—A complete neurologic and urologic examination was performed in 78 men, aged 23–40 years, who had spinal cord injuries. All patients were initially treated with penile vibratory stimulation. If this treatment was unsuccessful, rectal probe electroejaculation was performed. The ejaculate was used with cervical self-insemination, intrauterine insemination, in vitro fertilization, or gamete intrafallopian transfer.

Results.—Vibratory stimulation was successful in 20 of 37 patients who had a cervical lesion. It was also successful in 14 of 26 patients who had a thoracic lesion at T10 or above. The procedure was unsuccessful, however, in 15 patients with a lesion below T10. Thirty-two of 34 patients who underwent rectal probe electroejaculation had an antegrade or retrograde ejaculate. For 6 patients who had very poor semen quality, assisted fertilization was not performed. Conception was achieved in 17 of 27 couples.

Conclusions.—To obtain semen and achieve pregnancy, penile vibratory stimulation should be the initial therapy in patients who have spinal cord injuries above T10, or lower extremity spasticity. For patients who have injuries below T10, or lower extremity flaccidity, rectal probe electroejaculation should be the initial therapy.

▶ Ninety percent of men who have spinal cord injuries cannot ejaculate and require assistance if they desire to father children. This paper presents a good summary of the current state of the art for treatment of these men. Vibratory ejaculation was introduced in 1965 by Sobrero et al.[1] However, the use of assisted ejaculation has only recently gained notice as a method of rendering these patients fertile. The initial phase emphasized electroejaculation. More recently, several publications have emphasized that vibratory ejaculation is less expensive and is effective for many of these patients. Indeed, in some series, the success rate for this technique is significantly higher than that noted by the authors. The algorithm provided in this paper and the fertility statistics should prove very useful in advising and treating patients with spinal cord injury who wish to father children.

S.S. Howards, M.D.

Reference

1. Sobrero AJ, Stearns HE, Blair JH: Technic for the induction of ejaculation in humans. *Fertil Steril* 16:765, 1965.

Bilateral Varicocele: Impact of Right Spermatic Vein Ligation on Fertility
Grasso M, Lania C, Castelli M, Galli L, Rigatti P (Scientific Inst H San Raffaele, Milan, Italy)
J Urol 153:1847–1848, 1995   22–6

Introduction.—Primary left varicocele is the most common cause of male infertility, and most cases of grade 2–3 varicocele are treated surgically. There is lack of agreement, however, regarding the therapeutic approach to grade 1 disease. Patients who had grade 2–3 varicocele on the left side and grade 1 on the right were assessed for outcome after unilateral or bilateral ligation of the spermatic vein.

TABLE 2.—Mean Values Plus or Minus Standard Error Relative to
Percentage Increase in the 2 Groups of Patients

Change in	Group 1	Group 2	p Values
% Sperm count/ml.	36.52 ± 6.37	23.10 ± 5.05	0.11
% Normal morphology	73.22 ± 14.34	64.12 ± 11.77	0.98
% Fast linear motility at 60 mins.	109.07 ± 14.29	81.62 ± 11.22	0.20

(Courtesy of Grasso M, Lania C, Castelli M, et al: Bilateral varicocele: Impact of right spermatic vein ligation on fertility. *J Urol* 153:1847–1848, 1995.)

Methods.—During a period of 3 years, 248 patients underwent surgery at 1 institution for left or bilateral varicocele. All had different grades of oligoasthenoteratospermia. Seventy-four patients had a grade 2–3 left varicocele and a grade 1 right varicocele. Thirty-seven of these patients were randomly selected to undergo bilateral ligation, and 37 to undergo left spermatic vein ligation only. Retroperitoneal ligation was performed in all patients.

Results.—Nine patients found to have persistent intermittent basal reflux on the left side at Doppler velocimetry were excluded. In the remaining patients, bilateral and unilateral groups did not differ statistically in fertility parameters measured before and after treatment: sperm count per milliliter, percent normal morphology, and percent fast linear motility 60 minutes after ejaculation. Each parameter showed a positive increase after treatment, but mean values were always greater in the bilateral than in the unilateral ligation group (Table 2).

Conclusion.—Although most cases of primary varicocele involve the left side, subclinical right varicocele may be a frequent finding. The most reliable test for subclinical varicocele is Doppler ultrasound. Bilateral ligation offered no advantages over unilateral ligation in patients with ogligoasthenospermia who have grade 2–3 left varicocele and grade 1 right varicocele. Because bilateral surgery involves twice the operating time and a longer convalescence, the unilateral approach is recommended in such cases.

▶ This important paper supports our point of view on the issues of bilateral and subclinical varicoceles. We have always believed that there are no data to substantiate the repair of subclinical varicoceles. Indeed, there is no documented method for making the diagnosis. Further, we have been mystified by the very high frequency of bilateral varicoceles reported in the literature by "experts." Some authors report that as many as 85% of their patients have bilateral lesions. We have always found a much lower incidence. This well-designed, controlled study shows no benefit in bilateral repair if there is not a significant varicocele on the right side.

S.S. Howards, M.D.

Management of the Epididymal Tubule During an End-to-Side Vasoepididymostomy

Marmar JL (Univ Med Ctr, Camden, NJ)
J Urol 154:93–96, 1995   22–7

Objective.—Microsurgical techniques for repairing epididymal obstruction have greatly improved in recent years. A single epididymal tubule can be directly sutured to the mucosa of the vas. A number of modifications were evaluated in 51 men who had end-to-side vasoepididymostomy on at least 1 side. Forty-five patients required vasectomy reversal, and 6 required relief of inflammatory obstruction.

Technique.—After delivering the testis and cord structures through a scrotal incision and selecting an area for anastomosis where dilated tubules can be seen through the tunic, a 15-degree microsurgical blade with a 1.5-mm tip is used to create a 1 × 2-mm window laterally in the epididymal tunic (Fig 1). Its final diameter equalled the outer diameter of the vas. A distended tubule is forced out the window and punctured with a needle

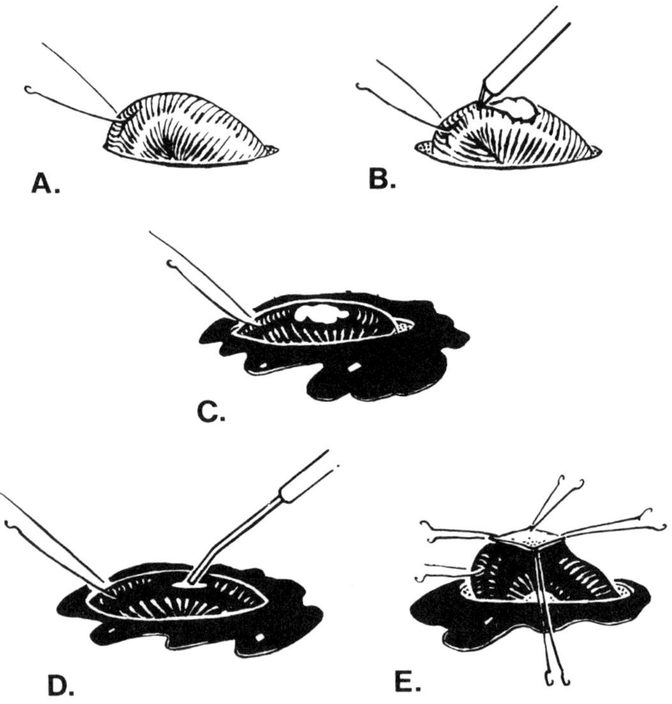

FIGURE 1.—**A,** after lateral window is cut in epididymal tunic, specific distended tubule protrudes, which is marked with closed tubule fixation using 11-0 nylon suture with a 30-μ needle. **B,** sharp tubulotomy is created with 15-degree microsurgical blade to open epididymal tubule. **C,** tissues are stained with methylene blue, but epididymal fluid remains pink at tubulotomy site. **D,** epididymal fluid is removed by continuous microsuction, and edges of tubule are visible. **E,** individual microsutures are placed through epididymal tubule and separated by 90 degrees to avoid entanglement (Courtesy of Marmar J: Management of the epididymal tubule during an end-to-side vasoepididymostomy. *J Urol* 154:93–96, 1995.)

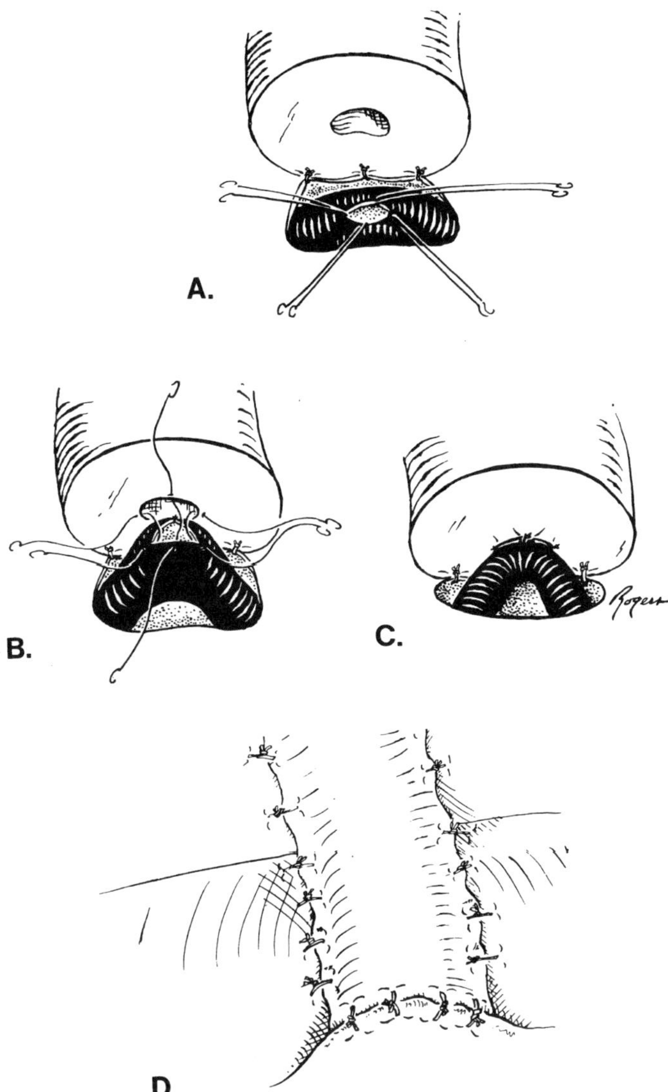

FIGURE 2.—**A**, marker stitch is removed, and epididymal sutures are rotated clockwise to expose edge of tunic. Sutures are separated by 60 degrees to avoid entanglement. Suture from leading edge of epididymal tubule is always maintained on extreme right of field. Vas is secured to tunic by individual sutures of 9-0 nylon. **B**, to begin anastomosis, suture from anterior edge of epididymal tubule is secured to 6 o'clock position of vas lumen and tied. Other epididymal sutures are placed in corresponding positions through vas lumen. **C**, each epididymal suture is individually tied to complete anastomosis. **D**, anterior wall of vas is secured to remaining tunic, and lateral sutures are placed through vas and epididymal tunic or fascia of spermatic cord to stabilize anastomosis. (Courtesy of Marmar J: Management of the epididymal tubule during an end-to-side vasoepididymostomy. *J Urol* 154:93–96, 1995.)

for closed tubule fixation. A sharp tubulotomy is made by directing the cutting edge of the blade upward and advancing its point into the distended tubule under direct vision. Epididymal fluid is removed by microsuction before securing the tubule with 1-inch sutures of 10-0 nylon attached to double-armed, bicurved needles. Finally, the vas is attached to the exposed tunic with three 9-0 nylon sutures (Fig 2). Additional lateral sutures are placed through the epididymal tunic and/or spermatic cord fascia.

Results.—Patency, as defined by more than 10 million sperm per milliliter and 35% motility at 18 months, was achieved in 11 of 19 men (58%) who underwent pure end-to-side vasoepididymostomy. Another 3 (16%) gained partial patency. Eight of 19 couples (42%) achieved pregnancy within 30 months after surgery.

Conclusion.—These modifications have proved helpful in enhancing the results of end-to-side vasoepididymostomy.

▶ Epididymal vasostomy is a difficult operation that requires microsurgical skills and patience. The technique described by Marmar is reasonable. We also like to mark the selected epididymal tubule with a small suture on a noncutting needle. There is an advantage in placing all the 10-0 mucosal sutures before tying them. The field can become cluttered, however, and it can be difficult to determine which is which. To alleviate this problem, we use microclips on 2 or 3 of the sutures. We also prefer to place the back muscular row before doing the mucosal anastomosis.

S.S. Howards, M.D.

Intracytoplasmic Sperm Injection: A Major Advance in the Management of Severe Male Subfertility
Harari O, Speirs AL, Bourne H, Johnston WIH, McDonald M, Baker HWG, Richings N (Royal Women's Hosp, Carlton, Australia; Melbourne IVF, East Melbourne, Australia; Univ of Melbourne, Australia)
Fertil Steril 64:360–368, 1995   22–8

Background.—Male infertility has proved more difficult to treat than other types of infertility. Intracytoplasmic sperm injection is a promising new technique that involves injection of a single sperm into the egg cytoplasm. The results of intracytoplasmic sperm injection during 119 treatment cycles between July and December 1993 at a tertiary infertility service were reported.

Patients.—One hundred fourteen patients were included. Thirty-one had severe oligospermia, 21 had oligoasthenoteratospermia, 22 had asthenoteratospermia, 19 had genital tract obstructions, and 21 had a low fertilization rate in vitro.

Results.—A total of 1,185 oocytes were treated by intracytoplasmic sperm injection. Normal fertilization and cleavage occurred in 717 of the 1,073 that survived the procedure, which represents a normal fertilization rate of 67%. Abnormal fertilization occurred in 11%, and 10% of the oocytes did not survive the procedure. The implantation rate was 7.4%. There were 36 clinical pregnancies, of which 24 were delivered or ongoing. Patients with genital tract obstruction had a higher fertilization rate than did patients with sperm defects.

Conclusions.—These results confirm that intracytoplasmic sperm injection is a valuable technique in the treatment of men who have various types of severe infertility.

▶ Intracytoplasmic sperm injection is unequivocally a major advance in the treatment of male infertility, just as stated in the title of this paper. The 1995 YEAR BOOK OF UROLOGY[1] included several abstracts on this subject. The unique and remarkable aspect of this technique is that the results have been equally good regardless of semen quality. This is not true for any other form of treatment of male infertility, including standard in vitro fertilization. In fact, overstated claims not withstanding, the delivery rate after standard in vitro fertilization for severe male factor infertility was miserable. The authors obtained delivery or ongoing pregnancy in 24 of 114 couples (21%). Although this is a good success rate, it is actually lower than that reported by other centers, including ours.

S.S. Howards, M.D.

Reference

1. 1995 YEAR BOOK OF UROLOGY, pp 243–245.

Simplified Sperm Retrieval and Intracytoplasmic Sperm Injection in Patients With Azoospermia

Tsirigotis M, Pelekanos M, Yazdani N, Boulos A, Foster C, Craft IL (London Gynaecology and Fertility Centre)
Br J Urol 76:765–768, 1995   22–9

Introduction.—Assisted fertilization and intracytoplasmic sperm injection (ICSI) have made treatment possible for patients who have azoospermia. The rate of recovery of spermatozoa from the epididymis, with the use of percutaneous epididymal sperm aspiration (PESA), was assessed. Subsequent fertilization was also observed.

Methods.—Forty-two patients (mean age, 34.9 years) underwent PESA to recover sperm for ICSI. Sperm was suitable for microinjection in 28 patients for 32 cycles. Six patients underwent microepididymal sperm aspiration (MESA). Spermatozoa was extracted from testicular tissue in the remaining 8 patients in whom PESA yielded no sperm or unsuitable sperm for ICSI.

Results.—Two hundred eighty-six of 362 collected oocytes were subjected to ICSI. Forty-nine of the injected oocytes (17.2%) were damaged, and 138 (48.3%) achieved normal fertilization. Of those that achieved fertilization, 112 (81.2%) cleaved. Sixty-seven embryos were transferred, and 18 additional ones were suitable for cryopreservation. Of 32 PESA-ICSI cycles, fertilization failed in 4 patients. In 2 patients who achieved fertilization, there was no cleavage. The pregnancy rate was 25% per cycle and 32% per embryo transfer. There was a 12% transplantation rate. Ultrasonography confirmed pregnancy in 7 of 25 patients who underwent embryo transfer. There were 6 singleton pregnancies and 1 set of twins. There was 1 early miscarriage. No postoperative complications occurred.

Conclusion.—Findings indicate that PESA can be used successfully to retrieve sperm in patients who have azoospermia. Recovery is rapid, postoperative complications are unlikely, and the procedure is cost-effective. This technique could become the method of choice for retrieving sperm in patients who have obstructive azoospermia.

▶ It is still not clear whether PESA or MESA is the preferred technique for obtaining sperm for ICSI from men who have azoospermic obstruction. Percutaneous epididymal sperm aspiration has the advantage of requiring less anesthesia and being less invasive. On the other hand, it is less frequently successful, may obtain lower quality sperm, and may cause permanent damage to the epididymis. We currently use MESA but probably will try PESA in the near future. The authors' ongoing pregnancy rate for PESA was only 17% (7 of 42 patients who underwent PESA). This rate does not compare favorably with the 21% to 33% delivery rate for ICSI. Because the cost of an in vitro fertilization cycle is $8,000 to $10,000, MESA will clearly be the approach of choice if the success rate remains significantly lower with PESA. The fact that a technique can be successful does not mean that it should be used if there are more cost-effective alternative methods.

S.S. Howards, M.D.

Pregnancies After Testicular Sperm Extraction and Intracytoplasmic Sperm Injection in Non-obstructive Azoospermia

Devroey P, Liu J, Nagy Z; Goossens A, Tournaye H, Camus M, Van Steirteghem A, Silber S (Brussels Free Univ, Belgium; St Luke's Hosp, St Louis)
Hum Reprod 10:1457–1460, 1995   22–10

Background.—Intracytoplasmic sperm injection results in high fertilization and pregnancy rates among couples who have extreme oligoasthenoteratozoospermia. Testicular sperm extraction with intracytoplasmic sperm injection will allow viable embryos to develop, even in the absence of epididymis. The efficacy of testicular sperm extraction and intracytoplasmic sperm injection was assessed in patients who had nonobstructive azoospermia.

Methods.—Before intracytoplasmic sperm injection with testicular sperm extraction was carried out, testicular biopsy was performed in 15 men who had nonobstructive azoospermia. Ovarian stimulation and oocyte retrieval were carried out in the women. Fertilization and embryonic development were assessed.

Results.—In 13 patients, spermatozoa were available for intracytoplasmic sperm injection. Of 182 metaphase II–injected oocytes, 2-pronuclear fertilization occurred in 87; 57 embryos were either transferred or cryopreserved. Three ongoing pregnancies were established: 1 singleton, 1 twin, and 1 triplet gestation. The ongoing implantation rate was 18.75%.

Conclusions.—These findings and those from related studies indicate that patients who have nonobstructive azoospermia, elevated levels of follicle-stimulating hormone, and small testes are potentially fertile. By using testicular sperm extraction and intracytoplasmic sperm injection, the fertilizing potential of these patients is similar to that of patients who have normal spermatogenesis. A follow-up study of the children is planned.

▶ This paper details yet another exciting development in the treatment of male factor infertility by assisted reproductive technology. Since this pioneering report, other groups have had similar experiences.

S.S. Howards, M.D.

Optimum Abstinence Time for Cryopreservation of Semen in Cancer Patients
Agarwal A, Sidhu RK, Shekarriz M, Thomas AJ Jr (Cleveland Clinic Found, Ohio)
J Urol 154:86–88, 1995

22–11

Objective.—A significant number of young men who have malignant diseases and wish to preserve their sperm have poor quality semen. The World Health Organization has recommended abstinence periods between ejaculates for normospermic men of 48–96 hours. Studies in men who have oligospermia suggest, however, that a second successive ejaculate carries a higher number of motile sperm than does the first. Results of an investigation of the optimum abstinence period and the prefreeze and post-thaw semen qualities in ejaculates of patients who had malignant diseases were presented.

Methods.—Ninety-five patients who had malignant disease but no history of chemotherapy or radiation treatments were included. Thirty-six patients had testicular cancer, 39 had Hodgkin's disease, and 20 had other cancers. The patients were divided into 3 groups. Group 1 (n = 15) abstained for 24–48 hours, group 2 (n = 53) abstained for 48–72 hours, and group 3 abstained for longer than 72 hours between ejaculates. Prefreeze and post-thaw motility, velocity, linearity, amplitude of lateral head movement, and motility index of sperm were compared and analyzed.

Results.—There were no significant differences between groups for any prefreeze or post-thaw semen variables. Post-thaw sperm motility and motion variables decreased significantly in all groups from pre-freeze values.

Conclusion.—Because there is no significant difference in semen variables between 24 to 48–hours and 48 to 72–hour abstinences, shortening the abstinence period would speed sperm collection and decrease the treatment delay period.

▶ The authors have conducted a simple but useful study. The data support their conclusion that shorter abstinence periods are appropriate in this setting. There is, however, a caveat. Group 1 (abstinence period, 24–48 hours) had only 15 individuals. There was an arithmetic difference between group 1 and group 2 in media prefreeze (6.2×10^6 vs. 12×10^6) and post-thaw motile (1.7×10^6 vs. 2.8×10^6) sperm count. The reason for the lack of a statistically significant difference may be the well-known variability in semen quality of patients who have cancer and the small number of men in group 1. Thus, if a larger study were conducted, there might indeed be statistically significant higher motile sperm counts pre- and post-thaw in group 2.

S.S. Howards, M.D.

Hormonal Protection From Cyclophosphamide-induced Inactivation of Rat Stem Spermatogonia

Meistrich ML, Parchuri N, Wilson G, Kurdoglu B, Kangasniemi M (Univ of Texas, Houston)
J Androl 16:334–341, 1995
22–12

Introduction.—Hormone treatment has been shown to protect stem spermatogonial survival from the effects of procarbazine and radiation in rat models. Cyclophosphamide is another commonly used chemotherapeutic agent that induces long-term azoospermia. Studying the protective effects of hormone treatment against cyclophosphamide has been complicated by the inability to produce detectible stem spermatogonial damage in a rat model at nonlethal doses. Bone marrow transplantation, sodium 2-mercaptoethanesulfonate (Mesna) treatment, and irradiation were used to increase the lethal dose of cyclophosphamide in rats to investigate the protective effects of hormone treatment.

Methods.—Adult rats were irradiated with 2.5 Gy 14–15 days before administration of cyclophosphamide in some experiments. After intraperitoneal injection of cyclophosphamide at a dose of 0.8 mL/100 g body weight, groups of rats were given either 2 saline injections at 15 minutes and 3 hours or 4 injections between 15 minutes and 4 hours 45 minutes. Some rats were injected with bone marrow cells 24 hours after injection of cyclophosphamide. The protective effects of 2 methods of hormone treatment were investigated. Some rats were given testosterone and estradiol-17β for 6 weeks before injection of cyclophosphamide. Others were treated with the gonadotropin-releasing hormone antagonist Nal-Glu and the antiandrogen flutamide for 14 days between irradiation and cyclophosphamide injection. The rats were killed 9 weeks after administration of cyclophosphamide, and stem spermatagonial survival was assessed.

Results.—Pretreatment of the rats with irradiation, bone marrow transplantation, and Mesna resulted in a 50% increase in the lethal dose of cyclophosphamide in the rats, while increasing spermatogonial toxicity by a factor of 60. Treatment with testosterone and estradiol provided a slight, nonsignificant protective effect. Treatment with Nal-Glu and flutamide, however, significantly reduced the effects of cyclophosphamide on sperm counts, testis weights and repopulation, and body weight, but did not affect these indices in rats not treated with cyclophosphamide.

Conclusions.—A 2-week period of hormonal treatment protected stem spermatogonia against cyclophosphamide in a rat model. Hormonal pretreatment may effectively prevent prolonged azoospermia in patients treated with chemotherapy protocols that incorporate cyclophosphamide.

▶ Preserving fertility in men who require therapy for cancer is an important goal. One option, freezing semen obtained before treatment, is described above. This animal study gives more insight into another option, inhibiting spermatogenesis during chemotherapy. The authors developed a new model to study this issue in rats treated with cyclophosphamide. The obvious question is, Will this approach work in human beings? There is actually a modestly extensive literature on the subject of preservation of spermatogenesis in experimental animals during radiation treatment or chemotherapy. Thus far, none of the methods developed have been practical enough for clinical use.

S.S. Howards, M.D.

Effect of Platelet-activating Factor on Motility and Acrosome Reaction of Human Spermatozoa
Krausz C, Gervasi G, Forti G, Baldi E (Univ of Florence, Italy)
Hum Reprod 9:471–476, 1994   22–13

Background.—Two characteristics of spermatozoa essential for fertilization are progressive motility and the acrosome reaction. Several components of follicular fluid appear to cooperate to activate spermatozoa at the time of fertilization. Recent studies have shown that platelet-activating factor (PAF) is present in human follicular fluid and is produced by mammalian spermatozoa. The effect of PAF on motility parameters and induction of the acrosome reaction in human spermatozoa was assessed.

Methods.—Thirty-six men who were undergoing semen analysis for couple infertility were included. Motility parameters were examined in 25 men, and the acrosome reaction was examined in 27. Men who had leukocytes and/or immature germ cell concentrations of 10^6 mL or greater were excluded. Sperm motility was assessed by computer-assisted sperm analysis (Hamilton-Thorn Motility Analyser). The percentage of acrosome-reacted spermatozoa was evaluated after 1 hour of incubation with PAF (10 nmol/L) and staining with fluorescent peanut lectin.

Results.—Short-term incubation (up to 4 hours) with PAF significantly enhanced both total and progressive sperm motility and the acrosome reaction. Sixteen of 25 men showed an increase in sperm motility in response to PAF and were considered responders, whereas 9 showed no enhancement of motility parameters. In 9 responders, the effect of PAF was apparent during the first hour of incubation. Responders and nonresponders were similar in the conventional parameters of semen analysis, but basal motility was slightly higher in the nonresponder group. The increase of motility in response to PAF was inversely correlated with basal motility. Long-term (overnight) incubation with PAF caused an increase in sperm motility in both responders and nonresponders to short-term incubation. Twenty of 26 participants exhibited an increase in numbers of acrosome reactions in response to 10 nmol/L PAF; this response was inhibited by the PAF receptor antagonist L659 989.

Conclusion.—In 65% to 75% of participants, PAF induced an increase of motility parameters and acrosome reaction in spermatozoa. The effect of PAF was inversely correlated with basal motility. Cases of reduced sperm motility may benefit from PAF during in vitro fertilization.

Suggested Reading

Brucker C, Lipford GB: The human sperm acrosome reaction: Physiology and regulatory mechanisms. *Hum Reprod Update* 1:51–62, 1995.

Mulhall JP, Albertsen PC: Hemospermia: Diagnosis and management. *Urology* 46:463–467, 1995.

Ohl DA, Rajesh KN: Infertility due to antisperm antibodies. *Urology* 46:591–602, 1995.

23 Urethral Strictures

A Prospective Randomized Study of Self-dilatation in the Management of Urethral Strictures
Matanhelia SS, Salaman R, John A, Matthews PN (Univ Hosp of Wales, Cardiff)
J R Coll Surg Edinb 40:295–297, 1995   23–1

Background.—Direct vision internal urethrotomy is currently the treatment of choice for urethral strictures. However, 20% to 50% of patients have recurrent strictures, which are probably caused by fibrosis and cicatrization preceding complete epithelization. Self-intermittent dilatation (SID) has been shown to prevent recurrent strictures, but it is unknown how long SID should be continued. The management of urethral strictures after optical urethrotomy was assessed in patients who had postoperative SID vs. those who did not in a prospective controlled randomized study.

Methods.—During a 3-year period, 51 patients who underwent urethrotomy were randomly assigned to either a 3-month course of postoperative SID or no SID. The patients in the SID group were shown how to insert a 16F catheter beyond the stricture but not through the external sphincter (to prevent ascending infection). They performed SID twice a day for 2 weeks, once a day for 3 weeks, twice a week for 3 weeks, and once a week for 4 weeks. After 3 months, SID was discontinued. All patients were evaluated 6 weeks, 3 months, 6 months, and 1 year after surgery.

Results.—Forty-four patients completed the study. New strictures occurred in 17 who had performed SID and in 15 who had not. Six patients in each group had recurrent strictures. Among the patients who had new strictures, a satisfactory peak flow rate was achieved by 76% in the SID group and 80% in the non-SID group. Among the patients who had recurrent strictures, a satisfactory peak flow rate was achieved by 66% in the SID group and 17% in the non-SID group. Further analysis of peak flow rates among the treatment failures showed significantly higher values in the SID group than in the non-SID group for the first 3 months; thereafter; the flow rates deteriorated significantly in the SID group. In patients who had strictures, the degree of narrowing did not correlate well with the flow rate.

Conclusions.—Performance of SID for 3 months did not significantly affect the rate of new or recurrent strictures or the peak flow rate at 1 year after a single optical urethrotomy. Although regular, sustained SID allowed the patients to maintain satisfactory flow, the benefit of SID was minimal after it was discontinued.

▶ Previous studies have suggested that SID improves the results after internal urethrotomy for urethral strictures.[1, 2] The authors present a carefully designed, randomized, prospective study to determine whether 3 months of self-catheterization improves long-term results of internal urethrotomy. Their data showed no effect of self-catheterization. This useful paper strongly indicates that, to be useful, self-catheterization after treatment of urethral strictures must be continued indefinitely.

S.S. Howards, M.D.

References

1. Lawrence WT, MacDonagh RP: Treatment of urethral stricture disease by internal urethrotomy followed by intermittent "low friction" self-catheterization: Preliminary communication. *J R Soc Med* 81:136–139, 1988.
2. Robertson GSM, Everitt N, Lamprecht JR, et al: Treatment of recurrent urethral strictures using clean intermittent self catheterization. *Br J Urol* 68:89–92, 1991.

Scrotal Flap Epilation in Urethroplasty: Concepts and Technique
Gil-Vernet A, Arango O, Gil-Vernet J Jr, Gelabert-Mas A, Gil-Vernet J (Univ of Barcelona)
J Urol 154:1723–1726, 1995
23–2

Introduction.—Because of the presence of abundant hair follicles, the use of scrotal skin flaps in urethral reconstructive surgery has been discredited. However, the unique qualities of the scrotum, such as its rich vascularization, excellent elasticity, and noncheloid scarring, make it suitable for urethral reconstructive surgery. Shaving, superficial local radiation therapy, direct electrocautery of the hair rod, and photocoagulation with a surgical laser have been used in scrotal epilation. A new method for the destruction of the dermal papilla using a depilatory needle was described.

Technique.—The disposable depilatory needle is 6 × 0.3 mm in diameter. It is made of copper wire and is coated with insulating varnish The tip is uncoated for 0.5 mm. The scrotal skin is stretched to reveal each hair root. Following the direction of the hair, the needle is introduced through the pilosebaceous canal. When the hair root becomes transparent and looks like a small, whitish papule at the tip of the needle, the thermal effect is complete. After the current has been switched off, the needle should be withdrawn.

Results.—The optimal schedule was an average of 3 epilatory sessions with a 4-week interval between treatments. Patient discomfort was reduced by a topical scrotal anesthesia of a eutectic mixture of lidocaine and prilocaine. Magnifying lenses or a surgical microscope provided excellent detail. After more experience, however, greater technical perfection was attained, and the procedure could be performed with the naked eye. There was no cutaneous infection.

Conclusion.—For the treatment of complex urethral stenosis in the postpubertal male, pedicle urethroplasty with scrotal skin has become the standard procedure. The best results were yielded with the scrotal flap epilation.

▶ There is no doubt that vascularized scrotal skin flaps are very useful for repair of urethral stricture, because of their proximity, blood supply, and elasticity. We have had considerable difficulty, however, with hair growth. The authors describe a method of epilation that is tedious but, they claim, successful. Unfortunately, they do not present any data, so it is difficult to evaluate their approach. We believe that the spiral penile vascular skin graft described by McAninch is preferable to scrotal skin grafts.

S.S. Howards, M.D.

24 Fistula

Early Versus Late Repair of Vesicovaginal Fistulas: Vaginal and Abdominal Approaches
Blaivas JG, Heritz DM, Romanzi LJ (New York Hosp-Cornell Med Ctr; St Luke's/Roosevelt Hosp, New York)
J Urol 153:1110–1113, 1995   24–1

Background.—The literature regarding surgical repair of vesicovaginal fistula reveals 2 major controversies of management: the use of a vaginal vs. an abdominal repair and the timing of the surgery. The practice of using a vaginal approach preferentially and performing surgery as soon as possible was examined by retrospectively analyzing the outcome of patients treated between 1989 and 1993.

Methods.—The records of 24 consecutive women who had vesicovaginal fistulas and were treated surgically between 1989 and 1993 were reviewed. All patients were evaluated preoperatively with pelvic examination, urinalysis and urine culture, excretory urography, cystoscopy, and bilateral retrograde pyelography. The repairs were performed with the vaginal approach whenever possible. The abdominal approach was used if the circumferential induration at the fistula site was greater than 2 cm, adequate vaginal exposure could not be obtained, the fistulas involved the ureters, or the patient preferred the abdominal approach.

Results.—All patients had fistulas caused by gynecologic, urologic, or obstetric surgery. Six patients were not seen until 6–12 months after their surgery; the remaining 18 underwent repair 5–22 weeks after their surgery. Surgical repair was not delayed to decrease induration in any patient. Sixteen patients underwent vaginal repair, although 1 procedure was switched to the abdominal approach because adequate exposure could not be achieved and the induration was greater than 2 cm. No major surgical complications occurred. Two patients have persistent urge incontinence, and 1 has mild persistent stress urinary incontinence.

Conclusions.—Delaying surgery does not produce outcome benefits but does seriously compromise quality of life and functioning in patients awaiting fistula repair. Successsful repair outcome depends on the surgeon's familiarity with both the vaginal and abdominal approaches and adherence to sound principles of fistula repair, which should determine the approach.

▶ We repair vesicovaginal fistulas as soon as it is convenient and prefer, whenever possible, a vaginal approach. We therefore agree with Blaivas et al. and are pleased that they have reported excellent results with this approach.

S.S. Howards, M.D.

25 Erectile Dysfunction

Efficacy of Prilocaine-Lidocaine Cream in the Treatment of Premature Ejaculation
Berkovitch M, Keresteci AG, Koren G (Univ of Toronto)
J Urol 154:1360–1361, 1995
25–1

Introduction.—Many attempts at treating premature ejaculation have been disappointing or too expensive. Lidocaine-prilocaine cream was used for penile desensitization in healthy men who had normal erection to determine whether this approach could prevent premature ejaculation.

Methods.—Eleven men, aged 36 years, were instructed to apply 1 tube (2.5 gm) of lidocaine-prilocaine cream on the glans penis and penile shaft, then cover the penis with a condom 30 minutes before intercourse. Patients were asked to keep a diary and rate effectiveness of the cream.

Results.—All men were involved in a constant heterosexual relationship and had sought help for what they considered premature ejaculation. Five patients who applied cream a mean of 8.4 times graded results as excellent, with ejaculation occurring 15–20 minutes after vaginal penetration. Four men who applied cream an average of 5 times graded the result as better, with ejaculation occurring 5–10 minutes after vaginal penetration. All female partners gave positive responses regarding effectiveness of the cream. Two patients were not pleased with the cream. One man complained of penile numbness with 5–8 applications and reported that he did not enjoy sexual activity. He could delay ejaculation for more than 20 minutes. His wife, however, gave a favorable response. The other patient reported no improvement with use of the cream.

Conclusion.—Ejaculation was delayed for most patients in a trial of lidocaine-prilocaine cream. Further investigation with a randomized, double-blind, placebo-controlled trial is recommended. If effective, this approach may be a breakthrough in the treatment of the most common form of male sexual dysfunction.

Sertraline Treatment for Premature Ejaculation

Mendels J, Camera A, Sikes C (Philadelphia Med Inst; Pfizer Inc, New York)
J Clin Psychopharmacol 15:341–346, 1995   25–2

Background.—Premature ejaculation affects up to 30% of men. Various neurotransmitters have been implicated as important mediators of ejaculation. Research suggests that the serotonergic system is a primary means through which ejaculation is controlled and modified. Sertraline, a highly potent and selective inhibitor of serotonin reuptake, has recently been approved for the treatment of depression. The value of inhibition of serotonin reuptake in the treatment of premature ejaculation was assessd in a controlled, double-blind study of sertraline.

Methods.—Fifty-two heterosexual men who had self-reported premature ejaculation were included. Sertraline or placebo was given by random assignment. After a 1-week washout period with placebo, the sertraline dose was titrated in weeks 1–3 from 50 to 200 mg daily until optimal clinical response was achieved or dose-limiting events occurred. The level of medication was maintained through week 8. Patient assessment of time from penetration to ejaculation, number of successful attempts at intercourse, and incidence of ejaculations during foreplay were the main outcome measures.

Findings.—Compared with placebo, sertraline significantly improved time to ejaculation and number of successful attempts at intercourse, as reported by the patients and their partners. Overall clinical judgments of improvement were also superior with sertraline. Most men tolerated the medication well.

Conclusions.—Sertraline titrated between 50 and 200 mg is safe, effective, and tolerable in the treatment of premature ejaculation. Patients given active treatment had significant increases in the estimated latency to ejaculation and in the number of successful attempts at intercourse when compared with baseline values and patients given placebo. In addition, fewer patients who received sertraline ejaculated prematurely during foreplay.

▶ Premature ejaculation, a common sexual problem, is estimated to occur in as many as 30% of men. The incidence depends on the definition of the entity. One definition is ejaculation within 1 minute of penetration. The American Psychiatric Association defines it as "persistent ejaculation with minimal sexual stimulation before, upon, or shortly after penetration and before the person wishes it." Many treatments have been tried for this condition, including topical anesthetics, neuroleptics, antidepressants, α-blockers, and the pause-squeeze technique. None of these has proved to be uniformly helpful. These 2 papers review the authors' experience with 2 techniques. The Toronto experience, although limited in numbers, is rather impressive. The Sertraline data show a significant, but rather modest, effect.

We have had reasonable results with gradually increasing doses of α-blockers such as sertraline hydrochloride (Zoloft).

S.S. Howards, M.D.

Sexual Function of Men Ages 40 to 79 Years: The Olmsted County Study of Urinary Symptoms and Health Status Among Men
Panser LA, Rhodes T, Girman CJ, Guess HA, Chute CG, Oesterling JE, Lieber MM, Jacobsen SJ (Mayo Clinic, Rochester, Minn; Merck Research Labs, Blue Bell, Pa; Univ of Michigan, Ann Arbor)
J Am Geriatr Soc 43:1107–1111, 1995
25–3

Background.—Because of the lack of current data from population-based studies, knowledge of male sexual function is somewhat limited. Sexual function and satisfaction among men were investigated in a population-based sample.

Methods.—A total of 2,115 men, aged 40–79 years, were randomly selected from the population of Olmstead County for a prospective study that was begun in 1989 and 1990. The men completed questionnaires on sexual concerns, performance, satisfaction, drive, and erectile dysfunction.

Findings.—The prevalences of problems and dysfunction increased with advancing age. Men aged 70–79 years were more worried about sexual function than were men aged 40–49 years (46.6% vs. 24.9). Thirty percent of the older age group and 10.4% of the younger group had worsened sexual performance compared with that in the preceding year. In addition, 10.7% of the older men, compared with only 1.7% of the younger men, said they were extremely dissatisfied with their sexual performance. Sexual drive was reportedly absent in 25.9% of the older group and in 0.6% of the younger group. Complete erectile dysfunction when sexually stimulated was reported by 27.4% of the older men and 0.3% of the younger men. In a logistic regression analysis, sexual dissatisfaction was significantly correlated with erectile dysfunction, reduced libido, and the interaction between erectile dysfunction and libido but not with age (Table 1).

Conclusions.—These findings are consistent with previously reported reduction in sexual function related to aging. The age-related increase in dissatisfaction may be explained mainly by the age-related increase in erectile dysfunction and reduced libido and the interaction between the 2.

▶ This study presents useful prospective, population-based data on sexual function in a significant number of men. It is unfortunate that the baseline response rate was only 55%. It is noteworthy that, although as many as 25% of men aged 40–49 years were concerned about sexual function, more than 50% of the men aged 70–79 years were not worried about theirs. Surprisingly, in the previous year, 10% and 30% of each age group, respectively, had experienced a significant decline in function. As the population ages, there will be very large numbers of men who will benefit from proper advice

TABLE 1.—Cross-sectional Association Between 5 Sexuality Variables Among White Men, by Age*

	Age 40–59 Years					Age 60–79 Years				
	Sexual Satisfaction	Sexual Drive	Erectile Function	Sexual Performance	Worry About Sex	Sexual Satisfaction	Sexual Drive	Erectile Function	Sexual Performance	Worry About Sex
Sexual drive	0.18	1.0				0.25	1.0			
Erectile function	−0.33	−0.24	1.0			−0.47	−0.58	1.0		
Sexual performance	0.32	0.23	−0.32	1.0	0.0	0.44	0.19	−0.35	1.0	
Worry about sex	−0.40	−0.21	0.45	−0.43	1.0	−0.52	−0.06	0.33	−0.50	1.0

* Spearman correlation coefficients. All P values were < 0.0001 for the associations between pairs of sexuality variables within 20-year age groups (except for the correlation between worry and libido among men aged 60–79 years [$P = 0.15$]).

(Courtesy of Panser LA, Rhodes T, Girman CJ, et al: Sexual function of men ages 40 to 79 years: The Olmsted County study of urinary symptoms and health status among men. *J Am Geriatr Soc* 43:1107–1111, 1995.)

regarding their sexual performance. It is very important that we be certain, by providing excellent sophisticated care, that the physicians delivering this service are urologists.

S.S. Howards, M.D.

Erectile Function Following Transurethral Prostatectomy
Hanbury DC, Sethia KK (Norfolk and Norwich Hosp, England)
Br J Urol 75:12–13, 1995
25–4

Introduction.—Some men experience loss of erections after transurethral prostatectomy (TURP). Although the reason for this impotence is unknown, perforation of the prostatic capsule during TURP may damage the neurovascular supply to the corpora carvernosa. The incidence of impotence after TURP and its relation to capsular perforation were determined.

Patients and Methods.—Two hundred sixty-eight men (mean age, 72 years) scheduled to undergo TURP for clinically benign disease were recruited for a prospective study. Data recorded included operative details and level of potency before surgery. Patients were interviewed again about their sexual function 3 months after TURP. Excluded from further study were men whose histology showed prostatic carcinoma.

Results.—Twenty-two patients were excluded for various reasons; 246 were therefore available for analysis. Before TURP, 137 had been fully potent, 43 partially potent, and 66 impotent. The incidence of impotence was age related: 63.8% of patients younger than 80 years, but only 9.1% of those older than 80, were potent. After TURP, potency was completely lost in 20 of the 180 men who had some preoperative erectile function and reduced in an additional 20 (Table 1). Total impotence occurred more often in men who had only partial potency before TURP (37.2%) than in those with full potency (2.9%). The risk of impotence was not related to patient age, size of gland resected, or operative time. Breach of the prostatic capsule at surgery was associated with an increased risk of impotence (28.1% vs. 10% in patients without capsular perforation).

Conclusion.—The risk of impotence after TURP was higher in men who were partially impotent before surgery. Capsular perforation occurred

TABLE 1.—Changes in Potency After Transurethral Prostatectomy
(n = 246)

	After operation		
Before operation	Fully potent	Partly potent	Impotent
Fully potent	113	20	4
Partly potent	1	26	16
Impotent	0	0	66

(Courtesy of Hanbury DC, Sethia KK: Erectile function following transurethral prostatectomy. *Br J Urol* 75:12–13, 1995.)

more often when the procedure was performed by less experienced surgeons and carried a statistically significant risk of causing impotence. Erectile function was recovered in some patients who sought postoperative treatment for impotence.

▶ This is an interesting prospective study of the incidence of impotence after TURP. It provides an analysis that had not been available previously, in that the authors categorized the men preoperatively as impotent, partially impotent, or potent. The partially impotent men were much more likely to be affected by the surgery than were the potent men. Among the latter group, there was only a 2.9% incidence of total impotence at 3 months. Three months may be too early, however, to evaluate these men. It would have been useful if the authors had provided us with the ages of the men who lost their potency, because, as the previous abstract documents, there is a 30% incidence per year in decreased potency in men, aged 70–79 years, who do not undergo surgery. It is also not possible to determine whether the observed decline in sexual function was on an organic or psychogenic basis. Thus, in previously potent men, TURP may have no effect on sexual function.

S.S. Howards, M.D.

Comparison of RigiScan and Sleep Laboratory Nocturnal Penile Tumescence in the Diagnosis of Organic Impotence
Licht MR, Lewis RW, Wollan PC, Harris CD (Mayo Clinic, Rochester, Minn)
J Urol 54:1740–1743, 1995   25–5

Background.—The RigiScan is now a well-accepted, commonly used tool for obtaining information on nocturnal penile tumescence (NPT) before the initial classification of erectile dysfunction as organic or psychogenic. The accuracy of the RigiScan device, however, has recently been questioned. RigiScan measurement of radial rigidity was compared with sleep laboratory measurement of axial rigidity and trained observer assessment of erectile function in diagnosing organic impotence.

Methods.—Twenty-eight patients underwent simultaneous 2-night RigiScan monitoring and formal sleep laboratory NPT. Standard normal values for radial and axial rigidity were assessed for accuracy in predicting normal NPT compared with determinations made by a trained observer of the adequacy of an erection for penetration.

Findings.—RigiScan tip measurements were poorly associated with buckling pressure. The correlation with base measures, however, was strong. Observer assessments were strongly associated with tip, base, and buckling pressure measurements. Using observer assessments as the gold standard, receiver operating curves were produced to select RigiScan base and buckling pressure measurements that could predict functional erections with the greatest sensitivity and specificity.

Conclusions.—RigiScan is a useful device for determining NPT. Base measures are more accurate than tip measures for determining erectile function. The level of rigidity currently used to define a normal erection, 70% or greater, overestimates organic erectile dysfunction.

▶ The authors clearly demonstrate that base measurements with RigiScan compare favorably with NPT monitoring. They also point out that a standard of 55% gives greater precision than the current standard of 70% established by Kessler.[1] This paper is somewhat dated, at least from our perspective. For the most part, we use NPT monitoring only in legal cases, because it is too expensive and other methods, such as clinical evaluation, diagnostic intracorporal injections, RigiScan, and even the stamp test, compare well with this approach.[2]

S.S. Howards, M.D.

References

1. Kessler WO: Nocturnal penile tumescence. *Urol Clin North Am* 15:81, 1988.
2. Saypol DC, Peterson GA, Howards SS, et al: Impotence: Are the newer diagnostic methods a necessity? *J Urol* 130:260–262, 1983.

Recovery of Erectile Function by the Oral Administration of Apomorphine
Heaton JPW, Morales A, Adams MA, Johnston B, El-Rashidy R (Queen's Univ, Kingston, Ont, Canada; Pentech Pharmaceuticals, Wheeling, Ill)
Urology 45:200–206, 1995   25–6

Introduction.—The search for a safe and effective oral treatment for impotence had led to interest in the dopamine agonist apomorphine, which has been reported to be effective in causing erections in animal and human studies. Apomorphine is associated with a variety of side effects, however, and has poor bioavailability in oral form. The effects of a formulation of apomorphine for sublingual absorption in men whose erectile dysfunction had no apparent organic origin were examined in 4 preliminary studies.

Patients and Methods.—The men who entered the therapeutic trial had a diagnosis of primary psychogenic dysfunction. Investigations were designed as single-blinded increasing dose studies, with patients tested on at least 3 separate days with at least a 3-day interval between doses. The 4 protocols used apomorphine preparations that consisted of a preliminary sublingual liquid, preliminary 5-mg tablets, an aqueous nasal spray, and new 3- and 4-mg controlled absorption tablets. Patients who aborted the trial because of nausea were asked to return the following week for retesting after pretreatment with the antinauseant domperidone. A Rigi-Scan ambulatory tumescence monitor was used to study erectile response to apomorphine with visual erotic or sexually neutral stimulation.

Results.—Although 7 of 10 evaluable patients responded to the sublingual liquid preparation of apomorphine, most experienced significant nausea. Neither the preliminary 5-mg tablet nor the aqueous forms of the drug produced a useful response free of side effects. Eight of 12 men (67%) who received the controlled absorption 3- and 4-mg tablets had erections. Compared with placebo, erectile activity during sexually neutral visual stimulation was significantly greater with this formulation of apomorphine. Seven of 11 patients who have used the tablets at home for 3–7 months report good erections, resumption of sexual intercourse, and an interest in continuing the medication.

Conclusion.—In this small, selected group of men with psychogenic impotence, 3 or 4 mg of apomorphine absorbed through the oral mucosa improved erectile function. The drug has no addictive potential, does not cause arousal, and was free from side effects in the special release formulation developed for this study.

▶ The authors have demonstrated that their special preparation of oral apomorphine has significantly fewer severe side effects than did other available preparations. In a very small number of patients, it also had a modest effect on erectile function. The men in this study, however, had psychogenic impotence. In addition, the agent used is not commercially available and therefore will not, at this time, affect clinical practice.

S.S. Howards, M.D.

Incidence of Penile Pain After Injection of a New Formulation of Prostaglandin E1
Chen J, Godschalk MF, Katz PG, Mulligan T (Med College of Virginia, Richmond; McGuire VA Med Ctr, Richmond, Va)
J Urol 154:77–79, 1995   25–7

Rationale.—The intracavernous administration of prostaglandin E_1 (PGE_1) is now a widely used treatment for erectile dysfunction because it infrequently causes priapism or penile fibrosis. Pain and burning do occur, however, and a new formulation of PGE_1 has been developed to eliminate these effects. The new formulation, which contains lactose and sodium citrate in addition to PGE_1 and is reconstituted in sterile water rather than in ethanol, was assessed.

Methods.—Sixty-three patients who had erectile dysfunction received 451 intracavernous injections of this preparation twice weekly in the office. Doses were increased until an adequate erection was achieved. Thirty-eight patients completed the home maintenance phase of the study.

Results.—Pain developed after 3.5% of office injections, and a burning sensation developed after 16%. At home, approximately 2% of injections were followed by pain or burning. In neither phase of the study were symptoms significantly associated with the dose of PGE_1 injected (Fig 1). The form of erectile dysfunction was unrelated to the production of symptoms.

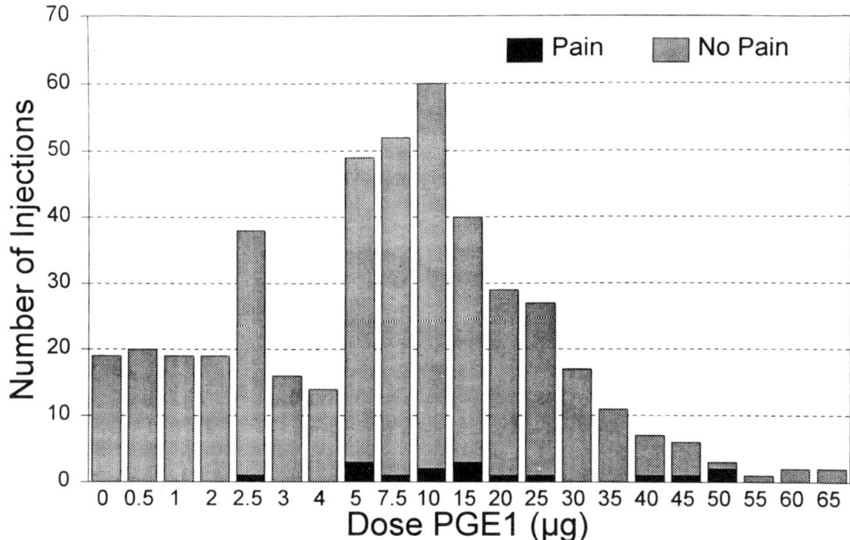

FIGURE 1.—Number of injections in office-based phase by dose of PGE_1. *Dark portions of bars* are injections that resulted in pain and/or burning. (Courtesy of Chen J, Godschalk MF, Katz PG, et al: Incidence of penile pain after injection of a new formulation of prostaglandin E1. *J Urol* 154:77–79, 1995.)

Conclusion.—An aqueous preparation of PGE_1 is less likely than an alcohol-based formulation to produce pain or burning when injected intracavernously in patients who have erectile dysfunction.

▶ This is a simple but useful study. The authors have documented that a new formulation of PGE_1, which is provided by the manufacturer in a freeze-dried state and reconstituted with sterile water rather than alcohol, dramatically reduces the amount of discomfort associated with intracorporal injection. The 12% to 80% incidence of pain or burning with the standard preparation reported in the literature was reduced to less than 5%.

S.S. Howards, M.D.

Double-blind Randomized Crossover Study Comparing Intracorporeal Prostaglandin E₁ With Combination of Prostaglandin E₁ and Lidocaine in the Treatment of Organic Impotence

Kattan S (King Saud Univ, Riyadh, Saudi Arabia)
Urology 45:1032–1036, 1995   25–8

Objective.—Pain during injection and during the induced erection remains the most frequent side effect of intracorporeal (IC) therapy with prostaglandin E_1 (PGE_1) for organic and psychogenic impotence. The efficacy of lidocaine 1% in relieving pain associated with IC PGE_1, as well as its effects on the pharmacologic erection, was evaluated.

Study Design.—Twenty-two patients who had organic impotence were included in a randomized, double-blind crossover study. The patients had experienced pain with a test dose of 20 µg of IC PGE_1. They received either 20 µg of IC PGE_1 alone or in combination with lidocaine hydrochloride 1%. The signed rank test for matched pairs was used to compare the effects of treatment.

Outcome.—Significantly fewer patients reported pain with the combination of lidocaine and PGE_1 (45.4%) than with PGE_1 alone (86.3%). In addition, 57.8% of patients who reported pain with PGE_1 alone experienced partial or complete relief of pain with combination therapy. Further, combining lidocaine with PGE_1 significantly improved the quality of erection from 27.2% to 63.6%. After combination therapy, 31.8% of patients had increased duration of erectile response, and 81.8% of patients who had improvement in pain also had improved erection. There were no significant side effects after either injection.

Conclusion.—The combination of PGE_1 and lidocaine can be safely used in the treatment of erectile dysfunction and provides relief of pain and enhanced erectile effect. This combination therapy should be used in patients who have pain only or pain associated with suboptimal erection with PGE_1 monotherapy. Further studies are warranted to substantiate these findings and to detect any long-term complications.

▶ This paper outlines another and previously described[1] method of reducing the pain associated with PGE_1 injections. Lidocaine clearly is not as effective at diminishing discomfort as is the preparation described in the previous abstract. It is interesting, if somewhat surprising, that lidocaine had such a significant effect on the erectile response. There may be cultural factors at work, because the author had only a 27% adequate response rate with PGE_1. That rate is much lower than the rate in the literature and in our experience.

S.S. Howards, M.D.

Reference

1. Schouman M, Lacroix P, Amer M: Suppression of prostaglandin E_1 induced pain by dilution of the drug with lidocaine before intra-cavernous injuection (letter). *J Urol* 148:1266, 1992.

Papaverine-Phentolamine and Prostaglandin E1 Versus Papaverine-Phentolamine Alone for Intracorporeal Injection Therapy: A Clinical Double-blind Study

Shenfeld O, Hanani J, Shalhav A, Vardi Y, Goldwasser B (Chaim Sheba Med Ctr, Tel Hashomer, Israel; Rambam Med Ctr, Haifa, Israel)
J Urol 154:1017–1019, 1995   25–9

Objective.—The effect of adding prostaglandin E_1 (PGE_1) to the combination of papaverine and phentolamine for intracorporeal injection in the treatment of impotence was assessed.

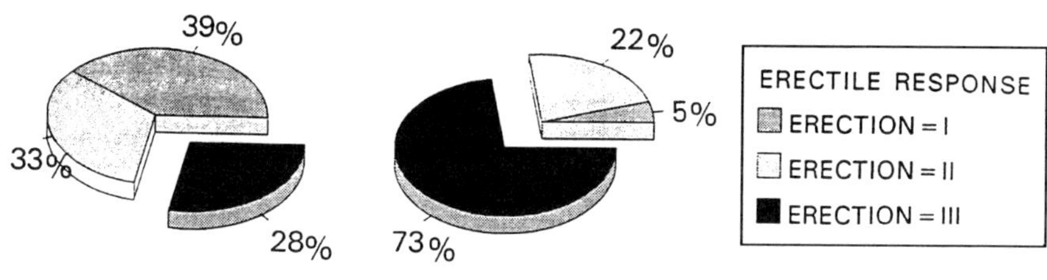

FIGURE 1.—Erectile response. (Courtesy of Shenfeld O, Hanani J, Shalhav A, et al: Papaverine-phentolamine and prostaglandin E1 versus papaverine-phentolamine alone for intracorporeal injection therapy: A clinical double-blind study. *J Urol* 154:1017–1019, 1995.)

Management.—Twenty patients, aged 44–71 years, were included. Twelve had arteriogenic impotence, 3 had neurogenic impotence, and 5 had other causes. Patients received 2 intracorporeal injections at a 2-week interval. One injection consisted of 9 mg of papaverine and 0.5 mg of phentolamine. The 3-drug combination included 4.5 mg of papaverine, 0.25 mg of phentolamine, and 5 µg of PGE_1. Both treatments were given in a volume of 0.5 cc. The quality of erections was determined by palpation 15 minutes after injection.

Results.—Seventy-three percent of patients achieved full erection when injected with the 3-drug mixture, but only 28% did after the 2-drug treatment (Fig 1). Penetration was possible in 95% and 61% of patients, respectively. No patient achieved a better result with the 2-drug injection. Erections lasted substantially longer with the 3-drug treatment (57 vs. 34 minutes). One patient who received the 3-drug injection had marked pain. Three patients had erections that lasted longer than 1 hour, 2 after the 3-drug injection.

Conclusions.—It is worthwhile to add PGE_1 to a combination of papaverine and phentolamine for intracorporeal injection in impotent men. A stronger erectile response is achieved without a substantial increase in complications.

▶ This well-done study unequivocally demonstrates that, at the doses used, papaverine, phentolamine, and PGE_1 are superior to papaverine and phentolamine alone. From our point of view, it would have been more interesting to compare PGE_1 alone with a combination of 2 drugs, because these are the alternatives we usually use.

S.S. Howards, M.D.

Papaverine Topical Gel for Treatment of Erectile Dysfunction

Kim ED, El-Rashidy R, McVary KT (Northwestern Univ, Chicago; Pharmedic Company, Wheeling, Ill)
J Urol 153:361–365, 1995   25–10

Background.—Intracavernous injection of vasoactive substances is effective in the treatment of organic erectile dysfunction. Up to 50% of men eventually discontinue treatment, however, because of discomfort and lack of spontaneity.

Study Design.—Twenty men were included in a phase I, placebo-controlled, nonblinded study to determine the efficacy and safety of a topical papaverine gel in the treatment of erectile dysfunction. Each patient was evaluated on 5 separate days with application to the penis, scrotum, and perineum of a 5.5% weight-in-weight papaverine hydrochloride gel; 7%, 15%, or 20% papaverine base gels; or placebo.

Results.—Seventeen men, including 13 who had spinal cord injuries, completed the study. After application of a 15% or 20% papaverine base gel, cavernous artery diameter significantly increased by 36%, and peak systolic flow velocity increased by 26%, as assessed by color flow Doppler ultrasound. However, only 3 patients achieved an increase in cavernous artery diameter of 75% or more, and only 2 had a peak systolic flow velocity of 25 cm/sec or more. Men who had spinal cord injury exhibited similar responses. The effect of a papaverine base in producing flow alterations to the penis was dose-dependent. Mean blood pressure decreased significantly at 15 and 30 minutes after application to the forearm, and mean heart rate decreased from 68 to 62 beats per minute after application to the genitalia. None of the patients were symptomatic, however, and serum levels of papaverine were not significantly increased compared with preapplication values. There were no hepatotoxic effects, and the rash that developed in 1 patient might have been related to prolonged application of the plastic wrap. Three patients exhibited full clinical erections with the papaverine gel for a mean duration of 38.7 minutes, as well as with the placebo for a mean of 8 minutes.

Conclusion.—Topical papaverine gel appears to be safe and well tolerated after application to the genitalia. It may not be as effective as intracavernous injection therapy for erectile dysfunction but may have promise at higher concentrations or when combined with different skin enhancers. Topical papaverine gel appears to augment reflex erections in men who have spinal cord injury and may be especially beneficial in this population.

▶ The data in this paper document that papaverine topical gel is safe. Previous studies of minoxidil and nitroglycerin[1,2] have shown that medications can be absorbed through the penile skin. This finding was confirmed by the authors, who demonstrated alteration in blood after the application of the gel. However, there was no significant clinical effect. The 3 men who had neurogenic impotence and had erections obtained similar results with placebo.

S.S. Howards, M.D.

References

1. Cavellini G: Minoxidil versus nitroglycerin: A prospective double-blind controlled trial in transcutaneous erection facilitation for organic impotence. *J Urol* 146:50, 1991.
2. Clark RV, Murray FT, Hirshkowitz M, et al: Treatment of erectile dysfunction in men with diabetes mellitus using a penetration-enhanced topical minoxidiol solution. *J Androl* 140:55A, 1994.

Long-term Results With Penile Vein Ligation for Venogenic Impotence
Kim ED, McVary KT (Northwestern Univ, Chicago)
J Urol 153:655–658, 1995   25–11

Background.—Most men who have organic impotence also have corporeal veno-occlusive dysfunction. The results of various surgical treatments have been unsatisfactory. Urologists can now identify impotent patients who have venous leak and sufficient arterial inflow. Patients with corporeal veno-occlusive dysfunction who will benefit from venous ligation cannot be selected conclusively. The long-term results of extensive penile vein ligation were evaluated.

Methods.—Penile vein ligation was performed in 15 patients, aged 29–68 years, who had venogenic impotence. Color flow Doppler ultrasound and dynamic infusion cavernosogram and cavernosometry with vasoactive substance injection, along with other evaluations, were done. Surgery was performed with use of the Lue technique. Patients underwent follow-up examinations 2 weeks to 12 months after surgery. Telephone follow-up was done 19–45 months after surgery.

Results.—Postoperative potency was defined as ability to have an erection sufficient for unaided coitus in more than 75% of attempts. By this definition, 9 patients were potent and 6 patients were impotent after surgery. Duration of erectile dysfunction before surgery was the only prognostic factor for success; longer duration of erectile dysfunction was less likely to result in postoperative potency. There was no correlation with systolic and diastolic arterial flow or resistive index, as assessed by color flow Doppler evaluation, leakage sites, or patient age at surgery. Nor was there correlation with preoperative dynamic infusion cavernosometry maintenance rates. Contracture of the penis, which was the most common complication, occurred in 6 patients but affected function in only 1.

Conclusions.—Favorable long-term results were observed in these patients after extensive venous ligation using the Lue technique. A follow-up period of at least 12 months is needed to assess surgical results. More knowledge about veno-occlusive pathophysiology is needed to develop future therapies.

Venous Leak Surgery: Long-term Follow-up of Patients Undergoing Excision and Ligation of the Deep Dorsal Vein of the Penis
Vale JA, Feneley MR, Lees WR, Kirby RS (St Mary's Hosp, London; St Bartholomew's Hosp, London; Middlesex Hosp, London)
Br J Urol 76:192–195, 1995   25–12

Introduction.—The idea of treating erectile disorders by occluding venous channels exiting the penis has a long history, but its efficacy remains uncertain. Apart from inadequate techniques and improper patient selection, some authors have proposed that venous leakage results from altered trabecular smooth muscle of a compliant tunica albuginea, thereby resulting in failed venous occlusion. The results of venous leak surgery were reviewed.

Methods.—Twenty-seven men, aged 26–63 years, with erectile failure in whom color Doppler imaging, pharmacocavernosometry, and cavernosography had demonstrated venous leakage. The patients had been impotent for 2 years on average. None of them responded to intracorporeal injection of papaverine or had vascular risk factors.

The deep dorsal vein was mobilized proximally via a transverse infrapubic incision under general anesthesia. Small tributaries and then the deep dorsal vein were ligated; a 5 to 10-cm vein segment was removed. Any dilated circumflex or accessory veins were also ligated and divided.

Results.—Nineteen patients (70%) could resume satisfactory intercourse within 3 months after surgery. Two of them required papaverine but had previously been unresponsive. Fourteen of 22 patients, whose status was followed for 1 year after surgery, were still able to achieve erections adequate for intercourse, but 4 in all required papaverine injection at this time. Penile numbness sometimes lasted up to 3 months after surgery, but there were no serious complications.

Conclusion.—Venous leak surgery is worthwhile for patients who have erectile failure caused by pure venous leakage. These patients are often desperate and prefer to try definitive surgery rather than receiving an implant or using a vacuum device.

▶ Venous leak surgery for impotence remains very controversial. Numerous abstracts describing extremely varied results of this procedure have been published in the YEAR BOOK during the past several years. Most authors who present well-done, long-term studies have had rather poor results. We are rather skeptical regarding venous leak surgery and use the technique only in highly selected and usually young patients. These 2 papers raise hope that, in carefully selected patients, the technique can achieve modest success. Both groups carefully screened their patients with duplex Doppler ultrasound, dynamic cavernosography after papaverine injection, and cavernosography. Only patients who had excellent arterial inflow were selected. The Northwestern group reports a success rate of 60%, but only 40% were potent by their definition without ever using a vacuum device or injections. They also report a disturbing 50% contracture rate. Considering the propensity of these patients to sue their urologists, this is worrisome. The London group reported a 46% potency rate with injection at 1 year. The status of 4 potent patients was followed for 2 years, at which time 1 patient required injections. If one assumes a similar pattern for the other patient, the 2-year unassisted potency rate would be 35%. Thus, these 2 papers document some venous surgery success in very carefully selected impotent patients.

S.S. Howards, M.D.

The Prosthesis Salvage Operation: Immediate Replacement of the Infected Penile Prosthesis
Brant MD, Ludlow JK, Mulcahy JJ (Indiana Univ, Indianapolis)
J Urol 155:155–157, 1996   25–13

Introduction.—The incidence of infection in penile prostheses is reported to range from 1% to 8%. Although this devastating complication can be treated successfully by removal of the device, irrigation, and antibiotics, reinsertion of a new device may be difficult or impossible. An experience with immediate salvage and replacement of an infected penile prosthesis was described.

Methods.—Since 1991, 139 inflatable and 46 semirigid prostheses were implanted at the study institution. Prostheses became infected in 7 patients. An additional 6 patients who had infected prostheses were referred from other centers. Infection had developed from 3 to 224 weeks after the initial prosthesis implantation. The salvage technique involved complete removal of all components of the prosthesis and any permanent foreign materials, thorough irrigation, and insertion of the new prosthesis. After surgery, patients were given ciprofloxacin, 500 mg twice a day for 1 month.

Results.—Two of the 13 patients were not considered candidates for salvage. Follow-up was a mean of 21.3 months, and results of the salvage operation were successful in 10 of 11 patients. The remaining patient is doing well after a second salvage procedure. *Staphylococcus epidermidis*, detected in 75% of patients, was the most frequent cause of prosthesis infection. The rate of infection and success of subsequent salvage did not appear to be influenced by etiology of impotence, initial prosthesis type, or route of prosthesis insertion. No wound infections occurred after the salvage procedure.

Discussion.—Signs of infection in a penile prosthesis include persistent pain, erythema, fever, adherence of the prosthesis components to overlying tissue, and purulent discharge. Preliminary results in this small series of patients support use of the immediate salvage procedure. Removal of the infected device serves to remove the encapsulated layer of infecting organisms, a particular problem with *Staphylococcus* species. Copious irrigation also contributes to the success of salvage.

▶ This significant paper has a useful take-home message. The authors have definitely shown that, contrary to standard surgical wisdom, one can remove an infected foreign body and replace it successfully at the same time. This "new surgical principle" may relate to modern oral antibiotics rather than to an inaccuracy in the former teaching. The administration of oral ciprofloxacin for a month may explain why the authors were successful with this approach.

S.S. Howards, M.D.

In Vivo Assessment of Trabecular Smooth Muscle Tone: Its Application in Pharmaco-cavernosometry and Analysis of Intracavernous Pressure Determinants

Hatzichristou DG, Saenz De Tejada I, Kupferman S, Namburi S, Pescatori ES, Udelson D, Goldstein I (Boston Univ)
J Urol 153:1126–1135, 1995

25–14

Background.—In animal studies, pharmacocavernosometric relationships are known to reflect relaxation and contraction of trabecular smooth muscle. Hemodynamic indicators of complete smooth muscle relaxation were assessed in impotent patients. In addition, the contribution of venous outflow and arterial inflow to intracavernous equilibrium was established. Vasodilators were used to override incomplete relaxation and produce linear flow–pressure relationships and uniform venous outflow resistance.

Methods.—Group 1 included 21 of 286 impotent men who had undergone previous pharmacocavernosometry. Flow-pressure and venous outflow resistance relationships were evaluated in this group to identify those who achieved complete trabecular smooth muscle relaxation after vasodilator administration. Group 2 included 123 impotent men, in whom trabecular smooth muscle tone was assessed in the second stage of the study. Five parameters were used to evaluate the patients hemodynamically: penile circumference, intracavernous pressure, blood pressure, Doppler ultrasound of arterial flow, and flow of saline. Venous outflow, outflow resistance values, and arterial values were determined. Vasoactive agents, such as papaverine, prostaglandins, and papaverine in combination with phentolamine, were administered. Patients in group 2 were given additional vasoactive agents if their flow-to-maintain values and pressure were not linear or if their resistance values were not constant. There were no redosing limits. Corporeal capacitance was determined.

Results.—In group 1, the mean intracavernous steady-state equilibrium pressure was equal to 78% of the ideal (87.9 ± 6.1 mm Hg). Group 1 patients had low flow-to-maintain values (0.5–2 mL/min). Phenylephrine was used to achieve detumescence. Despite redosing, 9% of patients in this

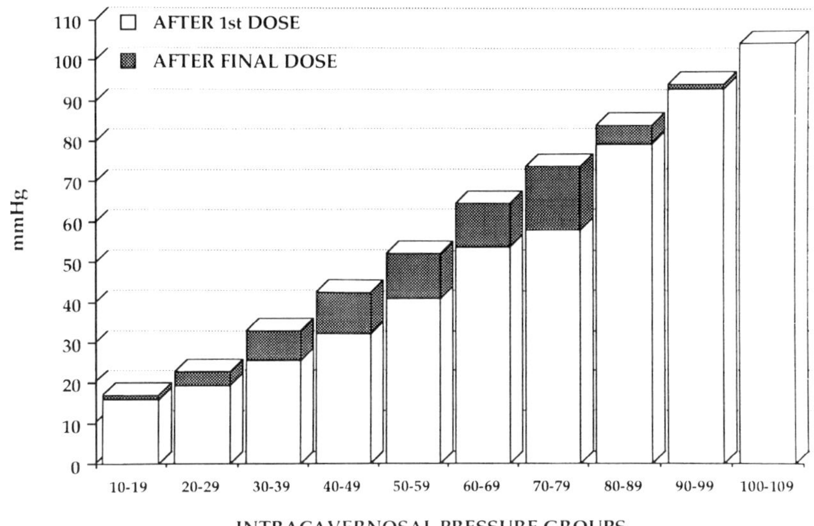

FIGURE 3.—Effects of redosing on steady-state equilibrium intracavernous pressure. Redosing induced greatest changes when, after first dose of vasoactive agents, equilibrium intracavernous pressure was 20–59 mm Hg. (Courtesy of Hatzichristou DG, Saenz de Tejada I, Kupferman S, et al: In vivo assessment of trabecular smooth muscle tone, its application in pharmaco-cavernosometry and analysis of intracavernous pressure determinants. *J Urol* 153:1126–1135, 1995.)

group did not achieve a linear relationship. Single dosing was required in 15% of patients, and 2–3 doses were required in the remaining 70%. No ill effects occurred from redosing. Redosing had the greatest effect when the equilibrium intracavernous pressure was 20–59 mm Hg (Fig 3). Two different capacitance states were identified on the basis of equilibrium pressures: pressures greater than 60 mm Hg were considered low capacitance, and pressures less than 50 mm Hg were considered high capacitance.

Discussion.—The relationship between venous outflow resistance and flow-pressure and complete trabecular smooth muscle relaxation was clearly identified. Redosing of intracavernous vasoactive agents is an effective method for assessment of smooth muscle tone.

▶ This is a very sophisticated study from an excellent research group. The authors' goal was to develop a method of distinguishing between the 2 causes of venous occlusive dysfunction: incomplete trabecular smooth muscle relaxation and corporal cavernosal structural changes. They had been able to do this in experimental animals, and this study is a successful attempt to do the same in patients. These findings can form the basis for reproducible methods of defining the pathophysiology in such patients, which might eventually lead to more rational treatment.

S.S. Howards, M.D.

Effect of Aging on Nitric Oxide–mediated Penile Erection in Rats

Garbán H, Vernet D, Freedman A, Rajfer J, González-Cadavid N (Univ of California, Los Angeles)
Am J Physiol 268:H467–H475, 1995

25–15

Background.—Production of nitric oxide stimulates vasodilation in the penis. This process, along with veno-occlusion, causes erection. The effects on penile erection of age, nitric oxide synthase (NOS) activity, pharmacotherapy, and histologic changes in the corpora cavernosa were studied in adult, old, and senescent male rats.

Methods and Results.—Anesthetized male adult (aged 5 months), old (20 months), and senescent (30 months) rats were studied. A significant decrease in penile response to electric field stimulation was seen as rats aged, with a 32% decrease for old rats and a 48% decrease for senescent rats. Administration of N^{omega}-nitro-L-arginine methyl ester, an NOS inhibitor, caused a fractional decrease in erectile response to 60% in adult, 30% in old, and 23% in senescent rats. Subsequent injection of L-arginine only partially reversed this effect in all age groups.

Papaverine yielded a decreased erectile response to 40% in old and to 18% in senescent males, compared with adults, and duration of erection was shorter. Nitroglycerine, a nitric oxide donor, elicited 20% less erectile response and a 50% shorter duration in adult rats and much less in old and senescent ones, which suggests decreasing responsiveness to nitric oxide with age. Nitric oxide synthase activity in penile homogenates was increased in old rats, compared with adults, but was significantly decreased in senescent tissue. Histology of old and senescent penises showed a progressive increase with age in collagen deposition, engrossed endothelium, and large lacunae, which suggests loss of elasticity with age.

Conclusions.—These results indicate that initial erectile failure with age is independent of nitric oxide production, because old rats respond to aging with increased NOS activity. In senescent rats, NOS activity is reduced remarkably, and hyalinization and sclerosis of the corpora cavernosa become marked.

▶ This is another excellent research paper. In the past year, we have seen an enormous increase in the number of research papers investigating the role of nitric oxide in normal physiology and the pathophysiology of disease. Indeed, nitric oxide was the "molecule of the year" in 1992. This paper shows that a decline in its availability is involved in the decreased potency of aging. Of course, the next question to be answered is why. Finally, treatments will need to be developed to prevent or reverse the change for the benefit of aging men who wish to be sexually active.

S.S. Howards, M.D.

26 Testis Tumor

Surgical Anatomy of the Lumbar Vessels: Implications for Retroperitoneal Surgery
Baniel J, Foster RS, Donohue JP (Indiana Univ, Indianapolis)
J Urol 153:1422–1425, 1995

26–1

Introduction.—Attention to the lumbar vessels in the retroperitoneal region is mandatory during a number of urological and vascular operations. Most available information is from cadaver and radiologic studies, many of which include select patients. Retroperitoneal lymph node dissection provides an opportunity to precisely map the lumbar vessels in young patients who usually lack vascular disease.

Objective.—The lumbar vessels were mapped in the course of 102 retroperitoneal node dissections, 45 of which were complete bilateral procedures. The vessels of 147 renal units were adequately demonstrated so that accessory arteries could be documented.

Observations.—A majority of patients had 3 lumbar arteries exiting the infrarenal aorta, most often coursing in pairs from the posterior aspect of the aorta. A common trunk was present in 15% of bilateral dissections. It was not uncommon for there to be 2–4 lumbar arteries exiting along the aorta. A few patients had a lumbar artery exiting the left common iliac artery. The number and topographic arrangement of the lumbar veins varied substantially. Most patients had 3 veins on the left side of the inferior vena cava and 2 or 3 veins entering the inferior cava on the right. Paired veins were present in a minority of cases. In 6 cases, 3 veins on the left upper side of the inferior cava formed a common branch that entered the cava as a trifurcation. More than 40% of patients had 1 or more lumbar veins entering the left renal vein.

Renovascular Anomalies.—About one fourth of patients had accessory renal arteries caudad to the main renal artery. Six patients had bilateral accessory renal arteries, and 2 patients had 2 accessory renal arteries on the same side. Three accessory right renal arteries passed anterior to the inferior vena cava. The only renal venous anomaly was a retroaortic left renal vein, noted in 3 cases.

Surgical Implications.—Branched lumbar arteries and veins and additional inferior renal arteries are encountered not infrequently during retroperitoneal lymph node dissection. There is a risk that a small accessory right renal artery will be damaged during dissection in the infrarenal area of the vena cava or the interaortocaval region. The "split and roll" technique of aortic dissection will accurately demonstrate the anatomy of the renal arteries.

▶ It is uncommon that a modern study of anatomy reveals anything new. However, Dr. Donohue's extensive experience in the retroperitoneums of young men with testis cancer has yielded some important insights in this paper. The predictable regularity of the arterial branches of the aorta and the frequent variation of the venous branches of the inferior vena cava are detailed in a very useful format. Because the urologist is the primary surgeon of the retroperitoneum, he or she must have a clear understanding of its vascular surgical anatomy.

M.S. Litwin, M.D., M.P.H.

Patterns of Metastatic Spread in Prepubertal Yolk Sac Tumor of the Testis

Grady RW, Ross JH, Kay R (Cleveland Clinic Found, Ohio)
J Urol 153:1259–1261, 1995   26–2

Introduction.—Testicular tumors are rare in the pediatric population, making it difficult to gather data at any 1 institution. The establishment of the prepubertal testicular tumor registry by the American Academy of Pediatrics in 1980 made it possible to make meaningful observations about this rare childhood disease. Records from the registry were reviewed of patients with metastatic yolk sac tumors to define the anatomical pattern of metastatic spread and clarify any role of retroperitoneal lymph node dissection.

Methods.—Records of 212 patients with yolk sac tumors were reviewed. Of these, 33 patients had metastatic disease on initial visit.

Results.—Of 33 patients with metastatic disease, 27% had retroperitoneal lymphatic spread of disease alone, 40% had hematogenous spread alone, and 19% had hematogenous and retroperitoneal lymphatic spread.

Of 14 patients who underwent initial CT, findings were consistent with metastatic disease in 3 patients, 10 patients did not have CT findings of metastatic disease, and 1 scan result was not recorded in the registry. Ultrasonography was performed initially in 6 patients. Of these, no evidence of metastases was detected in 5 patients. The 1 patient with positive findings did not have concurrent data about tumor location in the registry.

Of 11 patients who underwent retroperitoneal lymph node dissection, 5 had metastatic disease. One of 6 patients with negative findings on retroperitoneal lymph node dissection later had metastases to the lung. There was a 27% complication rate with the procedure.

All 6 patients with negative findings on retroperitoneal lymph node dissection had negative findings on CT. Three of 5 patients with proven retroperitoneal disease did not have CT findings in the registry. Of the 2 remaining patients, CT findings were positive in 1 patient and negative in the other.

Conclusion.—Findings suggest a hematogenous predilection in the spread of metastases in pediatric patients with metastases of yolk sac tumors of the testes. Therefore, routine retroperitoneal lymph node dissection as a part of initial treatment is not recommended in these patients.

▶ Because pediatric testis cancer is so rare, patterns of disease may be difficult to recognize. The prepubertal testis tumor registry of the American Academy of Pediatrics Section on Urology has now yielded important information about this tumor. The authors of this article present critical information about the common routes of spread of pediatric yolk sac testis tumors. In contrast to adult testis tumors, which usually spread initially to the retroperitoneal lymphatics, prepubertal patients with this tumor may harbor distant hematogenously spread lesions, obviating the need for routine retroperitoneal lymphadenectomy (RPLND). This is in sharp distinction to adult patients, in whom RPLND is an important component of management. Unlike adults, boys with yolk sac testis tumors must routinely undergo an exhaustive metastatic survey outside the retroperitoneum.

M.S. Litwin, M.D., M.P.H.

Late Relapse of Clinical Stage I Testicular Cancer
Baniel J, Foster RS, Einhorn LH, Donohue JP (Indiana Univ, Indianapolis)
J Urol 154:1370–1372, 1995   26–3

Introduction.—Relapses of testicular cancer typically occur within 2 years after treatment. A group of patients in whom clinical stage 1 testicular cancer was initially diagnosed and treated but who had late relapse were identified and studied retrospectively to analyze the management of early-stage carcinoma.

Methods.—Patients with recurrent testicular cancer 2 or more years after initial management of clinical stage 1 disease were studied. Follow-up status was determinied with patient or physician interviews or chart review.

Results.—Thirty-five patients were studied. Initial treatment included primary retroperitoneal lymph node dissection in 31, orchiectomy alone in 2, radiotherapy in 1, primary chemotherapy in 1, and adjuvant chemotherapy in 22. Late relapse most commonly occurred in the retroperitoneum. Chemotherapy was the initial management strategy in all the patients after late relapse, but only 17% had a complete response, and all 6 of these patients had a second relapse. Of the 29 patients who subsequently underwent additional surgery, 9 are continuously and 4 are currently disease-free. There was a trend toward better prognosis associated with minimal volume disease and teratoma at late relapse and relapse in the chest.

Conclusions.—Chemotherapy after late relapse does not appear to compensate for inadequate retroperitoneal lymph node dissection in the initial management of patients with clinical stage 1 testicular cancer. Therefore, precise surgical technique may be most predictive of the avoidance of late retroperitoneal relapse in these patients.

▶ Fortunately, late relapse of testis cancer is a rare event, especially in cases of clinical stage 1 disease. When recurrence does occur more than 2 years after diagnosis, this tumor that is typically responsive to multimodal therapy often becomes recalcitrant. Although the most common site of late relapses is in the retroperitoneum, the chest, liver, and neck must also be followed as well. This series provides further indictment of the use of primary observation for clinical stage 1 tumors.

M.S. Litwin, M.D., M.P.H.

Diagnosis and Follow-Up of Testicular Carcinoma In Situ by DNA Image Cytometry

Heidenreich A, Zumbé J, Engelmann UH (Univ of Cologne, Germany)
Eur Urol 28:13–18, 1995   26–4

Introduction.—Carcinoma in situ (CIS) of the testis is considered to be a precursor of all forms of germ-cell cancer other than spermatocytic seminoma. The diagnosis is based on light microscopic study of a testicular biopsy, but 2 recent cases were discovered by aspiration DNA image cytometry in azoospermic patients.

Cases.—Fifty infertile patients had both operative testicular biopsy and aspiration biopsy as part of an effort to evaluate spermatogenesis. In 2 patients CIS was diagnosed when DNA image cytometric analysis of the aspiration biopsy specimen revealed a typical aneuploid cell population consistent with malignancy. One of the patients had bilateral CIS, and 1 had embryonal carcinoma with CIS in the contralateral testis. The latter patient received local radiotherapy, and follow-up aspiration biopsy showed no haploid cells; the findings were consistent with the Sertoli-cell-only syndrome. The patient with bilateral CIS received no treatment, and continued to exhibit an aneuploid cell population. No invasive cancer developed within 4 years of initial diagnosis.

Conclusion.—The use of DNA image cytometry, applied to aspiration biopsies of the testis, is a sensitive means of detecting CIS, and also is a useful and minimally invasive means of following patients regardless of whether they are given radiotherapy.

▶ One obstacle to routine screening in patients at high risk for CIS is that surgical biopsy is invasive and not inexpensive. The authors confirm that DNA flow cytometry can establish the diagnosis of CIS, and it should be as accurate as surgical biopsy because CIS is a diffuse process that affects the entire testis. Although this could lead to more widespread screening if routinely adopted, its value might be even greater in patients known to have CIS who require follow-up. However, considerably more experience will be necessary to determine the extent to which the information obtained by a "minimally invasive" needle aspiration and flow cytometry can replace, or even complement the information obtained by what is now standard—the *noninvasive* ultrasound of the testis.

D.A. Swanson, M.D.

Evaluation of Reproductive Capacity in Germ Cell Tumor Patients Following Treatment With Cisplatin, Etoposide, and Bleomycin

Stephenson WT, Poirier SM, Rubin L, Einhorn LH (Indiana Univ, Indianapolis; Univ of Utah, Salt Lake City)
J Clin Oncol 13:2278–2280, 1995

26–5

Background.—First-line chemotherapy with cisplatin, etoposide (VP-16), and bleomycin ($PVP_{16}B$) has been found to be more effective and less toxic than cisplatin, vinblastine, and bleomycin (PVB) in patients with germ cell tumors. However, the incidence of infertility after $PVP_{16}B$ chemotherapy has not been thoroughly investigated.

Methods.—Thirty patients who had had chemotherapy with 2–4 cycles of $PVP_{16}B$ underwent a single semen analysis 24–78 months after chemotherapy was begun. All the patients were continuously free of disease. Eight had also had nerve-sparing retroperitoneal lymph node dissection.

Findings.—The patients had a median sperm concentration of 33.9 × 10^6. The median volume was 3.2 mL, and the median total sperm count was 86.4 × 10^6. Forty-three percent of the patients had oligospermia. Six of these 13 patients, or 20%, were azoospermic. The incidence of morphologically abnormal sperm was high. Only 1 patient had more than 50% normal spermatozoa. Only 43% of the patients had sperm motility exceeding 50%. Semen antisperm IgG was positive in 5 patients. Eight patients, including 3 with documented oligospermia, fathered children.

Conclusions.—A substantial risk for persistent semen abnormalities is associated with $PVP_{16}B$ chemotherapy in patients with germ cell tumors. However, some patients with oligospermia seem to recovery slowly, and others are still able to father children despite continued oligospermia.

▶ Most patients with germ cell testis tumors are oligospermic even before therapy, but chemotherapy makes it worse. This study, although based on a relatively small number of patients, supports the concept that higher doses and more courses of chemotherapy produce a higher incidence of oligospermia and azoospermia. However, because some patients with oligospermia can father children, anything that potentially reduces the amount of chemotherapy might have a positive impact on fertility. For example, if nerve-sparing retroperitoneal lymph node dissection were integrated into the therapeutic plan for patients with clinical stages I and II nonseminomatous germ cell testicular tumor, it might limit the amount of chemotherapy needed for cure.

D.A. Swanson, M.D.

A Review of Scrotal Violation in Testicular Cancer: Is Adjuvant Local Therapy Necessary?

Capelouto CC, Clark PE, Ransil BJ, Loughlin KR (Brigham and Women's Hosp, Boston; Beth Israel Hosp, Boston)
J Urol 153:981–985, 1995   26–6

Background.—Patients with suspected testicular cancer are conventionally managed by high inguinal orchiectomy. Nonstandard measures, termed "scrotal violations," include scrotal orchiectomy, open testicular biopsy, and fine-needle aspiration. These approaches have traditionally been assumed to compromise the outlook, and those managed in this way frequently undergo morbid or disfiguring local treatment. In addition, they usually are excluded from surveillance protocols.

Objective.—To determine whether these patients require adjuvant local treatment, a meta-analysis was performed that included 1,182 patients, 976 of whom were managed by standard radical inguinal orchiectomy. In the remaining 206 patients, there was a scrotal violation.

Findings.—Distant recurrences developed in 11.5% of patients who had inguinal orchiectomy and 12.7% of patients who had scrotal violation. The respective survival rates were 91.5% and 92.7%. Neither difference was statistically significant. Local recurrences were more prevalent in scrotal violation cases (2.9% vs. 0.4%). Comparable results were obtained when patients with stage I disease and those with seminoma were separately analyzed. Among patients subjected to scrotal violation, there were no significant differences in outcome between those given local adjuvant treatment and the others.

Conclusion.—Although the authors do not recommend scrotal orchiectomy as an approach to testicular cancer, scrotal violation does not in itself significantly compromise the outlook. When violation takes place, close monitoring may suffice unless there has been gross tumor spillage.

▶ The advantage of inguinal orchiectomy as opposed to scrotal orchiectomy in testis cancer is that surgical manipulation immediately adjacent to the tumor is minimized. This tends to minimize the risk of cutting into the tumor and spilling tumor in the operative wound. This meta-analysis is consistent with our experience at Indiana University.[1] The final lesson is that although scrotal orchiectomy increases the ultimate chance of patients requiring more intensive therapy such as chemotherapy, it has a minimal effect on the overall chance of cure.

R.S. Foster, M.D.

Reference

1. Leibovitch I, Baniel J, Foster RS, et al: The clinical implications of procedural deviations during orchiectomy for nonseminomatous testis cancer. *J Urol* 154:935–939, 1995.

Occupational Exposure to Extreme Temperature and Risk of Testicular Cancer
Zhang Z-F, Vena JE, Zielezny M, Graham S, Haughey BP, Brasure J, Marshall JR (Mem Sloan-Kettering Cancer Ctr, New York; State Univ of New York, Buffalo)
Arch Environ Health 50:13–18, 1995   26–7

Introduction.—The most common cancer of young men is testicular cancer. Risk factors of testicular cancer include cryptorchidism, inguinal hernias, genital trauma, mumps, orchitis, and selected genetic factors. Demographic risks include living in a rural area, marital status, religion, upper socioeconomic status, and "white collar" occupations. The extra-abdominal position of the testes also makes them susceptible to changes in environmental temperature. Whether occupational temperature is a risk factor of testicular cancer was determined.

Methods.—A total of 250 white males older than 15 years with confirmed testicular cancer were interviewed. Controls were from the neighborhood of the study patients. The interview was detailed, and information was collected about demographics, occupation, nutrition, medical history, residence, and other risk factors. The process took 1.5 hours. The individuals were asked in detail about exposure to extreme occupational temperatures. There were also questions regarding potential confounding variables such as illnesses with high fever; exposure to fumes, or smoke, fertilizers, or phenols; fertility problems; and atrophic testes.

Results.—Low occupational temperature ($\leq 60°F$) was associated with an odds ratio of 1.84 for testicular cancer and high occupational temperature ($\geq 80°F$) was associated with an odds ratio of 1.68. If the patient was exposed to extreme occupational temperature, ($\leq 60°F$ or $\geq 80°F$), the odds ratio was 2.25. When 16 potential confounding variables were controlled, the odds ratio of testicular cancer was 1.71 for exposure to extreme temperatures, 1.20 for exposure to high temperature, and 1.70 for exposure to low temperature.

Conclusion.—When multiple confounding variables are controlled for, the exposure to high, low, or both extremes of occupational temperature is associated with an increased risk of testicular cancer. Long durations of exposure, which may occur in the occupational setting, appear to affect this temperature-sensitive organ. Knowing that occupational temperatures can affect the testes offers 1 direction to pursue in the primary prevention of testicular cancer.

▶ I have an inherent distrust of this type of methodology. Self-reporting of exposure to extreme temperatures may have very little to do with the actual temperature within the testis itself. Experimentally, temperature clearly has an effect on spermatogenesis. The hypothesis that temperature may have an effect on the development of germ cell neoplasia is therefore very reasonable. However, because of the limitations of this type of methodology, I will not begin telling my patients to avoid working in an environment associated with extremes of temperature as defined in this paper.

R.S. Foster, M.D.

A Surveillance Study of Clinical Stage I Nonseminomatous Germ Cell Tumors of the Testis: 10-Year Followup

Nicolai N, Pizzocaro G (Istituto Nazionale Tumori, Milan, Italy)
J Urol 154:1045–1049, 1995

26–8

Introduction.—Men with clinical stage I nonseminomatous germ-cell tumors of the testis either undergo retroperitoneal node dissection or have orchiectomy alone and are closely watched. Surveillence has become more popular as risk factors such as vascular invasion have been identified, but the nerve-sparing technique of retroperitoneal adenopathy now is an option.

Objective.—Surveillance results were examined in 85 consecutive patients with nonseminomatous germ-cell tumors who were clinically normal after orchiectomy alone. The patients were recruited in 1981–1984 and were followed up for at least 10 years. Bipedal lymphangiography, ab-

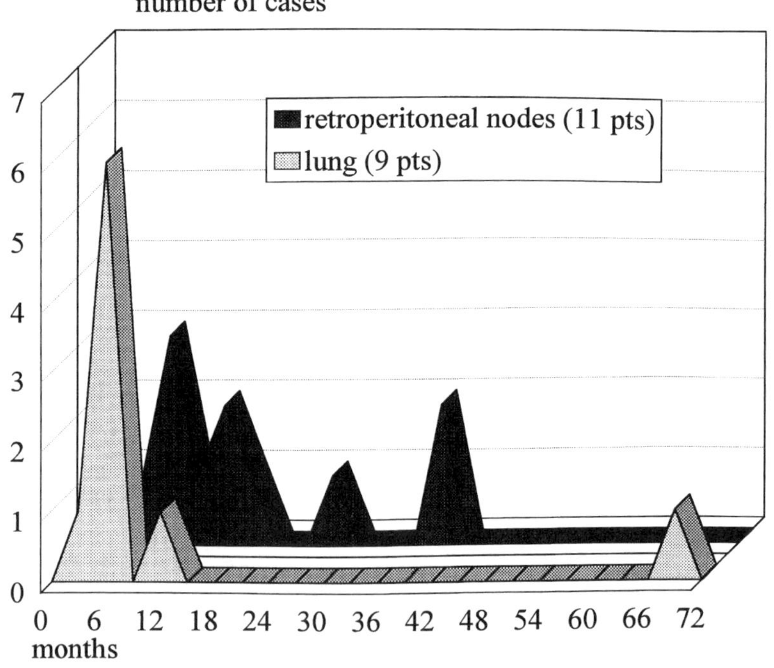

FIGURE 2.—Months at diagnosis of first relapse according to site in 20 patients with retroperitoneal or lung metastases only (*P* = 0.016, Mann-Whitney rank sum test). (Courtesy of Nicolai N, Pizzocaro G: A surveillance study of clinical stage I nonseminomatous germ cell tumors of the testis: 10-year followup. *J Urol* 154:1045–1049, 1995.)

dominal scans, and serum tumor marker estimates all were normal at baseline. A large majority of patients had had orchiectomy elsewhere. The median follow-up interval was 11 years.

Observations.—Twenty-five patients (29%) had relapses a median of 7 months after orchiectomy, 19 of them within the first year. About three fourths of relapses involved only the retroperitoneal nodes or the lung. The tumor-free interval differed with the site of relapse (Fig 2). Seven relapses (28%) were preceded by an elevation of α-fetoprotein or β-human chorionic gonadotropin. Embryonal carcinoma correlated with metastasis.

Current Status.—All but 3 of the 82 patients (96.5%) presently are free of disease. Most patients who relapsed received cisplatin-based chemotherapy, with or without subsequent surgery. Three patients (3.5%) died of disease, and 2 patients had secondary malignancies.

Suggestions.—Surveillance may be considered for good-risk stage I patients, but compliance with long-term follow-up must be ensured. High-risk patients may undergo nerve-sparing retroperitoneal lymphadenectomy, or may receive 2 courses of cisplatin-based chemotherapy. Definitive risk-benefit estimates will require studies that compare treatments in stratified-risk patients.

▶ Late recurrence of testicular cancer (greater than 2 years) has a much poorer prognosis compared with early recurrence. One of the fears of managing clinical stage I patients with surveillance has been late recurrence. This important paper provides 10-year follow-up of a group of patients managed by surveillance. It has become clear in clinical stage I nonseminoma that nerve-sparing retroperitoneal lymph node dissection and surveillance yield roughly equivalent results in the short-term. The decision as to which therapy to pursue is patient and physician dependent, however. Therefore, clinical stage I patients should be offered a choice of either surveillance or nerve-sparing retroperitoneal lymph node dissection.

R.S. Foster, M.D.

Secondary Tumours Following Etoposide Containing Therapy for Germ Cell Cancer

Boshoff C, Begent RHJ, Oliver RTD, Rustin GJ, Newlands ES, Andrews R, Skelton M, Holden L, Ong J (Royal London Hosp; Royal Free Hosp, London; Charing Cross Hosp, London; et al)
Ann Oncol 6:35–40, 1995   26–9

Background.—The regimen of cisplatin, etoposide, and bleomycin (BEP) is widely used in the management of metastatic germ cell cancer, based upon results of a randomized study comparing BEP with cisplatin, vinblastine, and bleomycin (PVB). Yet reports of secondary leukemia after chemotherapy including etoposide have raised questions about the wisdom of prescribing BEP rather than the more toxic and generally less efficacious PVB. A group of patients treated with etoposide for germ cell cancer was reviewed to determine the incidence of secondary cancer.

Methods.—At Charing Cross Hospital the POMB/ACE regimen, which incorporates 7 of the most active agents in germ cell cancer, has been used since 1978. The 679 patients whose records were reviewed received either the POMB/ACE regimen at Charing Cross Hospital (50.5%) or a regimen containing etoposide, platinum, and bleomycin at the Royal London Hospital (49.5%). The period reviewed extended from January 1979 until December 1992. Median follow-up for patients who were still alive was 68 months.

Results.—All but 31 of the 679 patients were available for follow-up; 529 were alive and 109 had died. Six patients treated with etoposide for germ cell cancer subsequently had acute myeloid leukemia (tAML) diagnosed. The median interval between the start of combination chemotherapy and the development of leukemia was 27 months. None of these patients had a primary mediastinal germ cell tumor, and only 1 had received previous radiotherapy. Four of the 6 cases exhibited the FAB M4 morphology. There were 4 solid cancers in addition to the cases of leukemia: squamous carcinomas of the lung, larynx, and esophagus, and melanoma.

Conclusion.—The relative risk of developing tAML was 150 for these men with germ cell cancer who were treated with etoposide as part of a combined regimen. Two of the patients had received more than 2,000 mg/m^2, but 4 had received a lower dose of etoposide. Overall, the benefits of protocols containing etoposide outweigh the risk of leukemia in patients with intermediate- or high-risk disease. For patients with low-risk disease, other regimens should be considered.

▶ Etoposide is clearly associated with secondary leukemia. This effect appears to be dose related. In poor-risk disseminated germ cell cancer, use of etoposide-containing regimens is justified to achieve disease control. In lower volume "good-risk" disease where alternative therapies are available (retroperitoneal lymph node dissection or different chemotherapeutic regimens), consideration should be given to avoiding the use of etoposide. However, because the leukemogenic effect is dose related, leukemogenesis in good-risk patients treated with etoposide is not a strong consideration because these patients characteristically receive lower doses. Nonetheless, this paper illustrates an important principle in oncology: As the probability of cure increases, side effects of therapy assume greater importance.

R.S. Foster, M.D.

27 The Penis

Priapism, Its Incidence and Seasonal Distribution in Finland
Kulmala RV, Lehtonen TA, Tammela TLJ (Univ of Tampere, Finland; Univ of Helsinki)
Scand J Urol Nephrol 29:93–96, 1995   27–1

Objective.—Priapism is an abnormal penile erection that is painful, persistent (longer than 6 hours), and not associated with sexual interest. The incidence of this rare disease, however, has not been reported. All cases of priapism in a homogeneous white population in Finland were analyzed to determine incidence.

Patients.—The records of white patients discharged from hospitals in Finland since 1967 with the diagnosis of priapism were studied. Patient characteristics, such as age, district of residence, and treatment with intracorporeal injections of vasoactive drugs for impotence, were also analyzed.

Results.—The incidence rate of priapism between 1975 and 1990 ranged from 0.3 to 1.1 cases/100,000 men/year (193 cases were recorded). This rate was stable during the entire period if cases caused by intracorporeal injections of vasoactive drugs were eliminated from the analysis. The average age of the patients with priapism was 43.5 years, and most patients were seen in eastern and central Finland. A significantly higher incidence of priapism was noted in the lightest 6 months of the year (March to August) than the darker months (September to February). The higher incidence during the lighter months may correlate with increased production of sex hormones during this time.

Conclusions.—Priapism is uncommon in whites in Finland. The incidence of priapism, however, remained stable for 16 years, and the disorder is more common during the lighter months of the year.

▶ This paper is of modest interest because, as the authors state, it is the only publication on the incidence of priapism. This investigation and, indeed, similar studies are possible in Finland and Denmark in particular, because of the excellent compulsory medical reporting system in those countries and the relatively small populations. Of course, the figures would be very difficult for a nation such as the United States, which has a significant black population. The fact that the frequency is higher during the lighter months is intriguing, but the rationale presented by the authors is completely speculative. There are many other possible explanations.

S.S. Howards, M.D.

Value of Magnetic Resonance Imaging in Patients With Penile Induration (Peyronie's Disease)
Vosshenrich R, Schroeder-Printzen I, Weidner W, Fischer U, Funke M, Ringert R-H (Univ Hosp, Göttingen, Germany)
J Urol 153:1122–1125, 1995   27–2

Background.—Peyronie's disease is characterized by the formation of fibrotic plaque in the tunica albuginea, erection pain, and potential loss of erection. It is typically diagnosed by the detection of a palpable plaque. High-resolution sonography is useful in determining the extent and location of the plaques. Magnetic resonance imaging is another noninvasive diagnostic procedure that produces precise imaging of the penile anatomy. The value of MRI was compared prospectively with palpation and high resolution sonography in the evaluation of patients who had Peyronie's disease.

Methods.—Thirty-four patients who had clinically suspected Peyronie's disease were evaluated with palpation, sonography, and MRI performed 5–10 minutes after intracavernous injection of 10 µg prostaglandin E[1]. Patients underwent MRI before and after the administration of gadolinium-diethylenetriaminepentaacetic acid (Gd-DTPA). Sonography was performed during the tumescence period.

Results.—Forty-five plaques were palpable. There was sonographic evidence of 30 plaques; 28 appeared as dense hyperechoic structures. Eight calcified plaques had a hyperechoic structure with an acoustic shadowing. Magnetic resonance imaging revealed 36 palpable lesions, a nonsignificant difference in detection from palpation and sonography. The lesions appeared as a thickening or irregularity of the tunica albuginea with a low-intensity plaque protruding into the corpus cavernosum. After administration of Gd-DTPA, 4 additional lesions, not detected by palpation or sonography, were found, which suggested questionable local inflammatory activity.

Conclusions.—Magnetic resonance imaging does not significantly improve the detection of fibrous plaques in patients who have Peyronie's disease and may provide questionable evidence of inflammatory changes when contrast is used. The combination of clinical examination and sonography should therefore be considered the preferred methods of diagnosis and follow-up.

▶ This paper presents a negative study. The authors appropriately conclude that MRI does not provide significantly more information than ultrasonography in patients who have Peyronie's disease. The finding is not unexpected but is useful in that it may prevent others from doing similar investigations or using this technique in clinical practice. Magnetic resonance imaging is very expensive. We almost never use MRI for Peyronie's plaques, because it is easy to make the diagnosis by history and physical examination, and imaging does not change our therapeutic approach.

S.S. Howards, M.D.

Evolving Concepts in the Diagnosis and Treatment of Arterial High Flow Priapism
Hakim LS, Kulaksizoglu H, Mulligan R, Greenfield A, Goldstein I (Boston Univ)
J Urol 155:541–548, 1996   27–3

Introduction.—Arterial high flow priapism occurs when an arterial-lacunar fistula from a lacerated cavernous artery caused by blunt or penetrating perineal or penile trauma allows blood to flow unabated through the erectile tissue. Limited study has been done on the diagnosis and treatment of arterial priapism. Two evolving concepts in the treatment of these patients were investigated: duplex Doppler ultrasound for diagnosis and watchful waiting as an alternative therapeutic option.

Methods.—Ten patients who had high flow arterial priapism were evaluated with concomitant perineal duplex Doppler ultrasonography and selective internal pudendal arteriography as the initial diagnostic procedure, as well as after initial embolization and before and after repeat embolization. The sensitivity and specificity of perineal duplex Doppler ultrasonography in the detection of a recurrent arterial-lacunar fistula were evaluated in comparison with follow-up physical examination. The ability of penile duplex Doppler ultrasonography to detect resolution of the autologous clot was examined. Morbidity and potency were evaluated in cases managed with watchful waiting by interviewing patients, reviewing medical records, and/or performing erectile function testing.

Results.—Twenty-one of the 24 concomitant initial diagnostic studies (88%) were in agreement. Of the 31 follow-up concomitant studies, 28 (90%) were in agreement. Normal bilateral antegrade cavernous artery flow was detected with penile duplex Doppler ultrasonography in 4 of 6 patients who underwent selective embolization. Four of these 6 patients had recurrent priapism, and 3 had changes in the quality of erection compared with premorbid levels. Of the 5 patients managed with watchful waiting, there were no morbidities aside from the annoyance of chronic erections, and potency was maintained during follow-up for up to 31 years.

Conclusions.—Perineal duplex Doppler ultrasonography is accurate in the internal pudendal arteriography findings in patients who have arterial priapism, with a sensitivity of 100% and a specificity of 73%. In documenting resolution of the arterial-lacunar fistula, this method has a sensitivity of 75% and specificity of 100%. Expectant management may have a role in the treatment of arterial priapism in sexually active men, as long as good erectile function and potency are maintained.

▶ These authors from Boston University have been leaders in the clinical evaluation and management of penile arterial disease. The topic of this paper is arterial high flow priapism, which is not to be confused with the more common high flow priapism. All these patients had a history of blunt trauma followed by prolonged priapism. The authors convincingly demonstrate that, in their expert hands, duplex Doppler ultrasound is comparable to the much more invasive arteriography as a diagnostic tool. In 3 cases in which there was disagreement between the 2 diagnostic techniques, the clinical situation correlated better with the ultrasonographic findings than with the arteriogram. The second point of the paper, that expectant management is safe, also seems to be substantiated by their experience. However, we recommend, and our patients prefer, a more aggressive approach using transcatheter embolization of autologous blood clots.

S.S. Howards, M.D.

The Nesbit Operation for Peyronie's Disease: 16-Year Experience
Ralph DJ, Al-Akraa M, Pryor JP (St Peter's Hosp, London)
J Urol 154:1362–1363, 1995   27–4

Objective.—The long-term outcome of patients who underwent the Nesbit operation to correct penile deformity resulting from Peyronie's disease was reported.

Patients and Methods.—Three hundred fifty-nine patients, aged 20–71 years, underwent the Nesbit operation between 1977 and 1992. Peyronie's disease had been present in all patients for at least 1 year, and penetration and coitus were difficult or impossible. The mean deformity angle was 68 degrees and the mean width of the ellipse of excised tunica was 7 mm. In 89% of patients, a single ellipse was excised; double ellipses were required in 10%, and multiple ellipses in 1%. Results were judged excellent when penile deformity was less than 10 degrees and erection and coitus were normal. Those with satisfactory outcome had a penile deformity of 10–30 degrees; erection was impaired, but coitus was possible.

Results.—Results were excellent or satisfactory in 295 patients, and the success rate of the procedure was improved in those treated after 1985. Forty-one patients experienced 61 complications, including urethral injury in 5, urinary retention in 5, and urinary infection in 2. Simple suture and catheterization managed the urethral injuries. Seventeen patients had significant penile shortening, and 1 required a penile lengthening procedure. Six patients underwent a repeat Nesbit operation, and 6 subsequently required a penile prosthesis.

Conclusion.—In this series of patients treated with the Nesbit operation for Peyronie's disease, 66% had an excellent result and 16% a satisfactory result. Most of the patients with a poor outcome before 1985 had impaired erectile capacity before surgery and should have received a penile prosthesis. Although some penile shortening is inevitable with the Nesbit operation, coital function is not affected.

▶ This paper documents very good results from the Nesbit procedure for the treatment of Peyronie's disease. The success rate after 1985 was 90%, which coincides with our experience. We use the Nesbit approach whenever possible and reserve plaque excision for very severe cases. Many types of grafting have been recommended for these patients. Dr. Tom Lue has recently recommended the use of venous grafts (see Abstract 25–8). The authors point out that many of their early patients in whom the procedure failed had inadequate erections; they now place a prosthesis for this group of patients. We do the same. It would have been helpful if the authors had told us how many patients had prostheses placed and/or plaque excision during the study period.

S.S. Howards, M.D.

Long-term Followup of Treatment of Peyronie's Disease With Plaque Incision, Carbon Dioxide Laser Plaque Ablation and Placement of a Deep Dorsal Vein Patch Graft
Kim ED, McVary KT (Northwestern Univ, Chicago)
J Urol 153:1843–1846, 1995   27–5

Introduction.—A number of operative procedures have been used to correct the fibrotic penile curvature characteristic of Peyronie's disease. Patients who have remained potent frequently do not wish to have a prosthesis implanted. Plication often is an inadequate approach to a large plaque.

Patients.—Seven patients aged 49–65 years, who had Peyronie's disease were included. The plaque was incised and ablated with the CO_2 laser, and a deep dorsal vein patch graft was placed. The status of 6 patients who were potent before surgery was followed 31 months on average after treatment.

Technique.—The penile root is delivered through an inguinoscrotal incision. The plaque is defined after an artificial saline-induced erection. The superficial layer of Buck's fascia is incised, and emissary and circumflex branches are then ligated or excised. The deep dorsal vein is removed from a site 1 cm proximal to the glans to near the pubic bone, and tributary veins are ligated. The dorsal neurovascular bundle is mobilized only if a transverse incision is needed to treat the plaque. Some patients require multiple incisions with grafting. Plaque substance is evaporated from its underside using the CO_2 laser. Finally, the harvested vein is opened, trimmed, and sutured to the edges so that its endothelial surface contacted spongy tissue.

Results.—The abnormal curvature was totally straightened in 4 of the 6 patients, but 2 of them had relapse to some extent. All patients remained potent and continued to have satisfactory erections. All patients but 1 claimed satisfactory intercourse. Voiding problems resolved in 2 patients. Three patients described a mild diminution in penile sensation.

Conclusion.—Combining plaque incision using the CO_2 laser with placement of a deep dorsal vein patch graft corrects the penile curvature in many patients who have Peyronie's disease and at the same time preserves potency.

▶ This is a small series with excellent results. All 6 patients remained potent. There is no way to determine whether this result is related to the skill of the surgeons or the use of lasers. More extensive trials in multiple groups will be necessary to make this determination. Vein grafting, rather than dermal or tunica vaginalis grafting, is currently in vogue. We very infrequently find it necessary to incise or excise the plaque, but the surgeon must have a technique for dealing with these complicated cases.

S.S. Howards, M.D.

Penetrating Trauma to the Penis: Functional Results
Goldman HB, Dmochowski RR, Cox CE (Univ of Tennessee, Memphis)
J Urol 155:551–553, 1996   27–6

Introduction.—Injuries involving penetration of the penis are rare. In these cases, the management goals are maintenance of function, restoration of urethral integrity, and preservation of cosmetic appearance. The functional and cosmetic results were reviewed in a series of patients who had penetrating penile trauma.

Methods.—The charts of 26 patients who had penetrating penile injuries treated between 1990 and 1994 were reviewed. The mechanism of injury, physical findings, urinalysis results, radiographic findings, associated injuries, surgical findings, and postoperative cosmetic and functional results were analyzed.

Results.—Twenty injuries were caused by handguns, 5 by shotguns, and 1 by stabbing. The sites of injury included the penile shaft in 22, the glans in 2, and the foreskin only in 2. Twenty patients had other associated injuries, most of which were in close proximity to the penis. Blood was found at the meatus in 3 of the 4 patients who had urethral injuries and in 1 of the 22 patients who did not have urethral injury. All 4 urethral injuries were evident with physical examination; 2 involved the glanular urethra, and 2 involved the distal urethra. Retrograde urethrograms were obtained for 21 patients, and contrast medium extravasation was seen in 3. Fifteen patients had corporeal body injuries. Sixteen patients underwent surgical exploration, and all corporeal and glanular urethral injuries in this group were repaired. One patient who had a close-range shotgun injury required multiple reconstructions. The condition of 1 patient who had a urethral injury became unstable during surgery; healing occurred by secondary intent after only Foley and suprapubic catheters were placed. The status of 16 patients was followed. All 11 patients who had corporeal body injuries in the follow-up group, all 9 patients injured with handguns, and the 2 patients who had minimal shotgun injuries had satisfactory erectile function. The 2 patients with close-range shotgun injuries had some erectile dysfunction at follow-up. Ten of the 11 patients considered the cosmetic results satisfactory.

Conclusions.—Penetrating penile injuries can generally be treated surgically with good functional and cosmetic results. Only cases involving close-range shotgun blasts that cause massive tissue destruction appear to have poor outcomes. Urethral injury should be ruled out with retrograde urethrography, and many patients will require surgical exploration to rule out or repair corporeal injury. Minimal or superficial wounds, however, may be adequately managed nonoperatively.

▶ This is the largest civilian series of penetrating wounds of the penis in the literature. Salvatierra et al. reported similar findings in 41 patients who had penetrating penile injuries during the Vietnam War (Management of urologic injuries. *West J Medicine* 122: 257–261, 1975). It is encouraging that the results are so good. The authors suggest that routine retrograde urethrograms may not be necessary, because they have only 1 patient with a urethral injury who did not have blood at the meatus. We would disagree. A retrograde urethrogram is easy to obtain, and, in most practices, these wounds are very infrequent. It would be unfortunate to miss an occult urethral injury.

S.S. Howards, M.D.

Outcome Prediction in Patients With Fournier's Gangrene
Laor E, Palmer LS, Tolia BM, Reid RE, Winter HI (Albert Einstein College, Bronx, NY)
J Urol 154:89–92, 1995   27–7

Background.—Despite advances in modern intensive care techniques and antibiotic treatment, the mortality rate associated with Fournier's gangrene continues to be as high as 50%. Possible prognosticators of outcome were determined.

Methods and Findings.—Thirty patients who had Fournier's gangrene and were treated during a 15-year period were included. Thirteen patients died. Survivors were significantly younger than those who died (mean age, 53 vs. 71 years). Admission laboratory parameters significantly associated with outcome were levels of hematocrit, blood urea nitrogen, calcium, albumin, alkaline phosphatase, and cholesterol. Outcome was also associated with white blood count and levels of platelets, potassium, bicarbonate, blood urea nitrogen, total protein, albumin, and lactic dehydrogenase 1 week after hospitalization. Nonsurvivors did not have a significantly different mean extent of involved body surface area than did survivors. Outcome was apparently unaffected by the number of surgical debridements. Compared with nonsurvivors, survivors had a lower mean Fournier's gangrene severity index, which was created by modifying the acute physiology and chronic health evaluation II severity score. These values were 6.9 for survivors and 13.5 for nonsurvivors. The index was highly correlated with mortality rate. The probability of death was 75% in those who had an index score greater than 9, and the probability of survival was 78% in those who had an index score of 9 or less.

Conclusions.—The most important general parameter in predicting outcome of patients who have Fournier's gangrene is deviation from homeostasis at initial examination. The Fournier's gangrene severity index, determined on admission, is an objective method for quantifying the extent of metabolic aberration and is useful for predicting outcome.

▶ Fournier's gangrene remains a very serious problem that most of us see from time to time. The authors' conclusion that the more severe the disease and the older the patient, the worse the prognosis seems self-evident, in spite of a debate in the literature regarding severity. Fournier first described the entity in 1883.[1] The clinical presentation is usually an early period of genital discomfort with fever, which progresses to the classic condition we all recognize, such as crepitus and a feculent odor. Most patients have a predisposing illness. We believe in early aggressive management with antibiotics and debridement. In addition, hyperbaric oxygen may be useful.

S.S. Howards, M.D.

Reference

1. Fournier AJ: Grangrene foudroyante de la verge. *Semaine Med* 3:345, 1883.

Radiation-induced Decrease in Nitric Oxide Synthase–containing Nerves in the Rat Penis
Carrier S, Hricak H, Lee S-S, Baba K, Morgan DM, Nunes L, Ross GY, Phillips TL, Lue TF (Univ of California, San Francisco)
Radiology 195:95–99, 1995   27–8

Objective.—There are many possible causes of erectile dysfunction after prostatic radiation therapy. To understand radiation-induced impotence further, several factors associated with erectile dysfunction after prostatic irradiation in the rat, including changes in nitric oxide–containing nerves in the penis, were examined.

Methods.—Three groups of adult male Sprague-Dawley rats were studied: 15 rats received no radiation (control), 15 rats were exposed to a radiation dose of 1,000 cGy (low-dose group), and 17 rats were exposed to a radiation dose of 2,000 cGy (high-dose group). Apomorphine was administered 5 months after irradiation to evaluate centrally mediated erection. Peripheral and pharmacologic erection were studied by cavernous nerve stimulation and reaction to papaverine. Proximal-shaft penile segments were stained at the completion of the study to determine the numbers of nitric oxide synthase–containing nerve fibers and cavernous smooth muscle fibers.

Results.—The number of erections in the apomorphine study was significantly lower in the high- and low-dose groups (0.6 and 2.5, respectively) than in control animals (4.5). Because apomorphine acts centrally and the radiation was delivered peripherally, these results suggest an impairment of the erectile pathway at the periphery. Significant differences in mean maximal intracavernous pressure were also noted. Mean pressure decreased from 104.8 cm H_2O in the control group to 19.7 cm H_2O in the high-dose group. The decrease in intracavernous pressure in the low-dose group, but not that in the high-dose, was eliminated by papaverine. These results suggest that damage of the smooth muscle of the corpus cavernosum is involved in erectile dysfunction after high-dose radiation, whereas nerve injury may play a stronger role in erectile dysfunction after low-dose radiation. Radiation also caused a dose-related reduction in nitric oxide synthase–containing fibers; 225.6 fibers in the control group compared with 156.3 in the low-dose group and 85.5 in the high-dose group. Radiation also decreased the number of cavernous smooth muscle fibers.

Conclusions.—Reduced erectile function after prostatic irradiation is caused by many factors, including damage to the nerves, arteries, and muscle.

▶ These authors are leading investigators of erectile dysfunction. They have provided us with many insights into the physiology of normal erection and the pathophysiology of erectile dysfunction. This paper extends their contribution to yet another aspect of the problem. The important clinical fact is that pelvic radiation causes a high incidence of impotence and is not necessarily, as some practitioners suggest, less morbid than surgery.

S.S. Howards, M.D.

28 Penile Cancer

Laser Treatment of Localized Squamous Cell Carcinoma of the Penis
Windahl T, Hellsten S (Örebro Med Ctr, Sweden; Gen Hosp, Malmö, Sweden)
J Urol 154:1020–1023, 1995   28–1

Background.—Traditionally, localized squamous cell carcinoma of the penis is treated with local excision or amputation with or without adjuvant radiotherapy and chemotherapy. However, recent studies have reported equally effective disease control with better cosmetic and functional results in patients treated with laser therapy. The efficacy of laser therapy was compared with that of conventional treatment in a series of patients with penile cancer.

Methods.—Between 1986 and 1994, 32 men with newly diagnosed squamous cell carcinoma of the penis were treated, 13 with conventional surgery and 19 with laser surgery. Indications for considering laser surgery were younger patients with carcinoma staged Tis to T2N0M0 and tumors less than 3 cm in diameter. Patients' ages ranged from 40 to 90 years (mean, 74 years) in the conventional surgery group and from 26 to 83 years (mean, 57 years) in the laser surgery group. Of the 19 patients in the laser therapy group, 8 were treated with only the carbon dioxide laser and 11 were treated with both the carbon dioxide (to excise macroscopic tumor or vaporize in situ cancer areas) and neodymium:yttrium-aluminum-garnet (Nd:YAG) lasers (to perform deep coagulation of the tumor bed). The patients in the laser group were reexamined with biopsies 3 months after treatment. The mean duration of follow-up was 35 months in the conventional surgery group and 31 months in the laser group.

Results.—All 19 patients in the laser group were survivors throughout follow-up, with no evidence of current disease, although 2 were retreated for recurrences. Only 5 of the 13 men in the conventional surgery group were long-term survivors, with 2 dying of cancer and 6 dying of cardiovascular disease. Four of these 6 patients had residual malignancy. Laser therapy produced a highly satisfactory cosmetic result, and all patients who were sexually active preoperatively maintained acceptable sexual function.

Conclusions.—Combined carbon dioxide and Nd:YAG laser therapy is effective in the management of stages Tis to T2N0M0, grades 1–2 penile squamous cell carcinoma. This therapy also has superior cosmetic and functional results and produces low morbidity rates.

▶ Patients treated by conventional surgery were a significantly higher risk group, as one might expect. The survival comparison is therefore meaningless. Nonetheless, the authors very nicely demonstrate that laser therapy can control small, low-grade primary tumors. The cosmetic result is excellent. This treatment is clearly an alternative to partial penectomy, especially in selected patients. My limited experience with radiotherapy for penile cancer suggests that laser therapy produces much more satisfactory cosmetic results with much less morbidity. Laser therapy should be considered in some of our patients with small tumors.

J.B. DeKernion, M.D.

Sentinel Lymph Node Dissection for Penile Carcinoma: The M.D. Anderson Cancer Center Experience
Pettaway CA, Pisters LL, Dinney CPN, Jularbal F, Swanson DA, von Eschenbach AC, Ayala A (Univ of Texas MD Anderson Cancer Ctr, Houston)
J Urol 154:1999–2003, 1995

28–2

Background.—Because approximately 20% of patients with invasive penile cancer and clinically negative inguinal lymph nodes subsequently have inguinal metastases, the management of these patients is controversial. Surgery is the most effective treatment for inguinal metastases, making early detection important. It has been proposed that there is a sentinel lymph node superomedial to the saphenofemoral junction and clustered about the superficial epigastric vein. The effectiveness of extended sentinel lymph node disssection in preventing subsequent metastatic disease was evaluated retrospectively.

Methods.—The records of 20 patients with penile squamous carcinoma who underwent extended sentinal lymph node dissection between 1985 and 1994 were reviewed. Extended sentinel lymph node dissection involved removal of all lymph node tissue medial to the saphenous vein between the inguinal ligament and superficial external pudendal vein. Patients with unilateral inguinal metastases underwent inguinal or ilioinguinal lymphadenectomy on the involved side and extended sentinel lymph node dissection on the contralateral side. The surgical specimens were evaluated histologically. All patients were followed for a median duration of 36 months (range, 13–117 months).

Results.—Of the 20 patients, extended sentinel lymph node dissection was performed bilaterally in 14 patients and unilaterally in 6. All the lymph nodes dissected were negative. Nevertheless, 5 patients had subsequent inguinal metastases ipsilateral to a negative extended sentinel lymph node dissection. All but 1 recurrence occurred within 1 year of dissection.

Conclusions.—Extended sentinel lymph node dissection had a 25% false-negative rate, possibly because of anatomical variation in the sentinel node position. Therefore, this procedure cannot be recommended for routine use.

▶ Sentinel node dissection has been shown to be unreliable. These authors showed that an extended sentinel node dissection is similarly unreliable. The entire concept should be abandoned once and for all. It is preferable to perform a total superficial groin dissection in patients without palpable nodes. This can easily be done with preservation of the main tributaries of the saphenous vein, leaving the deep femoral fascia intact over the vessels. It requires raising only a very small flap of skin and can be accomplished quickly. If a positive node is detected, it can easily be converted to a more extensive and definitive groin dissection.

J.B. DeKernion, M.D.

Penile Cancer: Is Lymphadenectomy Necessary in All Cases?
Srinivas V, Choudary R, Ravikumar R, Metha H, Kundargi P, Phadke AG
(Bombay Hosp, India; PD Hinduja Natl Hosp, Bombay, India)
Urology 46:710–712, 1995   28–3

Background.—Although the guidelines for managing the primary tumor in penile cancer are universally accepted, the management of regional lymph nodes is controversial. Records of patients with penile cancer seen by 1 physician during a 7-year period were retrospectively analyzed to learn whether lymphadenectomy is necessary in all cases of penile cancer and whether watchful waiting worsens the prognosis.

Methods.—All patients with initially clinically positive nodes underwent bilateral node dissection at the time of initial penectomy. Patients whose lymph nodes were initially clinically negative were seen monthly for follow-up; they underwent delayed lymphadenectomy only if the nodes became clinically positive.

Results.—Of the 36 patients (mean age, 58 years), 6 had a total penectomy, 29 had partial amputation, and 1 had radiotherapy. Of the 6 patients with total penectomy (all stage II, grade 2 or 3), 3 had positive groin nodes initially and underwent immediate node dissection. They all died within 3 years. Of the other 3 patients with initially clinically negative lymph nodes, 2 required delayed dissection. One died within a year and the other 2 are alive and well. Of the 6 patients with partial penile amputation and immediate lymphadenectomy for initially positive lymph nodes, 5 died within 10 months. Overall, of the 9 patients who initially had positive nodes and had immediate lymphadenectomy, 7 died of the disease. Of the 27 patients who initially had clinically negative lymph nodes, 17 have required follow-up only and 10 have had delayed lymphadenectomy. Of the 10 patients with delayed lymphadenectomy, 4 are alive and well, 3 have died, and 3 are lost to follow-up.

Conclusions.—Almost half the patients with penile cancer in this series did not require lymphadenectomy. Thus, lymphadenectomy may not be required in selected patients with penile cancer who agree to regular, close follow-up by the same physician.

▶ This is a small group of retrospectively studied patients with penile cancers. Of the 27 with initially negative groin nodes, 17 have never had recurrence and were spared lymphadenectomy. However, 10 patients required lymphadenectomy, and 3 have died. It is proper form to assume that the 3 patients who were lost to follow-up also died. One could turn the authors' argument around and say that rather having spared 17 patients an operation, some patients died who might have been cured by an early operation when the lymph nodes were small. A limited groin dissection is an easy operation to perform with low morbidity. We are more convinced that early node dissection is the best approach in patients with high-grade and/or invasive penile cancers and follow only the patients with very small, low-grade lesions, or those with some surgical risk factors.

J.B. DeKernion, M.D.

29 Hypospadias

Buccal Mucosal Urethral Replacement
Duckett JW, Coplen D, Ewalt D, Baskin LS (Children's Hosp of Philadelphia; St Louis Children's Hosp; Children's Med Ctr, Dallas; et al)
J Urol 153:1660–1663, 1995   29–1

Background.—Sometimes when hypospadiac repair fails there is not sufficient skin from the penis or preputial region to complete a secondary reconstruction. Extragenital skin and bladder mucosa are not satisfactory replacements, but promising early results have been achieved using buccal mucosa.

Patients.—Eighteen of more than 1,800 patients undergoing hypospadias repair and urethral reconstruction in an 8-year period lacked adequate local skin for urethroplasty. The patients, whose average age was 12 years, have been followed up for nearly 2 years on average after reconstruction. Twelve patients had had previous failed attempts at urethral reconstruction.

Technique.—As much as possible of the penile reconstruction is completed before harvesting buccal mucosa from the inner cheek. A full-thickness graft is dissected and fixed outside the body to remove excessive subcutaneous connective tissue. Most patients received a tubularized mucosal graft. The normal proximal urethra is fixed to the corporeal bodies, and a spatulated anastomosis with the buccal graft is made using the same suture. The distal graft is channeled through the glans by excising a core or onlayed onto the urethral strip and covered with the wings of the glans. The graft is tailored in place before closing the skin so as to ensure a good vascular supply.

Results.—Buccal mucosa was used in 12 complex hypospadiac repairs, 4 urethral interposition procedures for epispadias, and 2 urethral stricture repairs. Three patients have required further surgery. Meatal protrusion has not been a problem, but 5 patients (28%) had meatal stenosis and 2 of them required meatoplasty. One fistula developed after repairing a repeat hypospadiac procedure.

Conclusion.—Encouraging intermediate-term results have been achieved using buccal mucosa as a urethral replacement in patients with inadequate local skin.

▶ We and the authors, and most others prefer vascularized grafts whenever possible for the repair of hypospadias. It is extremely unusual that such tissue cannot be obtained. The authors who, because of their expertise and reputations must receive referrals of difficult cases, needed free grafts in only 1% of their patients. Bladder mucosal grafts have been popular, but there are problems with the neomeatus because of prolapse. The current vogue is to use buccal mucosa as reported in 1992 by Dessanti et al.[1] This abstract summarizes a series with satisfactory, if imperfect results, in these difficult cases. Six patients, or 33%, had either meatal stenosis or a fistula. Less experienced surgeons can anticipate a higher complication rate.

S.S. Howards, M.D.

Reference

1. Dessanti A, Rigamonti W, Merulla V, et al: Autologous buccal mucosa graft for hypospadias repair: An initial report. *J Urol* 147:1081–1084, 1992. (1993 Year Book of Urology, p 273.)

30 Pediatric Kidney

Outpatient Nephrectomy for Nonfunctioning Kidneys
Elder JS, Hladky D, Selzman AA (Case Western Reserve Univ, Cleveland, Ohio)
J Urol 154:712–715, 1995

30–1

Introduction.—Many pediatric urologic surgical procedures have become outpatient procedures. A novel approach to pediatric nephrectomy that can be safely performed on an outpatient basis was described.

Technique.—Patients are considered candidates for this surgical procedure if they are aged 4 months to 6 years and have a nonfunctioning kidney at least 3 cm long. After induction of general anesthesia, the patient is placed in the extended flank position. A regional block is usually performed. A 2.5-cm incision is made at the tip of the 12th rib and extended through the fascia until the retroperitoneum is identified. The kidney is grasped with an Allis clamp and mobilized into the wound. Any fluid is aspirated. The vascular pedicle and ureter are suture ligated. The kidney is removed, and the incision is closed. Children are discharged home after liquids are tolerated and they are comfortable.

Results.—From 1989 to 1994, 40 children, aged 4 months to 5 years, underwent outpatient nephrectomy at a hospital ambulatory surgical unit. The most common diagnosis was multicystic kidney disease. The kidney size ranged from 3 × 2 cm to 11.5 × 7.2 cm. The average operative time was 45 minutes with little blood loss or pain. Except for 1 child, all children were discharged on the same day. The 1 complication developed in a boy, aged 7 months, who had a multicystc kidney; the intraoperatively mobilized structure was determined to be a retrocecal appendix. Laparotomy and appendectomy were performed before nephrectomy, and the child was retained in the hospital overnight. There were no further complications. The average cost of the last 4 procedures was less than $5,500.

Conclusions.—A series of 40 pediatric patients underwent successful outpatient nephrectomy of a nonfunctioning kidney. The average duration of the surgery was 45 minutes, with little blood loss or pain. Discharge generally occurred on the day of surgery. These results justify a reexamination of the role of laparoscopic nephrectomy and nonsurgical management of nonfunctioning kidneys in pediatric patients.

▶ The authors have clearly demonstrated that, in their hands, outpatient nephrectomy for small nonfunctioning kidney is feasible. In the young child, there is very little postoperative pain after such a procedure. Therefore, as the authors suggest, there appears to be little reason to perform these operations laparoscopically. The question remains, however, whether most of the children needed any therapeutic procedure. We do not routinely remove multicystic kidneys and do not find the arguments relating to hypertension and malignant potential convincing.

S.S. Howards, M.D.

Outcome Analysis of Pediatric Pyeloplasty as a Function of Patient Age, Presentation and Differential Renal Function
Salem YH, Majd M, Rushton HG, Belman AB (George Washington Univ, Washington, DC)
J Urol 154:1889–1893, 1995
30–2

Introduction.—Dismembered pyeloplasty is the standard surgical treatment for ureteropelvic junction obstruction in children. There is considerable controversy, however, regarding the optimal time for surgical treatment and the optimal method of renal function assessment in neonates and young children. The outcome of pyeloplasty in children was analyzed to determine the prognostic importance of patient age, manner of presentation, and initial renal function.

Methods.—The charts of 98 patients who underwent pyeloplasty for the treatment of ureteropelvic junction obstruction in 100 kidneys were reviewed. Renal scans were done before and after surgery. Renal function and drainage was evaluated with diuretic renography. The patients were divided into groups according to preoperative differential renal function, age, and manner of presentation for analysis of outcome.

Results.—After surgery, differential renal function improved in 31% of the patients, remained stable in 68%, and deteriorated in 1%. A 5% or more increase in differential renal function occurred in similar proportions of all 4 age groups. A differential renal function improvement of at least 5% was most common in symptomatic patients, occurring in 50% of those who had an abdominal mass, 59% of those who had abdominal pain, and 36% of those who had a urinary tract infection. In contrast, asymptomatic patients, including those who had an abnormal prenatal sonogram (21%) or an incidentally discovered condition (9%), were less likely to show improvement. Improvement in differential renal function was seen in 11% of kidneys that had initial good function, 64% of those that had intermediate function, and 56% of those that had poor differential renal function at presentation. Of the 30 kidneys with postoperative functional improvement of more than 5%, 23 (77%) had a preoperative differential renal function of 40% or less. In logistic regression analysis of the 3 types of patient groups, only preoperative renal function was a statistically significant predictor of functional improvement after pyeloplasty.

Conclusions.—Pyeloplasty is highly successful for the treatment of ureteropelvic junction obstruction in neonates, infants, and children. It is particularly warranted in symptomatic patients and in those who have impaired renal function, regardless of age. Diuretic renography is a reliable method of evaluating renal function in patients of any age. Further study is needed to assess the value of pyeloplasty in asymptomatic children who have normal renal function.

▶ This is a thoughtful review of a significant number of pediatric patients who underwent pyeloplasty. Symptomatic patients who have ureteropelvic junction obstruction obviously require pyeloplasty. Almost everyone agrees that patients whose differential renal function deteriorates during observation should also undergo repair. For all other patients, however, there is no consensus. Although the authors state that all nonsymptomatic patients had a half-time of longer than 20 minutes, they do not give us their indications for surgery. Unlike some other authors, they did not find any effect of age on the potential for postoperative functional improvement. Some of their conclusions should be interpreted with caution. Of course, patients who have more than 40% differential function before surgery less frequently had a greater than 5% improvement, because it is unlikely that repair of an obstructed kidney would make it better (> 50%) than its mate. Also, although they make a big point of the different mean percent improvement in various groups, there is enormous overlap of the populations, so that the results in an individual appear unpredictable.

S.S. Howards, M.D.

Pediatric Laparoscopic Dismembered Pyeloplasty
Peters CA, Schlussel RN, Retik AB (Harvard Med School, Boston)
J Urol 153:1962–1965, 1995   30–3

Introduction.—The potential of pediatric laparoscopic surgery continues to evolve. The case of a boy who underwent dismembered laparoscopic pyeloplasty was reported.

> *Case Report.*—Boy, 7 years, had marked right hydronephrosis with calicectasis detected by abdominal ultrasound. He had no hematuria and did not complain of back or flank pain. Excretory urography showed delayed contrast medium excretion and severe ureteropelvic junction obstruction. Diuretic renography showed a markedly abnormal diuretic response in the right kidney. A laparoscopic approach was considered, because the boy was active in athletics and a rapid recovery was desired. A dismembering and

reanastomosis technique identical to that used in open pyeloplasty was performed using 4 cannula sites.

Results.—The boy could tolerate an oral diet 24 hours after surgery. He was discharged home 36 hours after the procedure. He underwent a nephrostomy study at 7 days that revealed free drainage of contrast material in the nephrostomy tube. He experienced pain with clamping. The nephrostomy tube was removed 3 days later, after he could tolerate 24 hours of clamping. At postoperative day 10, he had no symptoms. The cannula site wounds were well healed, and he returned to normal athletic activity. Six weeks after surgery, excretory urography revealed significant improvement from the preoperative examination. He had free drainage through a patent anastomosis.

Conclusion.—It is technically feasible to perform pediatric laparoscopic pyeloplasty with the use of a direct suturing technique identical to that used for open procedures. The favorable outcome and rapid return to normal activity provide encouragement for further development of pediatric reconstruction laparoscopy.

▶ The authors have demonstrated that they could perform a successful laparoscopic pyeloplasty. They have not documented, however, either the advisability or the cost-effectiveness of this approach. They state that the patient was discharged 36 hours after the operation, but, as noted in Abstract 28–1, children can be discharged the day of surgery after open renal operations.

S.S. Howards, M.D.

Evaluation of Pediatric Hydronephrosis Using Individualized Pressure Flow Criteria
Fung LCT, Khoury AE, McLorie GA, Chait PG, Churchill BM (Hospital for Sick Children, Toronto)
J Urol 154:671–676, 1995   30–4

Background.—A diagnostic technique that accurately quantifies urine transport efficiency of the collection system would be invaluable in the evaluation of hydronephrosis. Current diagnostic techniques do not allow for the substantial variations in size and physiology of pediatric patients. Results may be misleading if fixed pressure flow criteria are applied to all patients. Individualized pressure flow criteria were proposed, and results of conventional and individualized pressure flow studies were compared.

Methods.—Individualized pressure flow studies were performed in 37 renal units in 35 patients, aged 0.2–12 years, who had grade 3 or 4 hydronephrosis. Individualized infusion rates were based on estimated maximum physiologic urine output, adjusted for patient age and size. The upper limit of normal renal pelvic pressure was 14 cm H_2O.

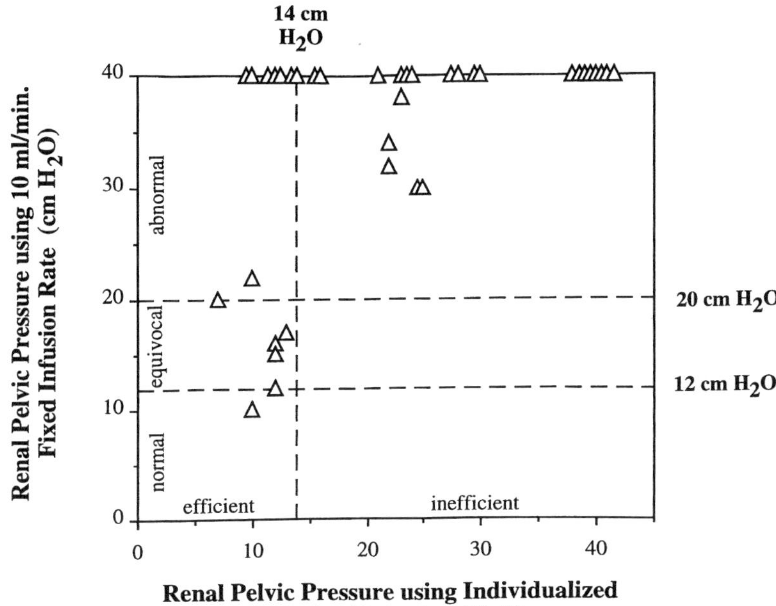

FIGURE 2.—Renal pelvic pressures resulting from fixed infusion rate of 10 mL/min vs. renal pelvic pressures resulting from using individualized infusion rates (37 U). Studies using pressures of 40 cm H_2O were generally still increasing in pressure but were terminated to avoid excessively high renal pelvic pressures. (Courtesy of Fung LCT, Khoury AE, McLorie GA, et al: Evaluation of pediatric hydronephrosis using individualized pressure flow criteria. *J Urol* 154:671–676, 1995.)

Results.—Individualized infusion rates were between 1.3 and 12.5 mL/min, and renal pelvic pressures ranged from 7 to more than 40 cm H_2O. In all patients, corresponding renal pelvic pressure from a fixed infusion rate of 10 mL/min was uniformly equal to or higher than corresponding individualized pressures. The correlation between renal pelvic pressure from individualized and fixed flow studies was weak in 37 renal units, with a correlation coefficient of 0.58 and a slope of a nonzero positive value (Fig 2). The difference between individualized and fixed flow studies was highest in younger patients. The correlation coefficient of 0.09 between diuretic nuclear renography half-times and individualized pressure flow indicated a random correlation between these 2 variables.

Conclusions.—Using individualized infusion rates, many falsely high pressures that result from fixed infusion rates are eliminated in these patients. The proposed individualized maximum physiologic urine output estimates may also be applicable to constant pressure and similar studies.

▶ This paper clearly demonstrates that individualized flow rates give different results from standardized flow in a Whitaker test. This is hardly surprising but definitely documented. These findings, however, have no clinical application. The critical evaluation of a new diagnostic technique, such as the one advocated by the authors, requires a gold standard. Otherwise, there is no criterion with which to judge the precision of the method. Unfortunately, not only is there no gold standard for obstructive hydronephrosis, but innumerable studies have shown a lack of correlation among diuretic renograms, pressure flow studies, and clinical results. Nevertheless, the clinician has to make decisions. We infrequently use passive flow studies for the reasons outlined above and because they are invasive and require anesthesia in young patients. We prefer to make these judgments on the basis of the clinical setting and a diuretic renogram, taking into consideration the differential renal function, the half-time, and trends.

S.S. Howards, M.D.

Suggested Reading

Peters CA: Urinary tract obstruction in children. *J Urol* 154:1874–1884, 1995.

Remuzzi G: The hemolytic uremic syndrome. *Kidney Int* 48:2–19, 1995.

31 Pediatric Reflux

Detrusorrhaphy for the Repair of Vesicoureteral Reflux: Comparison With the Leadbetter-Politano Ureteroneocystostomy
Ellsworth PI, Merguerian PA (Dartmouth-Hitchcock Med Ctr, Lebanon, NH; Stanford Univ Med Ctr, Calif)
J Pediatr Surg 30:600–603, 1995   31–1

Purpose.—The extravesical (detrusorrhaphy) and intravesical (Leadbetter-Politano ureteroneocystostomy) approaches for surgical repair of vesicoureteral reflux were compared. Measures of comparison were length of hospital stay, postoperative pain control, anticholinergic requirements, and postoperative results and complications.

Methods.—The extravesical approach was used in 29 patients (38 ureters), and the intravesical approach was used in 27 (43 ureters). All operations were performed by a single surgeon, and the 2 groups were similar in age and grade of reflux.

Results.—The success rate, as determined by postoperative absence of reflux, was similar for extravesical (94.7%) and intravesical (95.3%) approaches. Average hospital stay was shorter for patients who underwent detrusorrhaphy; this group had significantly fewer postoperative requirements for pain medication and anticholinergic therapy to control bladder spasm.

Discussion.—The extravesical approach causes less postoperative morbidity. Although this approach has not been widely used in the United States because of poor results, recent modifications have led to success rates of 93% to 98%. The bilateral extravesical approach may be associated with transient urinary retention, as seen in 2 patients in this study. The extravesical approach should therefore be limited to unilateral repair or to be performed with minimal dissection of the trigone.

▶ Detrusorraphy for the correction of vesicoureteral reflux, which was originally described many years ago, has become popular in the past few years, primarily because of the modified technique of Hodgson and the group from Children's Memorial Hospital in Chicago. Several series, like this small one, have demonstrated that the results are very good. The problem is that children occasionally have urinary retention after surgery, which can be very bothersome. In this series, 2 of 29 patients (7%) who had detrusorraphy required intermittent catheterization after surgery. Although this is a relatively low incidence, it is a very annoying complication for both the surgeon and the family and has been reported to last as long as 6 months. Various refinements in technique may reduce the incidence of urinary retention, but this complication remains our major concern regarding the procedure. It is particularly a problem when bilateral reimplantation is done.

S.S. Howards, M.D.

Endoscopic Subureteral Collagen Injection for the Treatment of Vesicoureteral Reflux in Infants and Children
Frey P, Lutz N, Jenny P, Herzog B (Centre Hospitalier Universitaire Vaudois, Lausanne, Switzerland; Univ Children's Hosp, Basel, Switzerland)
J Urol 154:804–807, 1995
31–2

Introduction.—Endoscopic subureteral injection, a noninvasive method, resolves vesicoureteral reflux in approximately 60% to 90% of children. The ideal substance for injection, however, remains a matter of controversy. Bovine collagen is biodegradable and well tolerated and does not provoke adverse host tissue reaction. The short-, mid-, and long-term results of subureteral glutaraldehyde cross-linked bovine collagen injection were evaluated.

Methods.—One hundred girls and 32 boys, treated between June 1988 and September 1994, were included. The mean age of the patients at first injection was 4.9 years. Follow-up was an average of 33 months. Primary reflux was present in 87.3% of the 204 injected ureters and secondary reflux was present in 12.7%. Voiding cystourethrography and ultrasonography were performed after injection, and clinical and radiologic evaluations were conducted at regular intervals. A second subureteral collagen injection was performed if grade 2 recurrent reflux was confirmed at 3-month follow-up voiding cystourethrography. Patients received prophylactic antibiotics for 3 months after injection.

Results.—The average collagen injected per refluxing unit was 1.5 mL; the average increased to 2.6 mL in the 66 ureters injected twice. All patients showed an absence of reflux when voiding cystourethrography was performed immediately after injection. Three months after a single injection, reflux was absent in 62.7% of patients; an additional 15.2% improved to reflux grades 1 and 2 and generally did not require further treatment. The overall cure rate after 1 or 2 injections was 79.4% with 3 months of follow-up. No correlation was found between initial degree of reflux and the risk of recurrent reflux (Fig 2). Only 11.3% of the 204 units had late recurrence of reflux after a reflux-free period. Sixty ureters had persistent reflux after 1 or 2 injections; 35% of these patients required no further treatment, 52% underwent reimplantation, and 13% received antibiotic prophylaxis again.

Conclusion.—Subureteral collagen injection was found to be a reliable, safe, and minimally invasive treatment for vesicoureteral reflux in children. The procedure has many advantages over reimplantation surgery, and a

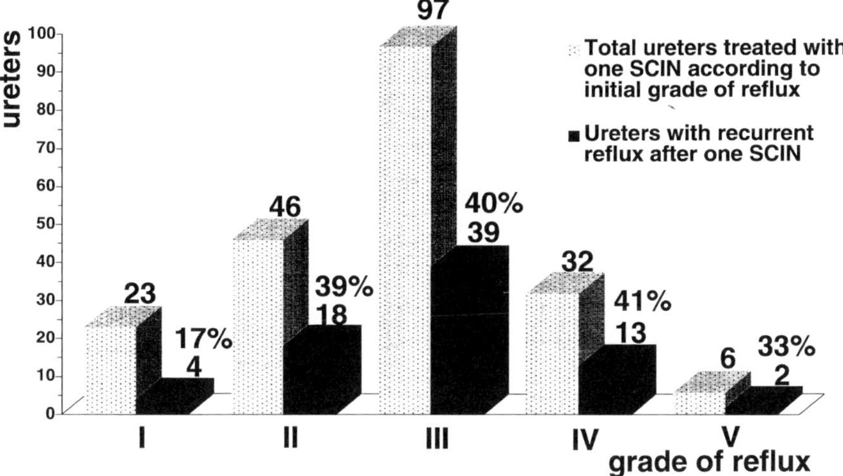

FIGURE 2.—Recurrent reflux as revealed by voiding cystourethrography after 1 subureteral collagen injection (*SCIN*) in 37.3% of 204 ureteral units 3 months after injection. Distribution of treated ureters and those with recurrent reflux after 1 SCIN according to grade of reflux. (Courtesy of Frey P, Lutz N, Jenny P, et al: Endoscopic subureteral collagen injection for the treatment of vesicoureteral reflux in infants and children. *J Urol* 154:804–807. 1995.)

second injection can be easily performed if necessary. There were no allergic reactions to the collagen injections.

▶ Over the years, we have presented many abstracts in the YEAR BOOK OF UROLOGY that described the results of injection therapy for vesicoureteral reflux.[1, 2] We have discussed the pros and cons of this approach, including the concerns regarding Teflon migration and the inflammatory reaction to Teflon. The use of collagen avoids these problems, but the long-term success rate, particularly for higher grade reflux, is lower. The authors had a failure rate of approximately 40%, and the follow-up was not long enough to document the long-term failure rate. Another problem with this approach is that it is not approved by the Food and Drug Administration; thus, the surgeon is legally and medically vulnerable. Nevertheless, it is definitely possible that this approach will become the treatment of choice.

S.S. Howards, M.D.

References

1. 1991 YEAR BOOK OF UROLOGY, pp 253–255.
2. 1994 YEAR BOOK OF UROLOGY, pp 273–275.

The Radiation Dose to Children From X-ray Examinations of the Pelvis and the Urinary Tract

Almén A, Mattsson S (Lund Univ, Sweden; Malmö Univ Hosp, Sweden)
Br J Radiol 68:604–613, 1995
31–3

Introduction.—Ninety-five children (average age, 3 years) underwent pelvic or urologic radiographs. Radiation exposure was measured with the use of a dose-area product meter and thermoluminescent dosemeters (TLD). The results were used to calculate the energy imparted, the effective dose, and the mean absorbed dose for various organs.

Results.—The male gonads absorbed more radiation than did female gonads across all age groups and all types of radiographs. Intravenous urographs (IVU), at least among children aged 6–15 years, seemed to show higher absorbed doses to a number of organs, probably because of the large number of exposures demanded. In general, the absorbed dose was highly dependent on body size. Like the mean organ dose absorbed, the effective dose per examination was consistently higher in boys than in girls, with highest levels seen in IVU, followed by micturating cysturethrograms and then pelvic bone films. Energy imparted, however, showed the highest levels in micturating cysturethrograms rather than in IVU, especially in the anteroposterior projection.

Conclusions.—As entrance surface dose and dose-area products are highly dependent on body size, reference values in the pediatric population might be better based on body size than on age range. It also appears that effective dose for pediatric pelvic and urologic radiographs can be estimated with reasonable accuracy with the use of a single conversion coefficient.

▶ This is a thoughtful analysis of radiation dose in children who undergo excretory urography or voiding cystourethrogram. The absorbed dose increases with increasing body size. Regardless of these calculations, the bottom line is to avoid all unnecessary radiation but to use radiologic studies when needed. We find that there is still an overuse of excretory urography in children in the urologic community. In many situations, ultrasound or radionuclide studies would not only expose the child to less radiation but also supply more information.

S.S. Howards, M.D.

Serum Intercellular Adhesion Molecule (ICAM-1), a Marker of Renal Scarring in Infants With Vesico-ureteric Reflux

Miyakita H, Puri P, Surana R, Kobayashi H, Reen DJ (Our Lady's Hosp for Sick Children, Dublin)
Br J Urol 76:249–251, 1995
31–4

Background.—The intercellular adhesion molecule (ICAM-1) has been implicated in inflammatory disorders and is induced in various cells by exposure to pro-inflammatory cytokines. It participates in leukocyte adhesion and in regulation of extravasation of leukocytes and their infiltration into inflamed tissues. Circulating levels of ICAM-1 were determined in 81 children who had vesicoureteric reflux (VUR).

Methods.—Fifty-two girls and 29 boys, aged 2 months to 13 years, were included. Thirty-four children were bilaterally affected, for a total of 115 refluxing ureters. Radionuclide scans demonstrated renal scarring in 33 of the 70 children examined. Serum levels of ICAM-1 were estimated by enzyme-linked immunosorbent assay.

Findings.—The mean serum level of ICAM-1 was 347 ng/mL in children who had Vur and 202 ng/mL in 24 urologically normal children. Serum levels did not correlate with the grade of reflux. In children younger than 2 years of age, however, the levels were substantially higher in those who had renal scarring (408 vs. 296 ng/mL).

Conclusion.—The serum level of ICAM-1 may be a useful marker of tubular damage in young children who have VUR, but further studies are needed to confirm a role for this molecule in the development of reflux nephropathy.

▶ This paper is of modest intellectual interest but no practical clinical value. As with many studies of this type, there is an overlap between the 2 tested populations. The assay therefore does not allow one to discriminate in a given individual whether scarring exists, even though the populations are statistically distinct.

S.S. Howards, M.D.

Subureteric Teflon Injection (STING): Results of a European Survey
Puri P, Ninan GK, Surana R (Our Lady's Hospital for Sick Children, Dublin; Royal Aberdeen Children's Hospital, Scotland)
Eur Urol 27:71–75, 1995   31–5

Objective.—The results of subureteric Teflon injection (STING) for the treatment of vesicoureteric reflux (VUR) in children were assessed in a large, multicenter survey.

Methods.—Twenty-two pediatric surgeons/urologists from 18 centers in Europe were surveyed regarding their experience with 6,216 refluxing ureters injected with Polytef paste in 4,166 children. There were 975 boys and 3,191 girls aged 2 months to 14 years. Primary VUR was present in 93% of ureters; reflux was in duplicated systems in 4% and secondary to neuropathic bladders in 3%. The reflux was grade I in 4.4%, grade II in 36.1%, grade III in 40.2%, and grades IV and V in 19.3%. Follow-up ranged from 3 months to 8½ years, with 90% followed up for more than 2 years.

Outcome.—The cure rate was 76.3% after a single injection of Teflon paste and increased to 84.9% after a second injection. Another 10.2% demonstrated significant improvement in the grade of reflux after 1 or 2 injections of Teflon paste, and needed no further treatment. Overall, 95.1% of all refluxing ureters were cured or improved significantly after 2 injections of Teflon paste; another 1.3% were cured after a third or fourth injection. Failure to correct or improve VUR was noted in 3.6% of ureters, necessitating reimplantation. Obstruction at the vesicoureteric junction developed in 0.32% after STING, but these ureters were reimplanted without difficulty. There were no clinically untoward effects from the use of Teflon as an injectable biomaterial.

Conclusion.—This multicenter survey confirms that STING is an effective day-case procedure for the treatment of all grades of VUR.

▶ This large multicenter survey found a high cure rate for the correction of reflux in which 93% of the ureters had primary reflux. Despite this, some authors continue to search for alternative injectable agents, citing the risks of migration of Teflon particles to the lungs and brain in experimental animal studies as a contraindication to the injection of Teflon in children.[1] Aaronson et al. have reported 15-μm particles in the brain after subureteric Teflon injection, suggesting that the brain may not always be adequately protected from particles that gain access to the venous circulation. Alternative autologous substances that can correct reflux have been developed and reported in the animal model.[2]

L. Stothers, M.D., M.H.Sc.

References

1. Aaronson IA, Rames RA, Greene WB, et al: Endoscopic treatment of reflux: Migration of Teflon to the lungs and brain. *Eur Urol* 23:394–399, 1993.
2. Atala A, Kim W, Paige KT, et al: Endoscopic treatment of vesicoureteral reflux with a chondrocyte-alginate suspension. *J Urol* 152:641–643, 1994.

Suggested Reading

Aaronson IA: Current status of the "STING": An American perspective. *Br J Urol* 75:121–125, 1995.

Puri P: Ten year experience with subureteric Teflon (polytetrafluoroethylene) injection (STING) in the tratment of vesico-ureteric reflux. *Br J Urol* 75:126–131, 1995.

32 Pediatric Testis

Evaluation of Acute Scrotum in the Emergency Department
Lewis AG, Bukowski TP, Jarvis PD, Wacksman J, Sheldon CA (Children's Hosp Med Center, Cincinnati, Ohio)
J Pediatr Surg 30:277–282, 1995   32–1

Background.—Children who have acute scrotal pain and swelling are commonly evaluated in the emergency department. Testicular torsion, torsion of the appendix testis (or other appendage), and epididymitis represent the most frequent diagnoses. The records of patients evaluated during a 2-year period for acute scrotal pain in a children's hospital emergency department were reviewed retrospectively to determine accuracy of diagnosis and treatment outcomes.

Patients and Methods.—Two hundred thirty-eight patients, aged 0–19 years, were included. Patients were treated according to a strict protocol. Those who had testes that were normal in size, shape, position, and consistency were discharged from the emergency department with appropriate therapy. Patients who had abnormal testicle(s) were treated on the basis of degree of clinical suspicion for testicular torsion. When suspected, immediate surgical exploration was performed. Imaging studies were performed when other diagnoses were suspected.

Results.—Sixteen percent of patients had testicular torsion, 46% had torsion of a testicular appendage, and 35% had epididymitis. Testicular salvage was highly dependent on the period between onset of pain and surgical intervention. No testis likely to have been viable at the time of evaluation was lost. The diagnostic error rate at first encounter was 7%, which led to a total of 10 negative scrotal evaluations. Both color Doppler ultrasound and radioisotope imaging proved to be highly specific diagnostic modalities, except for patients who had far-advanced necrotic testes. Twenty-eight children who had epididymitis underwent investigation; 39% had either structural or functional urinary tract abnormalities. Noninvasive urodynamic studies were useful screening tools for older children who had this condition.

Conclusions.—The primary goal of management of the acute scrotum in children is prevention of testicular loss. This goal necessitates a high level of diagnostic accuracy and prompt surgical intervention. Testicular salvage is achievable only if intervention is undertaken within 6 hours of onset of pain. Effective education of parents and primary care physicians may help increase the rate of testicular preservation.

▶ This paper does not add significantly to the medical literature but nevertheless contains some interesting information. The high incidence of torsion of the appendix testis is surprising. This diagnosis was much more common than it is in our experience. Two other relevant observations were noted. First, 39% of the patients with epididymitis had abnormalities of the urinary tract. It is well known that such findings are frequent, but it is also useful to document the incidence in a large series. Second, almost half the torsed testes that were seen 25–48 hours after the onset of symptoms were salvaged. This result fits with our bias but is at odds with the teaching in many textbooks.

S.S. Howards, M.D.

Color Doppler Ultrasound in Newborn Testis Torsion
Cartwright PC, Snow BW, Reid BS, Shultz PK (Univ of Utah, Salt Lake City)
Urology 45:667–670, 1995   32–2

Introduction.—Color Doppler sonography has been useful in the evaluation of testicular ischemia or torsion in older children and adults. Its usefulness in the assessment of suspected antenatal testis torsion was evaluated retrospectively.

Methods.—During a 4-year period, testis torsion was diagnosed clinically within 24 hours after delivery in 9 newborns who had a scrotal mass or swelling. All patients underwent real-time testicular ultrasonography with color Doppler imaging.

Findings.—Color Doppler ultrasound images revealed a dusky or deep red discoloration of each affected hemiscrotum. Intratesticular flow was absent on the affected side and normal in the contralateral testis in all 8 patients who had unilateral torsion and was absent on both sides in the 1 patient who had bilateral torsion. Two echo texture patterns appeared on gray-scale sonography. The 4 most enlarged testes had mixed echogenicity in the testicular parenchyma, with both hypo- and hyperechoic areas. The other 6 testes had a more consistently hypoechoic echo pattern with a distinct hyperechoic ring that corresponded to the tunica albuginea.

Discussion.—All 9 newborns who had testis torsion were accurately assessed with color Doppler ultrasound. Color Doppler settings should be optimally set to detect low flow and distinguish between intratesticular flow and flow within extracapsular vessels, the epididymis, or the surrounding structures. The 2 patterns detected by gray-scale sonography probably indicate the duration of the torsion in utero. Mixed echogenicity suggests late necrotic changes and minimal dystrophy calcification, and the more homogeneous echo pattern with an encircling hyperechoic ring suggests earlier torsion and more extensive necrotic change, parenchymal liquefaction, and dystropic calcium deposits.

▶ This paper addresses an important issue that is often critical during evaluation of potential newborn torsion of the spermatic cord. At the authors' institution, color Doppler ultrasound was very precise. We would warn, however, that both Doppler ultrasound and nuclear scan in most hands are not accurate in the newborn period. The precision of Doppler ultrasound depends on the sensitivity of the instrument. The latest versions can distinguish between ischemic and normal neonatal testis. Therefore, as always, good clinical judgment is necessary, and, when in doubt, exploration is indicated.

S.S. Howards, M.D.

The Chance for Fertility in Adolescent Boys After Corrective Surgery for Varicocele

Hadziselimovic F, Herzog B, Jenny P (Univ of Basel, Switzerland)
J Urol 154:731–733, 1995   32–3

Background.—Varicocele occurs in 10% to 15% of boys and on the left side in 90% to 95%. Pre-existing testicular atrophy resulting from varicocele is reversible only with successful surgery, but testicular atrophy in patients who have persistent varicocele is irreversible. Long-term results of men who underwent corrective surgery for varicocele during adolescence were reported.

Methods.—Spermiograms of 25 men (mean age, 23.6 years) were analyzed. All patients underwent surgery 10 years earlier to correct varicocele. At that time, bilateral testicular biopsy specimens were obtained.

Results.—In all patients, plasma levels of follicle-stimulating hormone, luteinizing hormone, and testosterone were normal. Patients were divided into 2 groups. Group 1 included 11 patients who had asthenoteratospermia. Group 2 included 14 patients who had normal spermiograms. The number of sperm per ejaculate was significantly different between groups. There was no difference between groups before surgery in testicular atrophy of the left testis compared with the right testis. There was also no preoperative difference in the comparative testicular histology of biopsy specimens, because the number of adrenal spermatogonia per tubule was significantly lower in all patients. At surgery, there was no difference in patient age or degree of atrophy of seminiferous tubules or Leydig cells in both testes. The left testis of patients in group 2 caught up in size to the contralateral testis, but the volume of the left testis in patients in group 1 was 80% of the right testicular volume. A second operation was performed in 1 patient because of a relapse.

Conclusions.—Testicular blood flow may be significantly atypical in these patients, but with a dramatic increase in testicular arterial blood flow rather than reduced blood flow. This finding may explain the differences in resolution. Early intervention for testicular atrophy is important. The persistent atrophy of the left testis in group 1 suggests that some patients may benefit somewhat from conventional surgery.

▶ This interesting paper demonstrates that boys who have catch-up growth of the left testis after varicocele repair have normal fertility potential, whereas those who do not have reduced fertility potential. The data support the authors' contention that early repair is indicated in any boy who has retarded growth of the left testis and in older young men who have reduced semen quality. The authors' speculation that blood flow is increased fits with our research findings but is not documented in this study.

S.S. Howards, M.D.

The Use of the hCG Stimulation Test in the Endocrine Evaluation of Cryptorchidism
Davenport M, Brain C, Vandenberg C, Zappala S, Duffy P, Ransley PG, Grant D (Hosp for Sick Children, London)
Br J Urol 76:790–794, 1995
32–4

Introduction.—The presence or absence of functional testicular tissue is commonly evaluated with the use of the human chorionic gonadotrophin (hCG) stimulation test. Some isolated reports have indicated that the testosterone response to hCG was absent with intra-abdominal testes or that persisting production of testosterone occurred with anorchia. The hCG stimulation test was reviewed in a series of 31 prepubertal boys who had impalpable testes to confirm or refute its value.

Methods.—All boys received age-dependent daily doses of hCG: younger than 1 year of age, 500 U; 1–10 years of age, 1,000 U; or older than 10 years of age, 1,500 U. Blood samples were obtained before the first dose and 24 hours after the final dose. All boys underwent a full surgical exploration.

Results.—Boys were grouped according to surgical findings. Group 1 included 8 boys who had anorchia. Group 2 included 14 boys who had bilateral intra-abdominal testes or normal volume. Group 3 included 9 boys who had either a unilateral intra-abdominal testis only or with bilateral dysplastic testes that were either intra-abdominal or intracanalicular (but impalpable) and were typically excised. The 8 boys who had anorchia and 1 who had bilateral atrophic intra-abdominal testes had no response to hCG. Findings indicated that 22 boys responded to hCG stimulation testing and had testes whose size was related to the degree of testosterone elevation. Positive and negative predictive values for the hCG test were 89% and 100%, respectively. There was a significant quantitative difference in testosterone response between the boys who had bilateral intra-abdominal testes of normal volume and those who had an otherwise reduced volume of testes.

Conclusion.—The hCG stimulation test is an accurate predictor of anorchia. A good response to hCG suggests bilateral intra-abdominal testes of sufficient size for orchidopexy. Patients who do not respond to hCG do not need formal surgical exploration for confirmation.

▶ This paper is puzzling. First of all, the hCG stimulation test is well known and not new. Second, it is also well established that one can rule out the presence of testis only if there is no testosterone response to hCG and the gonadotropins are elevated. The 1 patient reported who had no response to hCG but had testis had normal gonadotropins. The authors administered hCG on 3 successive days. We find that the test works well with just 1 dose of hCG.

S.S. Howards, M.D.

Clinical and Anatomopathological Study of 2000 Cryptorchid Testes

Gracia J, Gonzalez N, Gomez ME, Plaza L, Sanchez J, Alba J (Miguel Sevet Children's Hospital, Zaragoza, Spain)
Br J Urol 75:697–701, 1995

32–5

Background.—The morphologic lesions in cryptorchid testes may be the result of damage induced by the extrascrotal position or may represent a congenital lesion. Whether age at the time of surgery and location of the testes helped determine the anatomopathologic lesions was established.

Methods.—A total of 2,000 testes in 1,342 children, aged 0–14 years (mean age, 5.9 years), were studied. The tubular fertility index (TFI) and the tubular diameter (TD) were correlated with age at intervention and location of the testes.

Findings.—The most "normal" measured values were found in children younger than 2 years of age. The TFI was low in 24%, very low in 55%, and normal (> 60%) in 21%. The TFI did not differ significantly between children younger than 2 years of age and those older than 7 years, which suggests that the TFI did not deteriorate progressively with age. Only 8% of TDs were very low, 51% were low, and 41% were normal. The TD differed significantly between children younger than 2 years of age and those older than 7 years, but a higher mean was observed in the oldest age group. Parametric and nonparametric tests did not show a correlation between the TFI or TD and the time of surgery or testicular location.

Conclusion.—On the basis of these findings, no particular age can be recommended at which surgery should be performed for cryptorchid testes in relation to the anatomopathologic damage.

▶ This paper is of interest to us because the data and the conclusions drawn by the authors support our findings in experimental animals. Although it is often stated with great authority that early orchidopexy preserves fertility better than late surgery, there is no hard evidence to support this claim. There is evidence, however, that postpubertal surgery damages fertility potential. In spite of the above intellectual arguments, we perform our orchidopexies at age 9–14 months.

S.S. Howards, M.D.

Quantitative Histology of Germ Cells in the Undescended Testes of Human Fetuses, Neonates and Infants

Cortes D, Thorup JM, Beck BL (State Univ Hosp, Copenhagen)
J Urol 154:1188–1192, 1995

32–6

Objective.—Because germ-cell hypoplasia is a frequent finding in undescended testes of boys older than 3 years of age, germ cells were counted in 35 fetuses and 58 boys who had cryptorchidism. Ages ranged from 28 weeks' gestation to 3 years. The control series included 22 normal fetuses and 25 normal boys.

Findings.—The cryptorchid fetuses had a reduced number of germ cells per tubular cross-section and lower testicular weights than did control fetuses. These values were also reduced in the 34 cryptorchid boys who did have not a symptomatic inguinal hernia. In the 24 boys who had a hernia, values were normal in the first year of life but decreased from ages 1 to 3 years. Thirty-four percent of cryptorchid fetuses and 18% of cryptorchid boys without an inguinal hernia had malformations or dysplasia of the kidneys, ureter, or lower vertebrae.

Conclusions.—The number of germ cells in undescended testes is below normal from gestational week 28. Germ-cell hypoplasia appears to result when the testis remains undescended in postnatal life. Some cases of cryptorchidism may represent abnormal progression in the caudal developmental field.

33 Pediatric Oncology

Results of the United Kingdom Children's Cancer Study Group First Wilms' Tumor Study
Pritchard J, Imeson J, Barnes J, Cotterill S, Gough D, Marsden HB, Morris-Jones P, Pearson D (Univ of Leicester, England)
J Clin Oncol 13:124–133, 1995   33–1

Background.—Therapeutic advances have yielded steady improvement in the prognosis of Wilms' tumor during the past 3 decades. Radiation therapy and doxorubicin treatment can have late adverse effects; large collaborative studies have therefore been done to determine whether refined treatment protocols yield results comparable to those of standard treatment. The results of the first Wilms' Tumor Trial (UKW1) of the United Kingdom Children's Cancer Study Group were reported. The goals of the trial were to reduce treatment of patients who had low-stage tumors of favorable histology (FH) without impairing their survival and to use intensive chemotherapy to improve the prognosis of patients who had stage II and IV tumors of FH or unfavorable histology (UH).

Methods.—Three hundred eighty-four consecutive patients who had newly diagnosed Wilms' tumor were recruited from 1980 to 1986. Treatment was stratified by disease stage and histology, according to the criteria of the US National Wilms' Tumor Studies. Patients who had stage I tumors received vincristine only, whereas those who had stage II tumors received vincristine plus dactinomycin (Act-D). Three-drug chemotherapy was given to patients who had stage III tumors, and 4-drug regimens were given to those who had stage IV. The Act-D regimen was administered in pulsed doses of 1.5 mg/m^2 every 3 or 6 weeks. Patients who had stage IV disease did not receive lung irradiation. Because of the small sizes of the subgroups, no randomization was done. The patients were assessed at a median follow-up of 114 months for the main end points of survival and event-free survival.

Results.—Among patients who had FH, 6-year survival rates were 96% for those in stage I; 93%, stage II; 83%, stage III; and 65%, stage IV. For patients who had UH, 6-year survival rate was 50%, regardless of disease stage. Significant prognostic factors were age at diagnosis, histologic subtype, and disease stage. No second malignancies have been observed so far.

Conclusions.—The results of the UKW1 trial suggest that single-agent chemotherapy, without radiation, is as effective as previously reported

2-drug regimens for patients who have stage I FH Wilms' tumors. For those who have stage II and III disease, pulsed Act-D chemotherapy is effective, with no need for fractionation. Compared with studies in the United States, outcomes are worse for patients who have stage IV FH and UH disease, because of differences either in the use of lung irradiation or in case selection bias.

▶ The National Wilms' Tumor Study (NWTS2) has been very valuable, and the UKW1 adds more useful information. Because radiation therapy and doxorubicin cause serious late side effects such as irreversible hypoplasia of soft and bony tissues, and second tumors (see Abstract 31–2) and cardiomyopathy, respectively, both study groups have tried less aggressive therapies in favorable cases. The UKW1 had fewer patients with low-stage tumors. The most important difference between UKW1 and NWTS2 was the intensive use of vincristine alone in cases of stage I FH without exposing the patients to the risks and side effects of Act-D. Stages II and III were similar in the 2 studies, and the results were similar. Patients who had stage IV FH in UKW1 did worse than those in NWTS2.

S.S. Howards, M.D.

Second Malignant Neoplasms Following Treatment for Wilms' Tumor: A Report From the National Wilms' Tumor Study Group

Breslow NE, Takashima JR, Whitton JA, Moksness J, D'Angio GJ, Green DM (Univ of Washington, Seattle; Fred Hutchinson Cancer Research Ctr, Seattle; Univ of Pennsylvania, Philadelphia; et al)
J Clin Oncol 13:1851–1859, 1995   33–2

Introduction.—Approximately 90% of all patients with Wilms' tumor, and more than 95% of those with the best prognosis, are long-term survivors. Unfortunately, these results are accompanied by an increased risk of a second malignant neoplasm (SMN). A survey of 2,438 patients in the National Wilms' Tumor Study (NWTS) showed that SMN developed in 8.5 times the expected number of patients.

Patients.—The prevalence of SMN was determined in 5,278 patients enrolled by the end of 1993 in the NWTS. A total of 39,461 patient-years of follow-up were analyzed.

Findings.—Forty-three SMNs were observed, although only 5 were expected, for a standardized incidence ratio of 8.4. The cumulative incidence of SMN 15 years after Wilms' tumor was diagnosed was 1.6%; the incidence continued to increase steadily. The delivery of abdominal radiation as part of initial treatment increased the risk of SMN, and doxorubicin augmented this effect. Eight of 234 patients who received both doxorubicin and more than 35 Gy of abdominal radiation had SMN; only 0.2 were expected. Treatment for relapse increased the risk further by a factor greater than 4.

Conclusion.—Patients remain at increased risk of SMN many years after initial treatment for Wilms' tumor.

▶ It is a cruel reality that children cured of cancer are at risk for SMN. Thoughtful efforts to modify treatment have been undertaken to reduce the risk (see Abstract 31–1), but, of course, it remains necessary to treat the original tumor adequately. The original NWTS analysis of the risk of second tumors (published in 1988)[1] revealed an 8.5-fold increased risk of another malignancy in patients with Wilms' tumor. This risk is almost identical to the one uncovered by this study. The numbers are now more precise, because of the greater number of individuals at risk and the longer mean follow-up. The cumulative risk of 1.6% at 15 years is disturbing. One hopes that this risk will not increase significantly with longer follow-up, but it is very possible that it will. Radiation therapy clearly leads to SMNs, and drugs such as doxorubicin, which inhibit the activity of topoisomerase II, are leukemogens.[2]

S.S. Howards, M.D.

References

1. Breslow NE, Olshan A, Norkool P, et al: Second malignant neoplasms in survivors of Wilms' tumor: A report from the National Wilms' Tumor Study. *J Natl Cancer Inst* 80:592–595, 1988.
2. Long BH, Stringfellow DA: Inhibitors of topoisomerase II: Structure-activity relationships and mechanisms of action of podophyllin congeners. *Adv Enzyme Regul* 27:223–256, 1988.

34 Pediatric Incontinence

Primary Nocturnal Enuresis: A Comparison Among Observation, Imipramine, Desmopressin Acetate and Bed-wetting Alarm Systems
Monda JM, Husmann DA (Mayo Clinic, Rochester, Minn; Univ of Texas Southwestern Med Ctr, Dallas)
J Urol 154:745–748, 1995   34–1

Introduction.—Nocturnal enuresis is a common disorder that usually resolves spontaneously, although many patients seek medical attention. The treatment methods used most frequently are imipramine, desmopressin acetate (DDAVP), and bed-wetting alarm systems. These 3 methods were evaluated prospectively.

Methods.—Three hundred forty-five patients with primary nocturnal enuresis were included. Follow-up of 12 months was available for 261 patients, each of whom had at least 3 enuretic nights weekly. The patients and/or their families were advised of treatment options and selected observation or 1 of the 3 treatment methods. All were asked to keep a calendar to record the number of wet vs. dry nights. Patients who elected drug therapy were weaned at 6 months. Assessments took place at 3, 6, 9, and 12 months. Imipramine was given at doses of 1–1.5 mg/kg, taken orally before bedtime; DDAVP was administered intranasally before retiring, starting with 20 mg and increased if necessary to a maximum of 40 μg. The alarm systems (Sears or Palco) were abruptly discontinued after 6 months.

Results.—The observation group included 50 patients (mean age, 8 years); 8 patients (16%) became continent during follow-up. Imipramine was taken by 44 patients (median age, 9 years); a 16% rate of continence was achieved at 12 months. The median dose required was 50 mg daily. Although 68% of the 88 patients treated with DDAVP were continent at 6 months, only 10% had persistent continence at 12 months. Seventy-nine patients (mean age, 10 years) chose an alarm system. Forty-seven had discontinued use of the device before 6 months because of satisfactory urinary continence, and 44 (56%) remained continent at 1 year of follow-up (Fig 2). Seventy percent of patients who became continent with the alarm system were without nocturia when the alarm conditioning was completed.

Conclusion.—Both imipramine and DDAVP were more successful initially than observation alone in resolving nocturnal enuresis. When these

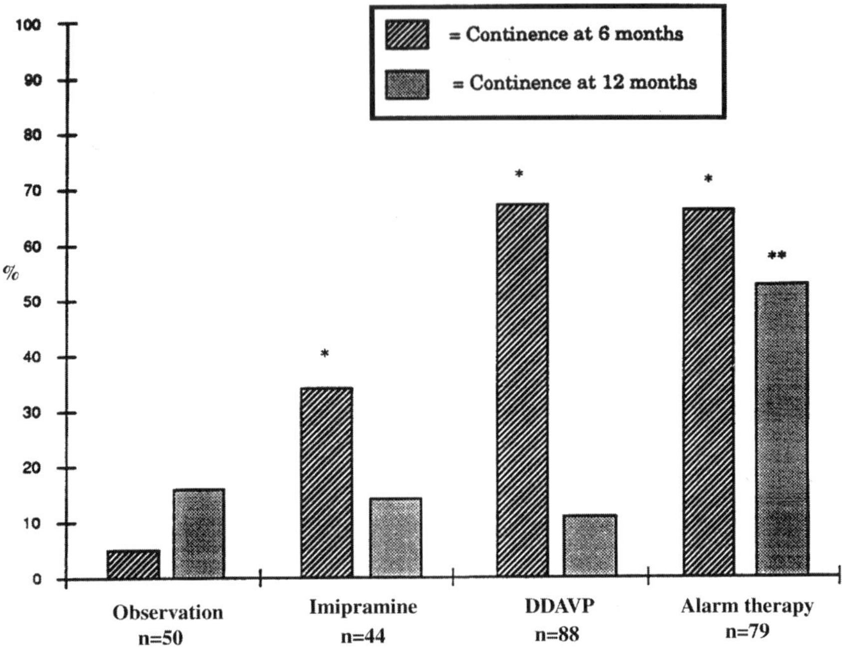

*p<0.001 compared to the observation study group at 6 months.
**p<0.001 compared to the observation, immipramine, and
DDAVP study groups at 12 months.

FIGURE 2.—Continence at 6 and 12 months. (Courtesy of Monda JM, Husmann DA: Primary nocturnal enuresis: A comparison among observation, imipramine, desmopressin acetate and bed-wetting alarm systems. *J Urol* 154:745–748, 1995.)

drugs were discontinued, however, the disorder returned in most patients. Persistent control of nocturnal enuresis was achieved only with the bed-wetting alarm systems. The alarm system was also considerably less costly than pharmacologic treatment.

▶ This is one of many investigations of nocturnal enuresis. The findings are not surprising but are nevertheless interesting. The study was prospective but not randomized. The continence rates of observation, imipramine, DDAVP, and alarm therapy were 6%, 32%, 68%, and 68%, respectively, at 6 months. It is our clinical impression that the success rate with imipramine is somewhat higher and that with DDAVP somewhat lower than observed in this study. The take-home message is that, at 1 year, the continence rate was significantly better with the alarm system than with either of the medical therapies. The high relapse rates with imipramine and DDAVP, as well as the much lower relapse rate with the alarm system, have been previously reported.

S.S. Howards, M.D.

Sexual Abuse: Another Causative Factor in Dysfunctional Voiding
Ellsworth PI, Merguerian PA, Copening ME (Dartmouth-Hitchock Med Ctr, Lebanon, NH; Stanford Univ Med Ctr, Calif)
J Urol 153:773–776, 1995   34–2

Background.—It has traditionally been believed that voiding dysfunction is learned. Domineering, intolerant parents and parental divorce or alcohol abuse have been implicated in this disturbance. In some patients referred for dysfunctional voiding, onset occurred after childhood sexual abuse. Results of evaluations of these patients were reported.

Methods.—Of 300 patients referred for dysfunctional voiding, it was determined that sexual abuse preceded the onset of urinary symptoms in 18. Gastrointestinal tract, genitourinary tract, and neurologic symptoms were evaluated. A history was obtained, and physical examination was performed.

Results.—Twelve of the 18 patients were younger than 6 years of age, and 6 were at least 18 years of age. Vaginal penetration was evident in 4 patients who had day and night enuresis. Most patients were first abused between the ages of 3 and 8 years. Of the 12 patients younger than 6 years of age, 5 had a history of urinary tract infections, 11 had day and/or night enuresis, 4 had encopresis, and 9 had frequent constipation. Of the 6 adults, 3 had a history of urinary tract infections, 5 had a history of enuresis, and 3 were frequently constipated. Results of cystometrography, electromyography, uroflowmetry, and voiding cystourethrography were also reported. Treatment included timed voiding, double voiding regimens, voiding diaries, behavior modification, improved bowel regimen, anticholinergics, and psychiatric counseling, which was encouraged for all patients.

Conclusions.—The possibility of sexual abuse should be considered when evaluating new onset of voiding dysfunction in children or long-term voiding dysfunction in adults. Any history of sexual abuse, evidence of abuse from patient history and physical examination, and urinary symptoms and urodynamic findings indicating a history of sexual abuse should be determined.

▶ The fact that 6% of patients with dysfunctional voiding have been sexually abused is hardly surprising. Nevertheless, it is helpful that the authors have documented this fact, and certainly their admonition that sexual abuse should be considered in children who have dysfunctional voiding is appropriate.

S.S. Howards, M.D.

Pelvic Floor Exercises for Children: A Method of Treating Dysfunctional Voiding

Wennergren H, Öberg B (Univ Hosp, Linköping, Sweden)
Br J Urol 76:9–15, 1995

34–3

Objective.—Pelvic floor exercises have been used successfully to treat women who have neurogenic stress incontinence. Incontinence in children, however, is usually the result of delayed or disturbed voluntary control of the bladder. To determine whether pelvic floor exercises could help incontinent children, the program was evaluated in a group of girls.

Methods.—Sixteen girls, aged 6–15 years, were enrolled in a training program that involved pelvic floor exercises and lasted at least 10 sessions. Voiding pattern and degree of incontinence were recorded at baseline and at the end of the study. Transurethral cystometry and surface electromyography were performed in 14 girls. Ultrasonography was performed at follow-up 3–4 years later. The girls were instructed on micturition and how and when to void. Electromyographic feedback was used to reinforce instructions.

Results.—All but 1 girl had daytime incontinence, and 8 were incontinent at night. Eleven girls were continent after treatment, but 1 had a relapse at 1 year and another had become dry. Seven girls improved after treatment, and 3 were cured at the 3–4 year follow-up. The 4 girls who remained incontinent were the youngest participants. Five of 6 girls with the most serious incontinence problems were cured.

Conclusion.—Pelvic floor exercises are easy to learn and are a satisfactory alternative noninvasive therapy for children who have dysfunctional voiding.

▶ Dr. Mikel Gray, our urodynamic nurse, believes that, in properly and highly selected patients, methods such as those outlined by the authors can be useful. The patients must have documented dyssynergia or pseudodyssynergia and have not responded to anticholinergic therapy. For those who have true Hinman's syndrome, a psychiatric consultation is essential. It is unlikely that the protocol used by the authors would be accepted in the United States. The patients had 10–12 visits. We find that most families will accept 3 or, for difficult situations, 6 sessions at most. This study also would have benefited from a control group. The complete success rate at 6 months, if one includes the dropouts as failures, is only 25%. This time-consuming, demanding approach may nevertheless be useful in selected patients, particularly if it is modified to make it more time- and cost-effective.

S.S. Howards, M.D.

Tethered Spinal Cord: The Effect of Neurosurgery on the Lower Urinary Tract and Male Sexual Function
Boemers TML, van Gool JD, de Jong TPVM (Univ Hosp, Utrecht, The Netherlands)
Br J Urol 76:747–751, 1995

Introduction.—Previous reports have suggested that neurosurgical treatment of tethered spinal cord syndrome can be beneficial. Early intervention has been recommended to prevent or improve lower urinary tract dysfunction. The outcome of neurosurgical correction in 36 patients who had tethered spinal cord was reported, with an emphasis on lower urinary tract function and sexual function in boys.

Methods.—Fifteen boys and 21 girls who had a tethered spinal cord or tight filum terminale underwent clinical and urodynamic evaluation of lower urinary tract function before and after neurosurgery. The children underwent neurologic evaluation every 3–6 months, with an emphasis on neurologic deterioration. All patients had visible cutaneous back lesions and could walk. Surgical intervention was prophylactic in 27 children. Nine children underwent surgery for neurologic deterioration and/or progression of an orthopedic foot deformity. Children in the latter group had myelomeningocele or lipomyelomeningocele. Sexual function was evaluated before and after surgery in 14 boys. In young boys, sexual function was assessed by parental observation and was considered normal if erections were observed regularly or if the child reported having erections. Pubescent and adolescent boys were asked whether they could achieve voluntary erections, orgasm, and ejaculation.

Results.—The 36 children underwent a total of 41 untethering operations. Eight children underwent surgical correction at a mean age of 6 months, and the remaining children underwent surgery at a mean age of 9 years. Two patients had permanent lower urinary tract function changes after surgery: 1 patient improved, and another became worse. Seven patients had temporary changes in bladder and sphincter function. After surgery, 2 girls with dermal sinus tracts had detrusor overactivity and dyssynergia but became normal within 1 month after surgery. Five children experienced signs of bladder denervation after surgery. Most symptoms gradually resolved and reverted to the preoperative urodynamic pattern within 6–10 months. Thirteen of 14 boys evaluated for sexual function were considered to have normal sexual function and could achieve erections. Five of these patients were older boys who could ejaculate (4 antegrade and 1 retrograde). One boy with a dermal sinus had a marked decrease in the frequency of erections before surgery. After surgery, this function improved remarkably. Another adolescent boy with lipomyelomeningocele had undisturbed erectile function but lost the ability to achieve erections totally until almost 6 months after surgery.

Conclusion.—All changes in bladder and sphincter function after untethering were usually transient in this cohort. The resultant denervation usually lasted less than 6 months. Definitive evaluation of lower urinary tract function should be delayed for 6 months after surgery. Some children benefited from untethering, and some became worse. Preoperative progression of neurologic symptoms and postoperative denervation occurred only in patients who had myelo- and lipomyelomeningocele. The natural history in these patients has not been determined. Controlled prospective trials are needed to determine whether these patients benefit from prophylactic untethering.

▶ There is controversy in the literature as to whether untethering of the spinal cord is beneficial to the urinary tract. The belief at our institution is that the procedure infrequently, if ever, has a major beneficial effect on the urinary tract but may nevertheless be useful vis-à-vis other neurologic functions. Eleven of the 36 children in this study did not have a urologic abnormality at the time of surgery. The authors found that only 2 patients had permanent changes in urinary function after untethering. One improved, and 1 deteriorated. This finding fits with our experience. Of course, there is no way to determine, whether the surgery prevented deterioration in some of the patients, because the study was not controlled.

S.S. Howards, M.D.

35 Bladder Exstrophy

Urinary Diversion in Bladder Exstrophy and Incontinent Epispadias: 25 Years of Experience
Stein R, Fisch M, Stöckle M, Hohenfellner R (Univ of Mainz, Germany)
J Urol 154:1177–1181, 1995   35–1

Objective.—Surgical management was analyzed in 115 patients who had bladder exstrophy or incontinent epispadias and underwent surgery between 1968 and 1994. All but 13 were available for follow-up after a mean of 16.7 years.

Management.—Thirty-nine previously untreated patients underwent urinary diversion. Another 3 patients had a sling plasty, and 1 had a modified Young-Dees procedure. The remaining 59 patients were referred after primary treatment elsewhere. Twenty-seven of these patients had urinary diversion after failed bladder closure–bladder neck reconstruction, and 7 had a modified Young-Dees procedure. Twenty-two patients who wished to regain continence underwent surgery. Three patients had genital reconstruction.

Results.—All patients with a functioning ureterosigmoidostomy have normal renal function, and none have upper tract dilation. Current continence rates are 96% for patients who had a rectal reservoir; 97% for those who had a Mainz pouch I; and 67% for those who underwent the modified Young-Dees augmentation procedure. No patient has had neoplastic disease of the bowel.

Conclusions.—The rectal reservoir is currently the urinary diversion procedure of choice. A Mainz pouch I is constructed if reconstruction has failed or the anal sphincter is deficient. If the upper tracts have deteriorated, a colon conduit is made.

▶ The authors report the results of a large series of patients who had bladder exstrophy and/or significant epispadias. Their approach to these children is distinctly different from that of most North American urologists, including the Johns Hopkins group, whose papers have been frequently abstracted in the YEAR BOOK OF UROLOGY. The authors acknowledge these differences and state that their patients are very satisfied and socially successful. Further, they argue that many patients who are categorized as successful results by their surgeons are actually rather disturbed by a marginal level of continence; this creates significant psychological problems for these individuals. These authors' position has merit, and clinicians should be certain that the options they choose are, in fact, in the best interest of their patients.

S.S. Howards, M.D.

36 Pediatric Reconstruction

Comparative Urodynamics of Appendiceal and Ureteral Mitrofanoff Conduits in Children
Watson HS, Bauer SB, Peters CA, Mandell J, Colodny AH, Atala A, Retik AB
(Harvard Med School, Boston)
J Urol 154:878–882, 1995   36–1

Background.—The Mitrofanoff principle is widely used in the construction of continent catheterizable urinary conduits. Although this procedure is generally successful, the mechanism of continence has never been defined, and a comprehensive urodynamic analysis has not been performed. The continence mechanism and causes of failure were examined and ureteral and appendiceal conduits were compared in children who had Mitrofanoff conduits.

Methods.—From July 1986 to April 1993, 24 patients were treated with Mitrofanoff conduits at 1 institution. Urodynamic evaluations were performed on 20 of these patients, aged 5–21 years. The conduits were created from ureter in 10 patients, appendix in 8, and other sources in 3. One patient had a ureteral conduit replaced with an appendiceal conduit, and both were studied. The urinary reservoir consisted of bladder with colon or stomach in 11 patients, an ileocolonic or colonic pouch in 7, and nonaugmented bladder in 2. Two patients were incontinent between catheterizations. The urodynamic examinations were done 1–76 months after the conduits were created. The examinations consisted of static conduit pressure profilometry, functional profile length, static profile maximal closure pressure, and cystometrography during dynamic filling.

Results.—All 20 patients had positive static and dynamic maximal Mitrofanoff closure pressures, with the dynamic pressure always greater than the static pressure. The functional profile length ranged from 1.5 to 7.5 cm and was correlated with both static and dynamic maximal closure pressures. The continent patients had significantly longer functional profile lengths. The incontinent patients had a conduit functional profile length of 2 cm or less. The average static maximal closure pressure and functional profile length were significantly greater for the appendiceal conduits than for the ureteral conduits. The longest functional profle and the highest static and dynamic maximal closure pressures were found with appendiceal conduits implanted to bowel or bladder segments.

Conclusions.—The results support the flap valve theory of Mitrofanoff conduit continence. The functional profile length, which is the length of the conduit intramural tunnel, was the most important factor in continence and was related to both static and dynamic conduit closure pressures. When continence rates and urodynamic profiles were compared, appendiceal conduits were preferable to ureteral conduits. Incidental appendectomy should therefore not be performed in children who have urinary dysfunction, as the appendix may be needed for Mitrofanoff urinary reconstruction. The urodynamic studies may be useful in improving the Mitrofanoff procedure and in correcting dysfunctional conduits.

▶ The Mitrofanoff procedure is widely applied and, in our experience, very successful. An additional advantage is that there is a very quick learning curve; the first one usually works. This urodynamic study is well done. It confirms what most surgeons have believed regarding the technique. Nevertheless, it is useful to document that appendix is better than ureter and that 2 cm appears to be a minimal functional length.

S.S. Howards, M.D.

The Physiology of Gastrocystoplasty: Once a Stomach, Always a Stomach

Bogaert GA, Mevorach RA, Kim J, Kogan BA (Univ of California, San Francisco)
J Urol 153:1977–1980, 1995   36–2

Introduction.—Gastrocystoplasty has been performed with excellent results. There have also been reports of significant complications, however, such as severe hypochloremic hypokalemic alkalosis and hematuria and dysuria. The physiology of these findings is not completely understood. The physiology of urinary acid excretion was determined in a prospective, standardized, 3-day investigation of children who had undergone a specific operative technique for bladder replacement and augmentation that excluded antrum.

Methods.—Thirteen patients (mean age, 12.5 years) were included. The median postoperative time was 2 years for 12 patients who had undergone bladder augmentation and 1 patient who had complete bladder replacement. Patients were placed on a low-salt diet for 2–3 days before testing and fasted for 2–3 hours after breakfast on the day of the test. Patients were fed a low-salt meal for 30 minutes. After gastric distention with a low-salt meal and bladder distention with urethral filling with a histamine-2 receptor antagonist or anticholinergic agent, urinary pH and titratable acid and serum gastrin levels were measured at baseline and after medication. Cystoscopy and biopsy of the gastric and native segments of the gastroplasty were performed in 5 children.

Results.—At the beginning of the test, all children had neutral urinary pH. Urinary pH decreased after the meal and the level of titratable acid increased to a maximum 1 hour after the beginning of the meal in all children. Serum levels of gastrin responded similarly. There were no significant changes observed in urinary secretion of sodium, potassium, or chloride after the meal. Two patterns of response were observed in the 7 children who received a histamine-2 receptor antagonist. Three children had no decrease in urinary pH and nearly no urinary titratable acid after the meal. The other 4 children had a decrease in urinary pH and level of titratable acid, but the magnitude of the change was less than without medication. Two patterns of response were also observed in 6 children who received the anticholinergic medication. Three had no decrease in urinary pH and no titratable acid after the meal, and the other 3 had a decrease in urinary pH and a level of titratable acid that was less than at baseline. Bladder distention did not elicit urinary acid secretion or gastrin secretion. Cystoscopic and histologic examination of the native bladder and stomach segment of the gastrocystoplasty were normal in the 5 patients examined.

Conclusion.—Significant urinary secretion of acid after gastrocystoplasty is regulated by the native stomach. This secretion can be reduced with a histamine-2 receptor antagonist and/or anticholinergic agent. Patients also benefit from reduction of gastrin release. After gastrocystoplasty, the gastric body continues to react as though it were still a part of the native stomach.

▶ This abstract, as the one above, describes a physiologic study in patients of a form of urologic reconstructive surgery. The study is well done, considering the limits involved in studying patients. Some of the results, however, are inconclusive. It is surprising that there were no significant changes in levels of sodium, potassium, and, particularly, chloride. This finding may be a result of the methodology. There were no long-term controlled metabolic balance studies. It is also curious that there were both responders and nonresponders to histamine-2 receptor and antihistamine treatment. It would have been interesting to have generated dose-response curves. Perhaps the selected doses were at the margin of efficacy?

S.S. Howards, M.D.

Subject Index*

A

Abdominal
  cramping during or after radiotherapy
    for prostate cancer, *95:* 176
  fluid collection after urinary
    reconstruction using stomach, in
    children, *94:* 278
  pain
    after radiotherapy for prostate cancer,
      95: 176
    in renal malacoplakia, *94:* 260
  repair of vesicovaginal fistulas, early *vs.*
    late, *96:* 293
  transabdominal *vs.* flank living donor
    nephrectomy, *96:* 92
  trauma, blunt, major renal lacerations
    with devitalized fragment after,
    94: 20
ABH
  antigen expression on vaginal and
    buccal epithelial cells and mucus, in
    women, *94:* 5
Abscess
  perinephric
    in malacoplakia, renal, *94:* 260
    after nephrectomy for combined renal
      and pancreatic trauma, *95:* 13
    after repair of coexisting
      intraperitoneal and renal trauma,
      94: 21
    after repair of renal gunshot wounds,
      94: 19
  prostate, transrectal ultrasound-guided
    perineal drainage for, *96:* 13
  renal, minimally invasive treatment of,
    96: 14
  subphrenic, after urinary reconstruction
    using stomach, in children, *94:* 478
Abstinence
  time, optimum, for cryopreservation of
    semen in cancer patients, *96:* 285
Abuse
  sexual, causing dysfunctional voiding,
    96: 363
ACE
  inhibitors in diabetes mellitus
    for nephropathy, *94:* 27
    type II, in normotensive, effect on
      plasma creatinine and proteinuria,
      94: 25

Acid
  -base changes after urinary tract
    reconstruction for continent
    diversion and orthotopic bladder
    replacement, *95:* 98
Acidification
  defect, renal, in urolithiasis, furosemide
    test for, *94:* 29
Acidosis
  metabolic
    gastroileoileal pouch and, *94:* 127
    hyperchloremic, after urinary tract
      reconstruction for continent
      diversion, *95:* 98
  renal tubular in recurrent stone formers,
    96: 35
Acquired immunodeficiency syndrome
  testicular tumor and, *95:* 270
Acrosome
  -reacted sperm selection with
    MH61-immunobeads, *95:* 247
  reaction
    of sperm, effect of platelet-activating
      factor on, *96:* 287
    sperm ionophore-induced, after
      overnight incubation with
      mycoplasmas, *95:* 248
Actinomycin D
  in rhabdomyosarcoma, bladder-prostate,
    in children, *94:* 297
  in sarcoma, genitourinary, in children,
    94: 297
Activity
  physical, prostate cancer, and ethnicity,
    96: 202
Acyclovir
  in herpes, recurrent genital, *94:* 17
Adenectomy
  pelvic, bilateral, for
    radio-recurrent/resistant prostate
    cancer, critical evaluation of,
    96: 233
Adenocarcinoma
  prostate (*see* Cancer, prostate)
Adenoma
  adrenal, hyperintense rim sign on
    fat-saturated MRI in, *95:* 26
  aldosterone-producing, outcome of
    adrenalectomy or enucleation for,
    96: 40
  prostate, effect of endothelin-1 on
    smooth muscle contractility of,
    94: 94

Q

U

Author Index